The facial nerve (VII) carries taste sensations from the anterior two thirds of the tongue, the glossopharyngeal nerve (IX) from the posterior third of the tongue, and the vagus nerve (X) from the epiglottis.

CHEWING
Function

Food taken into the mouth is chewed or masticated by the teeth.

Chewing breaks food into smaller food particles which increases the efficiency of digestion.

Reflex

Chewing is controlled mostly by a reflex integrated in the medulla oblongata called the chewing reflex.

Presence of food stimulates sensory receptors that cause muscles to relax.

As the mandible is lowered, muscles are stretched stimulating a reflexive contraction which closes the mouth.

The cycle is repeated.

The cerebrum influences the activity of the chewing reflex.

Muscles and Innervation

The muscles of mastication are the masseter, the temporalis, and the pterygoids (internal and external), all innervated by the trigeminal nerve (V).

SWALLOWING

Swallowing is a complex process requiring coordination of many muscles and structures in the head and neck.

The process of swallowing or deglutition has three phases as a bolus of food moves from the mouth to the stomach.

Oral or Voluntary Phase

A bolus of food is pushed by the tongue against the hard palate.

The bolus then moves posteriorly toward the oropharynx.

This first step is voluntary and under the control of the cerebral cortex.

Pharyngeal Phase

The bolus of food in the oropharynx stimulates tactile receptors, which initiates an involuntary swallowing reflex.

The soft palate is elevated to close off the nasopharynx.

The tongue is elevated to close off the mouth.

The larynx is blocked by muscle action that causes the larynx to elevate and the epiglottis to move posteriorly to cover and protect the larynx. The pharynx elevates to receive the bolus from the mouth, and three pharyngeal constrictor muscles contract in succession to force the bolus along with gravity toward the esophagus.

The swallowing center in the medulla oblongata sends motor stimuli that travel through the trigeminal (V), glossopharyngeal (IX), vagus (X), and accessory nerves (XI) to the soft palate and pharynx.

Esophageal Phase

The pharyngoesophageal constrictor and the cricopharyngeus muscle relax simultaneously, allowing the bolus of food to enter the esophagus.

This phase of swallowing is involuntary.

Reflexes of skeletal and smooth muscle in the wall of the esophagus move the bolus through the esophagus toward the stomach by successive constrictions (peristalsis).

SPEECH

Speech is a highly integrative function requiring many organs and processes in the head and neck.

Cerebrum

Speech area is located in the left cortex in most people.

Wernicke's area (sensory speech area) in the parietal lobe comprehends and formulates speech. Broca's area (motor speech area) in the frontal lobe receives input from Wernicke's area and sends impulses to the premotor and motor areas (cortex), which causes the muscle movements required for speech.

The ear and auditory cortex and the eye and visual cortex also send impulses necessary for communication by speech.

Larynx

Speech is produced in the larynx by air moving past the vocal cords, causing them to vibrate.

Pitch is controlled by the frequency of the vibrations.

Oral Cavity

The lips and cheeks help form words during the speech process.

The tongue is one of the major organs of speech.

The teeth and gums also play a role in speech.

Pharynx

The soft palate, pharynx, and larynx contain several muscles involved in speech.

COUGH REFLEX

The cough reflex is stimulated by foreign particles in the trachea or bronchi.

The trachea and bronchi contain sensory receptors that detect these particles and initiate nerve impulses.

These impulses pass along the vagus nerve (X) to the medulla oblongata, where the cough reflex is triggered.

The epiglottis and glottis reflexively close, and contraction of the expiratory muscles causes air pressure in the lungs to increase.

The epiglottis and glottis then open suddenly. The resulting upward burst of air that removes foreign particles is a cough.

HICCUP

Hiccup is a term used to describe an involuntary, spasmodic contraction of the diaphragm.

This contraction usually occurs at the beginning of an inspiration.

The glottis suddenly closes, producing the characteristic sound.

Hiccups can be caused by irritation of the phrenic nerve or sensory nerves in the stomach or by direct pressure on certain areas of the brain.

EAR, NOSE, AND THROAT DISORDERS

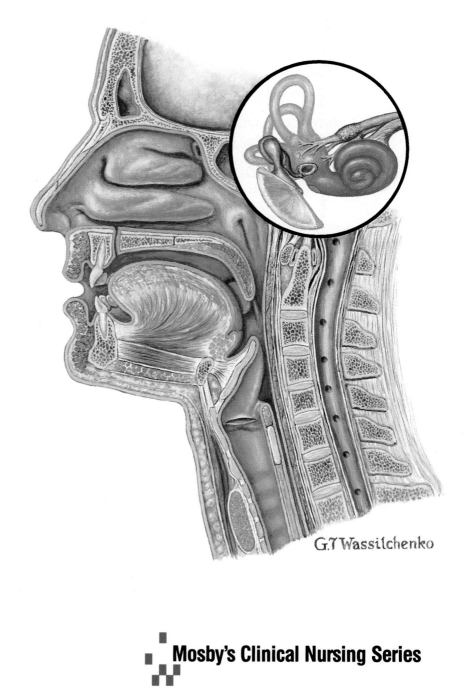

G.T.Wassilchenko

Mosby's Clinical Nursing Series

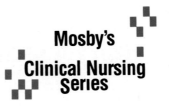

Mosby's Clinical Nursing Series

Cardiovascular Disorders
by Mary Canobbio

Respiratory Disorders
by Susan Wilson and June Thompson

Infectious Diseases
by Deanna Grimes

Orthopedic Disorders
by Leona Mourad

Renal Disorders
by Dorothy Brundage

Neurologic Disorders
by Esther Chipps, Norma Clanin, and Victor Campbell

Cancer Nursing
by Anne Belcher

Genitourinary Disorders
by Mikel Gray

Immunologic Disorders
by Christine Mudge-Grout

Gastrointestinal Disorders
by Dorothy Doughty and Debra Broadwell Jackson

Blood Disorders
by Anne Belcher

Ear, Nose, and Throat Disorders
by Barbara Sigler and Linda Schuring

Women's Health Care
by Valerie Edge and Mindi Miller

AIDS and HIV Infection
by Deanna Grimes and Richard Grimes

Skin Disorders
by Marcia Hill

EAR, NOSE, AND THROAT DISORDERS

BARBARA A. SIGLER, MNEd, RN, CORLN

Clinical Nurse Specialist
Otolaryngology and Head and Neck Surgery
Eye and Ear Institute of Pittsburgh
University of Pittsburgh Medical Center
Pittsburgh, Pennsylvania

LINDA T. SCHURING, MSN, RN

Nurse Director
Balance Disorder Clinic
Warren Otologic Group
Warren, Ohio

Original illustrations by

GEORGE J. WASSILCHENKO
Tulsa, Oklahoma
and

DONALD P. O'CONNOR
St. Peters, Missouri

Original photography by

Patrick Watson
St. Louis, Missouri

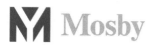 Mosby

St. Louis Baltimore Boston Chicago London Philadelphia Sydney Toronto

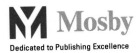

Mosby
Dedicated to Publishing Excellence

Publisher: Alison Miller
Editor: Sally Schrefer
Developmental Editor: Penny Rudolph
Project Manager: Mark Spann
Manuscript Editor: Christine O'Neil
Layout: Doris Hallas

Composition by The Clarinda Company
Printed by Von Hoffmann Press

Printed in the United States of America

Mosby—Year Book, Inc.
11830 Westline Industrial Drive
St. Louis, Missouri 63146

Library of Congress Cataloging-in-Publication Data

Ear, nose, and throat disorders / Barbara A. Sigler, Linda T. Schuring; original illustrations by George J. Wassilchenko and Donald P. O'Conner; original photography by Patrick Watson.
    p.   cm.—(Mosby's clinical nursing series)
    Includes bibliographical references and index.
    ISBN 0-8016-8011-5
    1. Otolaryngologic nursing.   I. Schuring, Linda T.   II. Title.
III. Series.
    [DNLM: 1. Otorhinolaryngologic Diseases—nursing.   WY 158 S577e
1993]
RF52.S54 1993
617.5′1—dc20
DNLM/DLC
for Library of Congress

93 94 95 96 97 CL/VH 9 8 7 6 5 4 3 2 1   93–23154
                                                                              CIP

Preface

Ear, Nose, and Throat Disorders is the twelfth volume in *Mosby's Clinical Nursing Series,* a new kind of resource for practicing nurses.

The *Series* is the result of the most elaborate market research ever undertaken by Mosby. We first surveyed hundreds of working nurses to determine what kinds of resources practicing nurses require to meet their advanced information needs. We then approached hundreds of clinical specialists—proven authors and experts—and asked them to develop a consistent format that would meet the needs of nurses in practice. This format was presented to nine focus groups composed of working nurses and refined between each group. In the later stages we published a 32-page full-color sample so that detailed changes could be made to improve physical layout and appearance, page by page.

In response to requests from scores of nurses participating in our research, a distinctive feature of this book is its usefulness for patient teaching. Background material increases the nurse's ability to answer common patient questions with authority. The illustrations in the book, particularly those in the structure and function, assessment, and diagnostic procedures chapters, are specifically designed to support patient teaching. Chapter 12 is a compilation of patient teaching guides that supplement the patient teaching sections of each care plan. The patient teaching guides are ideal for reproduction and distribution to patients.

We hope this book contributes to the advancement of professional nursing by providing a comprehensive resource that supports a scientific and holistic approach to professional nursing practice.

Acknowledgments

I acknowledge the following people for their assistance and support during the preparation of this book: My mother, Ann Sigler, for her support and encouragement; Dr. Eugene N. Myers, Dr. Jonas T. Johnson, and Heather Rebic, RN, BS for their review and editing of the manuscript; Mary Jo Tutchko for her overall assistance in the preparation of the text; my coauthor Linda Schuring; and the editors, Sally Schrefer and Penny Rudolph, for their guidance in the development of this book.

B.A.S.

I want to thank my husband, Arne Schuring, MD, for editing, suggesting, and encouraging the contents of this book. I would also like to acknowledge my friend, Bill Lippy, MD, for whom I've worked 25 years taking care of patients with ear disorders. Without these two men, my knowledge of otologic nursing would not exist. Finally, my heartfelt gratitude to my friend for life, Barb Sigler, for making this book a reality.

L.T.S.

The Society of Otorhinolaryngology and Head-Neck Nursing (SOHN) is a specialty nursing organization for the care of patients with ear, nose, throat and/or head and neck disorders. The purpose of SOHN is continuing education for all members. The authors wish to recognize this society for professional support, encouragement, and nurturing. Some of the impetus to write this book was to give back the accumulation of education that SOHN has given to us over the past seventeen years.

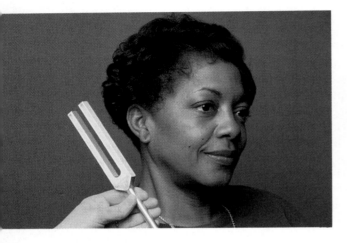

Contents

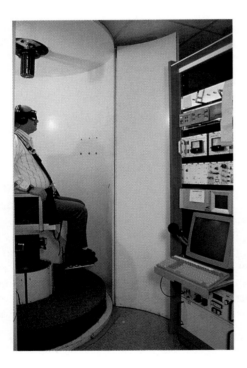

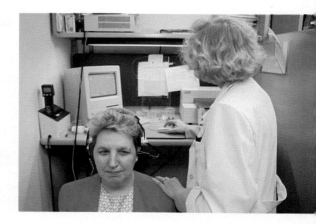
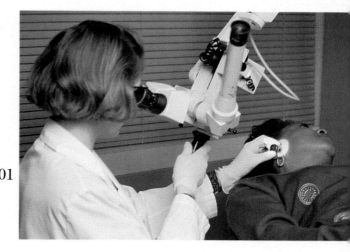
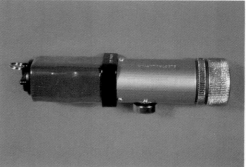

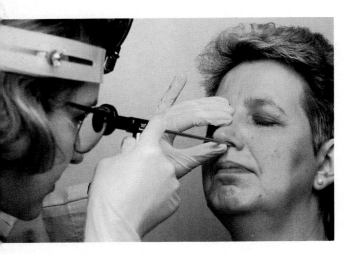

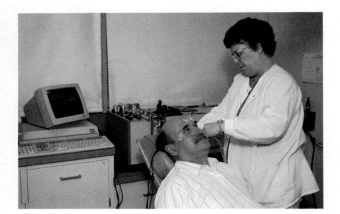

11 Tumors of the Head and Neck, 214

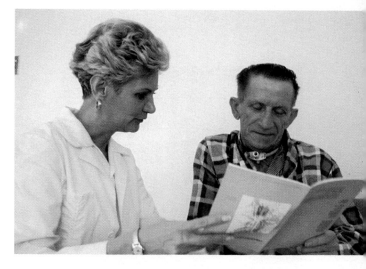

12 Patient Teaching Guides, 260

13 Ear, Nose, and Throat Drug Therapy, 269

Appendixes

Color plates

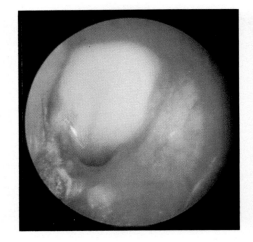

PLATE 1
PURULENT OTITIS MEDIA.

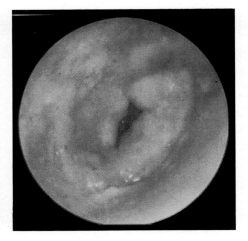

PLATE 2
EXTERNAL OTITIS.

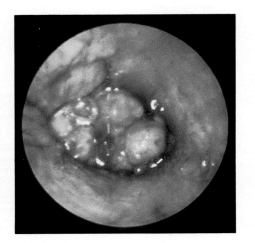

PLATE 3
SQUAMOUS CELL CARCINOMA.

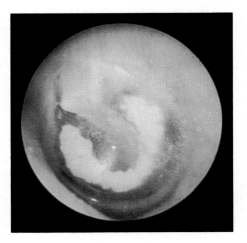

PLATE 4
TYMPANOSCLEROSIS.

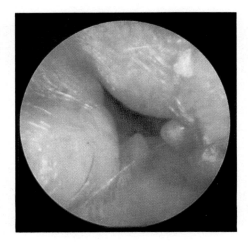

PLATE 5
EXOSTOSIS.

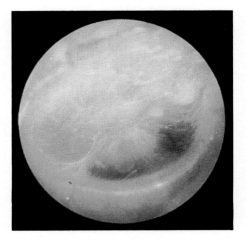

PLATE 6
GLOMUS TYMPANICUM.

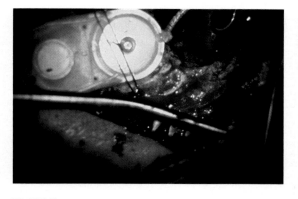

PLATE 7
INTRAOPERATIVE VIEW OF COCHLEAR IMPLANT.

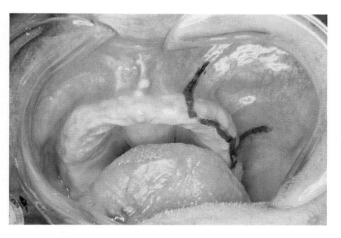

PLATE 8
CALDWELL-LUC INCISION.

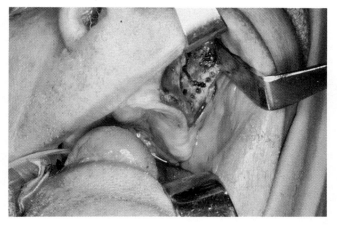

PLATE 9
CALDWELL-LUC INCISION (OPEN).

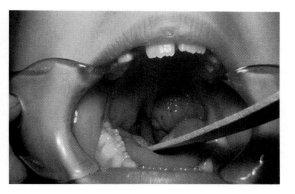

PLATE 10
ENLARGED TONSIL.

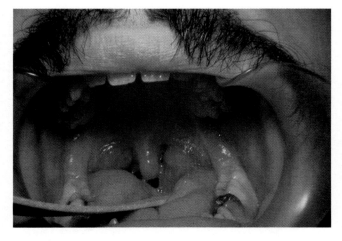

PLATE 11
CHRONIC TONSILLITIS.

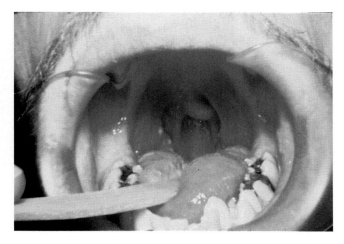

PLATE 12
ACUTE TONSILLITIS.

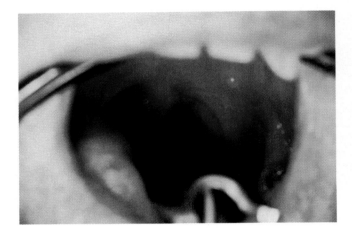

PLATE 13
SWELLING OF PERITONSILLAR ABSCESS.

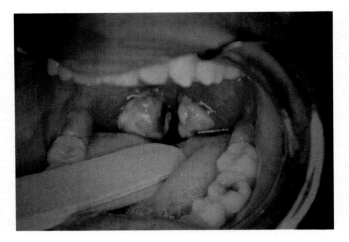

PLATE 14
TONSILS COATED WITH DEBRIS DURING MONONUCLEOSIS.

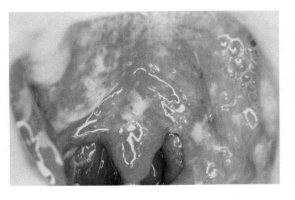

PLATE 15
CANDIDIASIS.

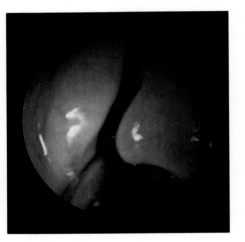

PLATE 16
VOCAL CORD POLYP.

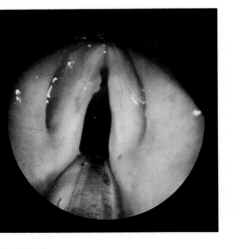

PLATE 17
VOCAL CORD NODULE.

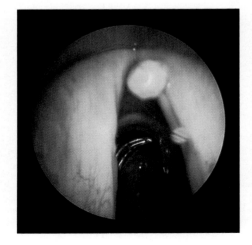

PLATE 18
UNILATERAL VOCAL CORD PARALYSIS.

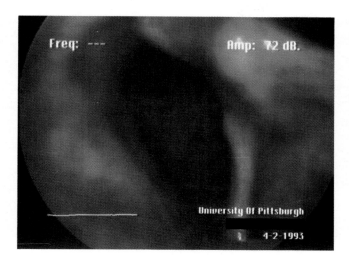

PLATE 19
X-RAY FILM DEMONSTRATING VOCAL CORD PARALYSIS.

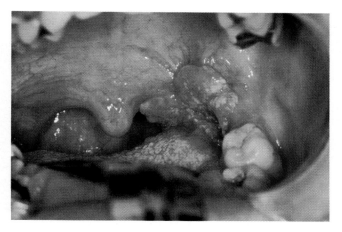

PLATE 20
CANCER OF THE TONSIL AND PALATE.

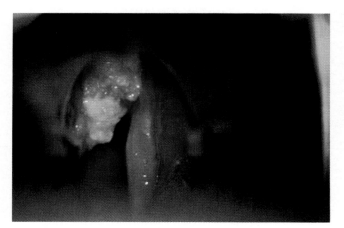

PLATE 21
CANCER OF THE VOCAL CORD.

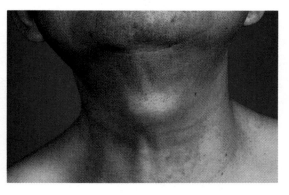

PLATE 22
THYROGLOSSAL DUCT CYST.

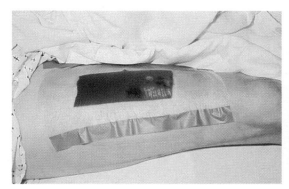

PLATE 23
SKIN GRAFT DONOR SITE.

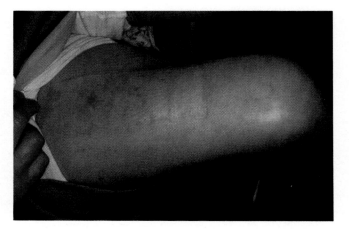

PLATE 24
HEALED SKIN GRAFT DONOR SITE.

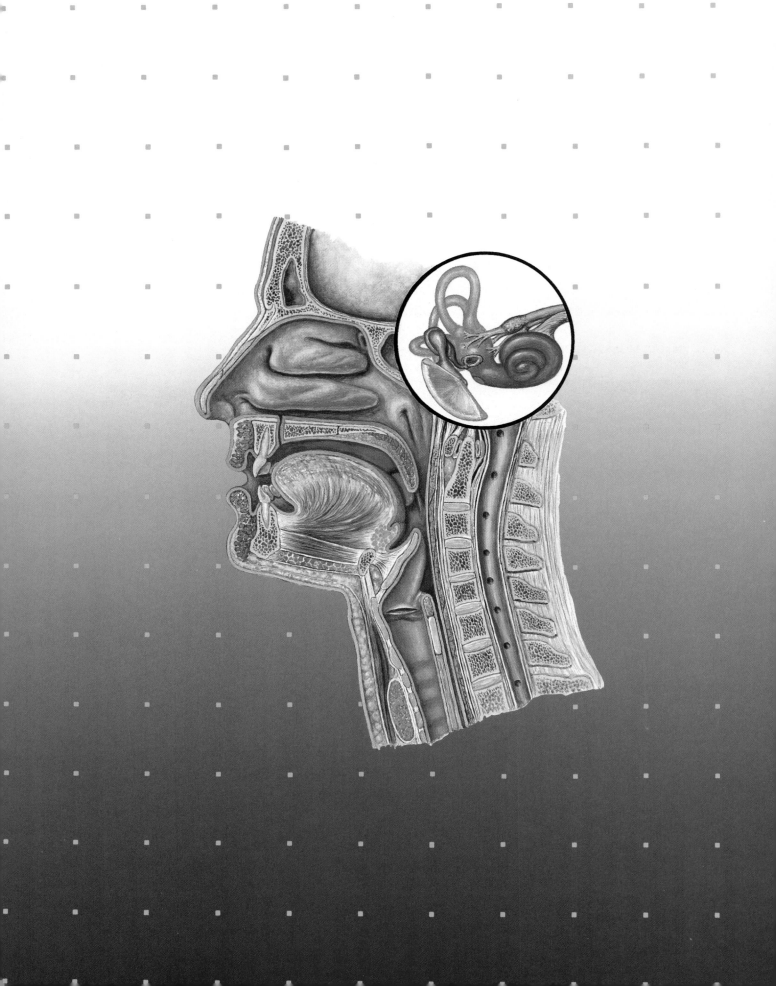

CHAPTER 1

Color Atlas of the Structure and Function of the Ear, Head, Neck, Nose, and Throat

In otorhinolaryngology (the study of diseases of the ear, nose, and throat) and disorders of the head and neck, the nurse faces three important challenges: (1) several body systems are involved; (2) the sensory symptoms often overlap; and (3) these disorders affect a wide range of individuals. This complex multisystem specialty can best be comprehended by examining the large supportive structures of the head and neck (the cranium, facial skeleton, and neck) before studying the important interior components: the temporal bones and ears; the nose and paranasal sinuses; the oral cavity; the pharynx; the larynx; the trachea; the thyroid gland; and the parathyroid glands.

HEAD AND NECK

Together the head and neck provide the bony housing and protective covering for the brain and special senses. An overview of these structures is important for clinical evaluation. The human skull consists of 22 bones, all of which are firmly interlocked along sutures (irregular lines or seams) except for the lower jaw, or mandible. Eight of the bones form the *cranium*, and 13 immovable bones make up the *facial skeleton;* the *mandible* is attached to the cranium by ligaments.

CRANIUM

The cranium encloses and protects the brain, and its surfaces provide the attachment for various muscles

that control jaw and head movements. The eight bones that form the cranium are the frontal bone, two parietal bones, the occipital bone, two temporal bones, the sphenoid bone, and the ethmoid bone (Figure 1-1). Some of the cranial bones contain sinuses, which are lined with mucous membranes and are connected to the nasal cavity. These sinuses, as well as the mastoid air cells, reduce the weight of the skull.

FACIAL SKELETON

The 13 bones that make up the facial skeleton are the two maxillae, two palatine bones, two zygomatic

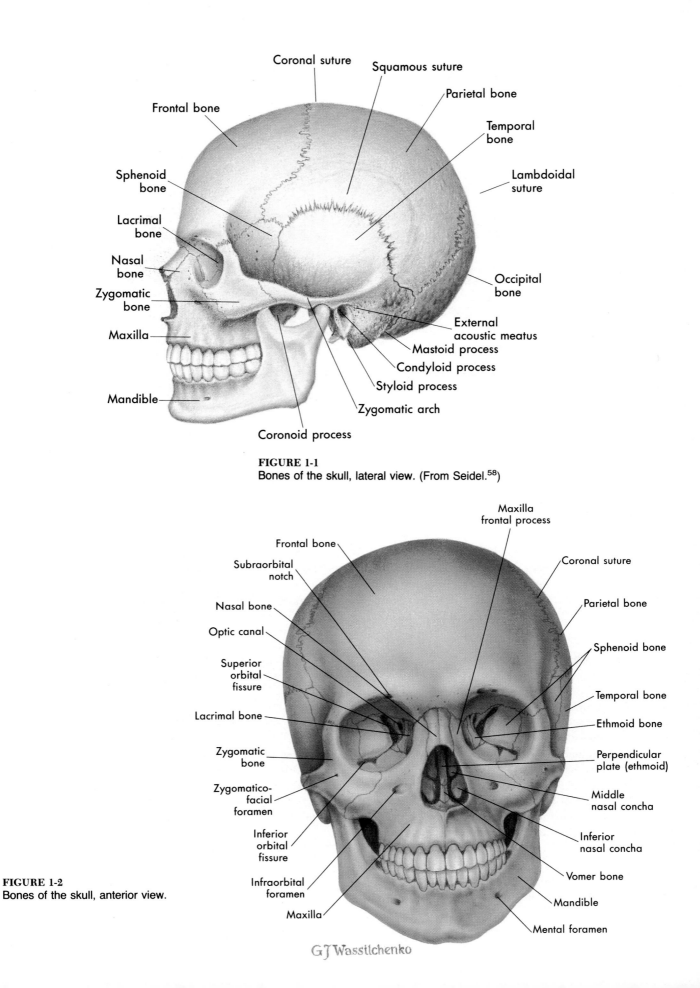

Coronal suture
Squamous suture
Frontal bone
Parietal bone
Temporal bone
Sphenoid bone
Lambdoidal suture
Lacrimal bone
Nasal bone
Zygomatic bone
Maxilla
Occipital bone
External acoustic meatus
Mastoid process
Condyloid process
Styloid process
Zygomatic arch
Mandible
Coronoid process

FIGURE 1-1
Bones of the skull, lateral view. (From Seidel.[58])

Maxilla frontal process
Frontal bone
Subraorbital notch
Coronal suture
Nasal bone
Parietal bone
Optic canal
Sphenoid bone
Superior orbital fissure
Temporal bone
Lacrimal bone
Ethmoid bone
Zygomatic bone
Perpendicular plate (ethmoid)
Zygomatico-facial foramen
Middle nasal concha
Inferior orbital fissure
Inferior nasal concha
Infraorbital foramen
Vomer bone
Maxilla
Mandible
Mental foramen

FIGURE 1-2
Bones of the skull, anterior view.

GJ Wasstlchenko

bones, two lacrimal bones, two nasal bones, two inferior nasal conchae, and the vomer bone, in addition to the movable mandible (Figure 1-2), or lower jawbone—the strongest facial bone. The facial skull has several cavities for the eyes, nose, and mouth and forms the basic shape of the face. It also provides the attachment for muscles that move the jaw and control facial expressions.

Facial muscles are innervated by cranial nerves V (the trigeminal nerve) and VII (the facial nerve). The major accessible artery of the face is the temporal artery, which passes in front of the ear and continues over the temporalis muscle and onto the forehead.

NECK

The structure of the neck is formed by seven cervical vertebrae, ligaments, and the sternocleidomastoid and trapezius muscles, which give support and allow movement. Mobility is greatest at the level of C4-5 or C5-6. The sternocleidomastoid muscle extends from the upper sternum and anterior third of the clavicle to the mastoid process. The trapezius muscle extends from the scapula, lateral third of the clavicle, and the vertebrae to the occipital prominence.

The relationship of these muscles to each other and to adjacent bones creates triangles that can be used as anatomic landmarks. The *posterior triangle,* which is formed by the trapezius and sternocleidomastoid muscles and the clavicle (Figure 1-3), contains the posterior cervical lymph nodes (Figure 1-4). The *anterior triangle,* which is formed by the medial borders of the sternocleidomastoid muscles and the mandible, houses the carotid artery and the internal and external jugular veins, among other features (Figure 1-3).

Posterior Triangle

In the posterior triangle, lymph nodes occur along the lower border of the mandible, in front of and behind the ears, and deep within the neck along the paths of larger blood vessels. These nodes provide drainage from the scalp, face, nasal cavity, and pharynx.

Anterior Triangle

The anterior triangle houses the carotid artery, internal jugular vein, and external jugular vein. Other structures contained within the anterior triangle are the hyoid bone, cricoid cartilage, thyroid cartilage, anterior cervical lymph nodes, thyroid and parathyroid glands, and trachea. The internal structures of the throat are discussed later in this chapter.

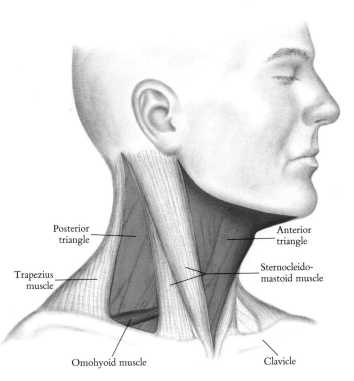

FIGURE 1-3
Anterior and posterior triangles of the neck. (From Seidel.[58])

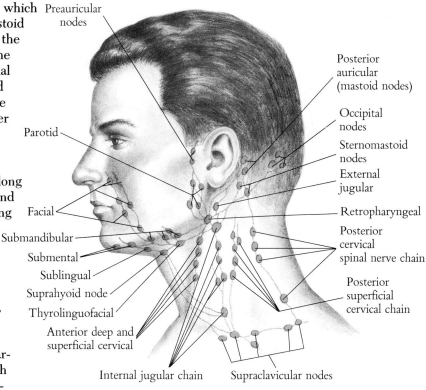

FIGURE 1-4
Lymphatic drainage system of head and neck. (From Seidel.[58])

The *carotid artery* and *internal jugular vein* lie deep and run parallel to the sternocleidomastoid muscle along its anterior aspect. The *external jugular vein* crosses the surface of the sternocleidomastoid muscle diagonally. The *hyoid bone* is located in the neck between the mandible and larynx. It is fixed into position by muscles and ligaments and does not articulate with any other bones. The hyoid bone supports the tongue and serves as an attachment for muscles involved in tongue movement and swallowing. The *cricoid cartilage* is the uppermost ring of the laryngeal cartilages and is the only complete ring of cartilage; the *thyroid cartilage* is shaped like a shield, its notch on the upper edge marking the level of bifurcation of the common carotid artery.

The cervical lymph nodes in the anterior triangle, like those in the posterior triangle, provide drainage from the head and neck.

TEMPORAL BONES AND EARS

The ears are complex sensory organs that provide both hearing and balance. Their location on either side of the head produces binaural hearing, allows determination of a sound's direction, and aids in maintaining equilibrium.

The ears are housed in the temporal bones, the most detailed part of the skull. If a half-dollar coin were superimposed on the external auditory canal, the tympanic ring and tympanic membrane, the three ossicles, the jugular vein, the carotid artery, the facial nerve, and the auditory and vestibular parts of the inner ear would all be within the coin's circumference.

TEMPORAL BONES

The temporal bones, which house the ears, are two of the eight cranial bones. The temporal bones are the hardest bones of the body, and form part of the base and lateral wall of the skull. The temporal bones can be divided into four parts: the squamous, mastoid, petrous, and tympanic portions. The temporal bone articulates with the sphenoid, parietal, and occipital bones (see Figure 1-1).

The temporal bone protects the external and internal auditory canals, the mastoid air cells, the blood vessels, the facial and auditory nerves, the labyrinth, and the cochlea.

Mastoid

The mastoid section of the temporal bone comprises the mastoid process, the mastoid antrum, and the mastoid air cells, which branch off from the mastoid cavity. The mastoid bone can be felt as a bony protuber-

ance behind the lower portion of the pinna (the outer, protruding portion of the ear). The mastoid cavity is surrounded by important cranial structures: the dura, the sigmoid sinus, and the internal carotid artery.

The cavity of the mastoid bone, in conjunction with the interconnected arrangement of the air-filled spaces, aids the middle ear in adjusting to changes in pressure. In addition, the system of cavities and air cells lightens the skull—an important factor for human posture.

EXTERNAL EAR

The external ear is divided into the pinna (or auricle), the external auditory canal (or ear canal), and the tympanic membrane (Figure 1-5). The ears are located on each side of the head at approximately eye level.

Pinna (Auricle)

The conspicuous part of the ear that projects outward is called the pinna, or auricle. The pinna is attached to the side of the head by skin and is composed mainly of cartilage, except for the fat and subcutaneous tissue in the lobule. The cartilage is held to the skull by the posterior, anterior, and superior auricularis muscles and is innervated by a branch of the facial nerve. The pinna collects and directs sound.

The parts of the pinna are illustrated in Figure 1-6. The helix, the outer rim of the pinna, leads inferiorly to the lobule. The concha, the deepest part, is bounded anteriorly by a triangular fold of cartilage called the tragus; the concha leads to the ear canal. Hair covers most of the ear, but it usually is rudimentary, except around the tragus and antitragus. Sebaceous glands also are found on the skin's surface. In front of the external opening of the ear is the temporomandibular joint. The head of the mandible can be felt by placing a fingertip in the external meatus while opening and closing the mouth.

External Auditory (Ear) Canal

The ear canal extends from the concha to the tympanic membrane. This S-shaped canal is approximately 2.5 cm long and follows an inward, forward, and downward path. The lumen of the ear canal is irregularly shaped, with a skeleton of cartilage in the outer third that is continuous with the cartilage of the pinna, and a bony skeleton in the inner two thirds. The lumen is narrowest where the transition from cartilage to bone occurs. The skin over the bony portion is very thin, but the skin that covers the cartilage is thick and contains sebaceous glands, ceruminous glands, and hair follicles. The secretion from the ceruminous glands and the fat from the sebaceous glands form cerumen (wax). The sticky consistency of the wax, along with

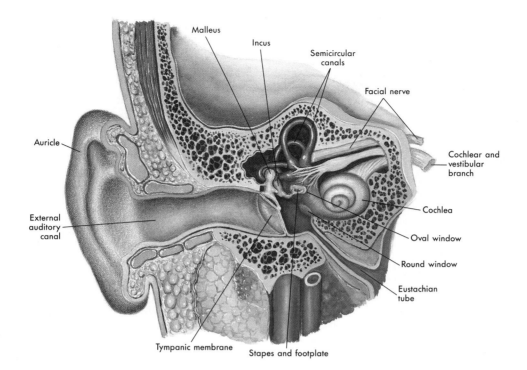

FIGURE 1-5
Anatomy of the ear. (From Seidel.[58])

the fine hairs of the ear canal, helps cleanse the ear canal of foreign matter.

Tympanic Membrane

The tympanic membrane, or eardrum, covers the end of the ear canal and separates the ear canal from the middle ear. The eardrum is a thin, oval membrane about 1 cm in diameter; it is translucent with a pearl gray color.

The eardrum is made up of three layers of tissue: an outer layer, which is continuous with the skin of the ear canal; a fibrous, supporting middle layer; and an inner mucosal layer, which is continuous with the mucosal lining of the middle ear cavity. About four fifths of the eardrum is made up of all three layers; this portion is called the *pars tensa*. The remaining one fifth of the eardrum, which is made up of only the outer epithelial layer and the inner mucosal layer, is called the *pars flaccida*. The absence of the fibrous middle layer makes the pars flaccida more vulnerable to pathologic disorders.

Some distinguishing landmarks of a normal eardrum (Figure 1-7) are the annulus, the fibrous border that attaches the eardrum to the temporal bone; the short process of the malleus, which protrudes into the eardrum superiorly; the long process of the malleus (the manubrium); the umbo of the malleus, which is found at the point of maximum concavity and attaches

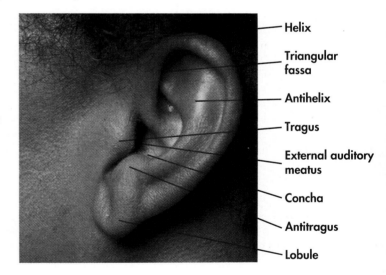

FIGURE 1-6
Anatomic structures of the auricle. The helix is the prominent outer rim, whereas the antihelix is the area parallel and anterior to the helix. The concha is the deep cavity containing the auditory canal meatus. The tragus is the protuberance lying anterior to the auditory canal meatus, and the antitragus is the protuberance on the antihelix opposite the tragus. The lobule is the soft lobe on the bottom of the auricle.

to the center of the eardrum; the pars flaccida, a small triangular area above the short process of the malleus; and the pars tensa, the remaining and largest portion of the eardrum.

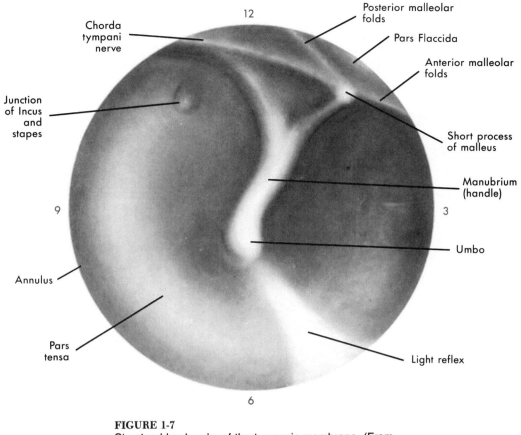

FIGURE 1-7
Structural landmarks of the tympanic membrane. (From Seidel.[58])

The tympanic membrane protects the middle ear and conducts sound vibrations from the external ear to the ossicles. The sound pressure applied to the stapes (the smallest ossicle) is 22 times greater than that exerted on the eardrum, as a result of transmission from a larger area to a smaller one.

MIDDLE EAR

The middle ear consists of the middle ear cleft and contents: the ossicles, the oval and round windows, and the eustachian tube. The middle ear cleft, or tympanic cavity, is a small, oblong, air-filled space with a mucosal lining found in the petrous section of the temporal bone. If this cleft is viewed in relationship to surrounding structures, it is above the jugular fossa, behind the carotid canal, and in front of the mastoid air cells.

Ossicles

The middle ear contains the three smallest bones of the body. These bones, the auditory ossicles, were given their particular names because of their appearance (Figure 1-8). The outermost and largest ossicle is the malleus (hammer), which is firmly attached to the tympanic membrane at the short process. The center

ossicle is the incus (anvil), which is shaped like a tooth with two roots. The innermost and smallest ossicle is the stapes (stirrup), which fills the oval window and is in contact with the perilymph of the inner ear.

The ossicles are held in place by joints, muscles, and ligaments, which also offer protection from loud sounds (Figure 1-9). The configuration and light weight of the ossicles provide an efficient means of transmitting sound vibrations from the air molecules of the external and middle ear to the fluid molecules of the inner ear. Because liquids offer more resistance than air and need more force to produce movement, the ossicular chain produces and magnifies the force needed to move the inner ear fluids.

Windows

The two windows in the middle ear also are named for their shapes (Figure 1-5). The oval window, which is filled by the footplate of the stapes, is the opening through which vibrations enter the inner ear. The round window also opens into the inner ear, serving as an *exit* for sound vibrations.

Eustachian Tube

The eustachian tube is a narrow channel about 35 mm long and only 1 mm wide at its narrowest end. It con-

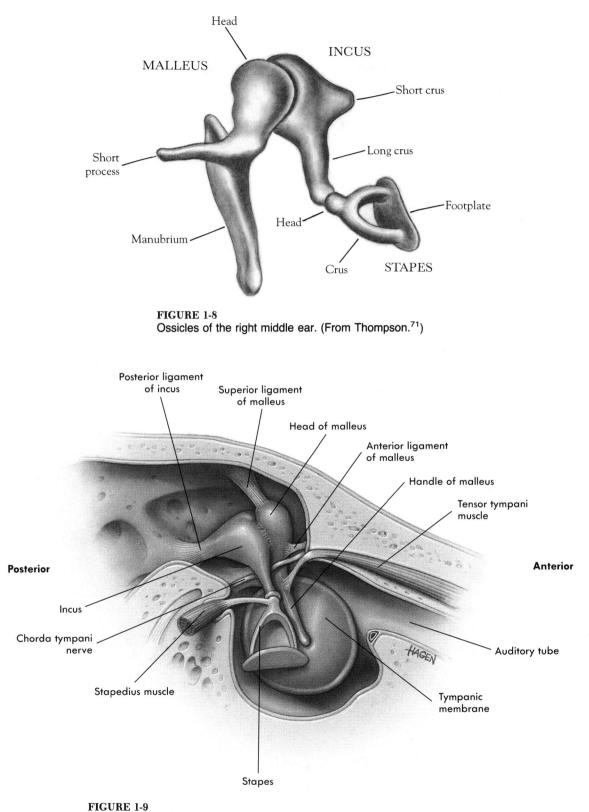

FIGURE 1-8
Ossicles of the right middle ear. (From Thompson.[71])

FIGURE 1-9
Muscles of the middle ear. Medial view of the middle ear (as though viewed from the inner ear) showing the three ear ossicles with their ligaments and the two muscles of the middle ear, the tensor tympani and the stapedius. (From Seeley, Stephens, Tate.[57])

nects the middle ear to the nasopharynx (see Figure 1-5). The eustachian tube is made up mostly of fibrous tissue, cartilage, and bone. It extends downward, forward, and inward from the middle ear. The eustachian tube is lined with mucous membrane, which is continuous with the lining of the middle ear at one end and with the lining of the nasopharynx at the other end. The walls of the tube touch each other lightly, closing the tube to both the throat and the ear. This closure prevents the sound of nasal respiration and of one's own voice from passing to the ear. However, during yawning, swallowing, and sneezing, the eustachian tube is opened by the tensor veli palatini muscle to equalize pressure.

The eustachian tube provides an air passage from the nasopharynx to the middle ear to equalize pressure on both sides of the eardrum for normal hearing. If the pressure is greater in the ear canal than in the middle ear, the eardrum retracts. If the pressure is greater in the middle ear than in the ear canal, the eardrum bulges. Malfunction of the eustachian tube leads to many middle ear disorders. The tube can be forcibly opened by increasing nasopharyngeal pressure, a technique called the Valsalva maneuver.

INNER EAR

The inner ear, or labyrinth, is located deep within the petrous section of the temporal bone. It contains the sense organs for hearing and balance and cranial nerves VII and VIII. The inner ear is a complicated system of intercommunicating chambers and connecting tubes composed of two major structures, the bony labyrinth and the membranous labyrinth. The membranous labyrinth lies within the bony labyrinth but does not completely fill it (Figure 1-10).

Bony Labyrinth

The bony labyrinth surrounds and protects the delicate membranous labyrinth. The bony labyrinth is made up of the cochlea and the semicircular canals. The cochlea looks like a snail shell with two and a half turns. It is about 7 mm in diameter at the widest part and is structurally divided into two compartments. The upper compartment is the *scala vestibuli,* and the lower compartment is the *scala tympani* (see Figure 1-10).

Bony Semicircular Canals

The three bony semicircular canals are at right angles to each other. Because of their positions, they have been named the superior canal, the posterior canal, and the lateral, or horizontal, canal (see Figure 1-10).

Membranous Labyrinth

The membranous labyrinth is bathed in a fluid called perilymph, which communicates with cerebrospinal fluid (CSF) via the cochlear duct. The membranous labyrinth consists of the utricle, the saccule, the semicircular canals, the cochlear duct, and the end organ for hearing, the organ of Corti. The membranous labyrinth holds a different fluid, called endolymph.

Membranous Semicircular Canals

The membranous semicircular canals are arranged to sense rotational positional movements. Each of the semicircular canals connects with the utricle by an enlarged portion, the ampulla. The ampulla contains a cluster of nerve hair cells called the crista, which helps maintain dynamic balance. When the head changes position, movement of the endolymph stimulates the hair cells, initiating impulses that travel to the brain via the vestibular division of the acoustic nerve.

Utricle and Saccule

The utricle and saccule are vestibular receptors that position the head as it responds to the pull of gravity and changes in position. Both the utricle and saccule contain structures called maculae, which are composed of nerve hair cells, and a membrane containing otoliths, or "ear stones." A change in head position or pressure causes the otoliths to move the hair cells. This initiates impulses that travel over the vestibular division of the acoustic nerve. The utricle is thought to be involved with linear movement; the function of the saccule is unknown.

Cochlea

The cochlea is a snail-shaped, bony tube about 3.5 cm long with two and a half spiral turns that contains the end-organ for hearing. Sound waves are transmitted by the ossicles to the oval window, moving the perilymph in the scala vestibuli (Figure 1-11). The perilymph of the scala vestibuli is continuous with that of the scala tympani. Sound vibrations enter through the oval window and exit through the round window. Vibrations in the perilymph are transmitted through the vestibular membrane, or Reissner's membrane, to the endolymph that fills the cochlear duct. The cochlear duct is located between the scala vestibuli and the scala tympani. The organ of Corti, which is bathed in the endolymph, lies on the basilar membrane. This organ transforms mechanical sound vibrations into neural activity and separates sound into different frequencies. This electrochemical impulse travels to the temporal cortex of the brain via the acoustic nerve. The acoustic nerve (cranial nerve VIII) reaches the brain via the internal auditory canal. The facial nerve (cranial nerve VII) travels through the same canal.

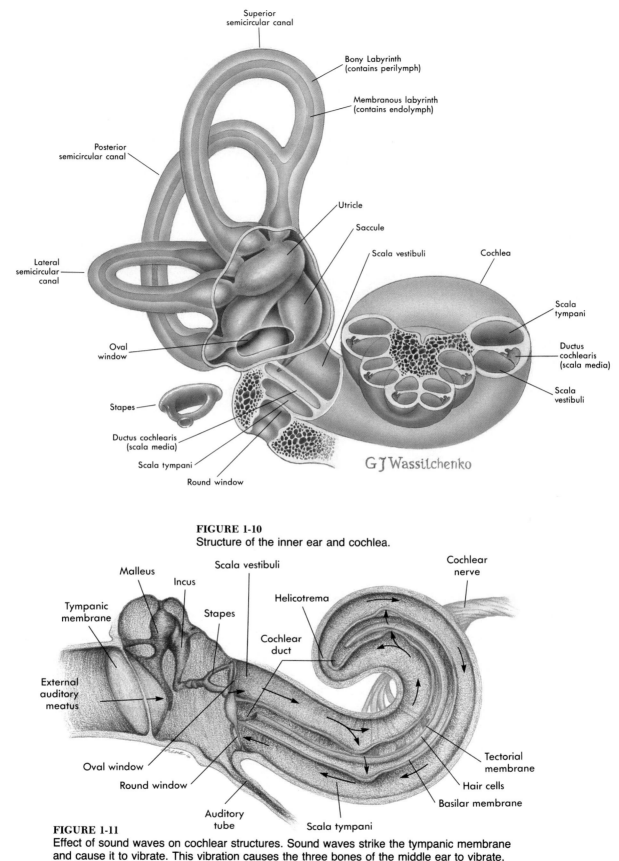

FIGURE 1-10
Structure of the inner ear and cochlea.

FIGURE 1-11
Effect of sound waves on cochlear structures. Sound waves strike the tympanic membrane and cause it to vibrate. This vibration causes the three bones of the middle ear to vibrate, causing the footplate of the stapes to vibrate in the oval window. This vibration causes the perilymph in the scala vestibuli to vibrate. Vibration of the perilymph causes stimultaneous vibration of the endolymph in the cochlear duct, which causes the basilar membrane to vibrate. Short sound waves (high pitch) cause the basilar membrane near the oval window to vibrate, and longer sound waves (low pitch) cause the basilar membrane some distance from the oval window to vibrate. Sound is detected in the hair cells of the organ of Corti, which is attached to the basilar membrane. Vibrations are transferred to the perilymph of the scala tympani and to the round window where they are dampened. (From Seeley, Stephens, Tate.[57])

NOSE AND PARANASAL SINUSES

NOSE

External Nose

The external nose consists of a framework made up of a bony section (the upper third) and a cartilaginous section (the lower two thirds) covered by skin. The midpoint where the nose joins the forehead is called the nasion, the bridge of the nose is called the dorsum, and the point where the nose joins the upper lip (which includes the nares) is called the base. The flaring, cartilaginous expansion that forms and supports the outer side of each naris is called the ala. The nares are separated by the columella. The nares allow air to enter and pass to the nasopharynx (Figure 1-12). The two nasal bones meet superiorly, where they are surrounded by the frontal bone. The frontal and maxilla bones form the nasal bridge. The nose is surrounded by the maxilla laterally and inferiorly at its base (see Figure 1-2).

Internal Nose

The internal nose, or nasal cavity, lies over the roof of the oral cavity. The palatine bones form the floor of the nasal cavity. The roof is separated from the cranial cavity by the cribriform plate, a portion of the ethmoid bone. This plate admits branches of the olfactory nerve, which enter and leave the cranial cavity.

The irregularly shaped nasal cavity is separated in the midline by the septum, which divides the internal nose into two anterior cavities called the vestibules. The lateral walls are formed by three turbinates, or conchae, which are curved, bony structures covered by vascular mucous membranes that run horizontally and protrude into the nasal cavity, increasing the surface area over which the air passes. In this way they aid filtration through three passageways, the superior, middle, and inferior turbinates (Figure 1-13). The superior and middle turbinates are processes of the ethmoid bone; the inferior turbinate is a separate bony plate. The nasolacrimal duct drains into the inferior meatus, and the paranasal sinuses drain through the medial meatus.

MOVEMENT OF AIR FROM NOSE TO NASO-PHARYNX
1. Anterior nares (nostrils)
2. Vestibule
3. Inferior, middle, and superior turbinates (simultaneously)
4. Posterior nares
5. Nasopharynx

Blood is supplied to the nose by the external and internal carotid arteries. The internal maxillary artery, a branch from the external carotid artery, supplies most of the posterior nasal septum and the lateral wall of the nose. The internal carotid artery, via the ante-

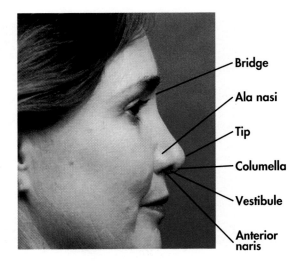

FIGURE 1-12
Anatomic structures of the external nose.

Labels: Bridge, Ala nasi, Tip, Columella, Vestibule, Anterior naris

rior ethmoidal artery, also supplies blood to the nose.

The muscles of the external nose are innervated by cranial nerve VII (the facial nerve), but the external skin receives its nerve supply from cranial nerve V (the trigeminal nerve). The internal nose is supplied by cranial nerve I (the olfactory nerve) and cranial nerve V.

Nasal Mucosa

The nares, or nostrils, open into an area called the vestibule, which is lined with stratified squamous epithelium. Coarse hairs (vibrissae), sebaceous glands, and sweat glands are found in the skin of the vestibule. The mucous membrane, or respiratory mucosa, that lines the nasal cavity has a pseudostratified, ciliated epithelium with goblet cells that secrete a thick layer of mucus. Olfactory nerve cells permeate the olfactory epithelium near the roof of the nasal cavity and over the superior turbinate, the uppermost part of the nasal cavity. The posterior nares are funnel-shaped openings that allow air to pass from the nasal cavity into the nasopharynx.

Functions of the Nose

The major functions of the nose are to warm, filter, and moisten inhaled air, to provide the sense of smell, and to serve as the primary passageway for air to the lungs (see box). Air entering the body through the nasal cavity is filtered first by the vibrissae and then the turbinates to remove particulate matter and bacteria. The respiratory membrane allows rapid warming and moistening of dry inspired air. Inspired air reaches the nasopharynx in one fourth of a second. During this short time the temperature of the air is warmed to 36.1° to 36.7° C (97° to 98° F) and the humidity becomes a constant 75% to 80%.

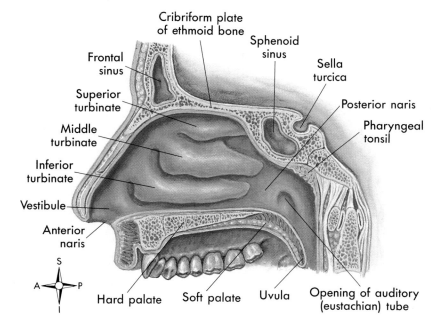

FIGURE 1-13
Cross-sectional view of the anatomic structures of the nose and nasopharynx. (From Seidel.[58])

Mucous secretions and fluid from the lacrimal ducts provide the final means of removing particulate matter and moistening inhaled air. The cilia on the surface of the mucous membrane sweep the mucus posteriorly to the nasopharynx, where it is expectorated or swallowed. Residual bacteria are destroyed by the hydrochloric acid and gastric juices of the digestive system.

The olfactory organs are located in the olfactory epithelium, which covers the roof of the nose. Deflection of air by the middle and superior turbinates over the olfactory epithelium makes the sense of smell possible.

PARANASAL SINUSES

The paranasal sinuses are air-containing spaces that open and drain into the nasal cavity. They lighten the weight of the skull and give timbre and resonance to the voice. The paranasal sinuses are named for the skull bones in which they are located; the four pairs are called the frontal, maxillary, ethmoid, and sphenoid sinuses (Figure 1-14). The paranasal sinuses are lined with respiratory mucosa and cilia, which move secretions. The openings of these sinuses into the middle meatus of the nasal cavity are easily blocked.

The frontal sinuses are located above the orbit of each eye. The maxillary sinuses, the largest of the sinuses, lie along the lateral wall of the nasal cavity and

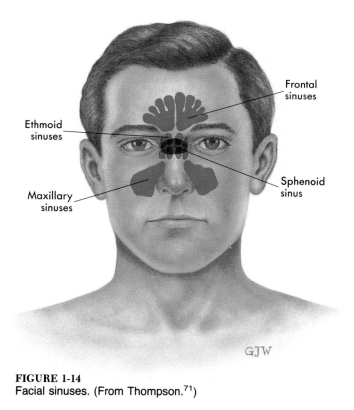

FIGURE 1-14
Facial sinuses. (From Thompson.[71])

extend into the maxilla. The ethmoid sinuses, a collection of small air cells, lie near the superior portion of the nasal cavity. The sphenoid sinuses are deep in the skull, behind the ethmoid sinuses.

PHARYNX

The pharynx (from the Greek word for throat) is a muscular, conical, tubelike structure approximately 12.5 cm long that extends from the base of the skull to the larynx. The pharynx conducts air between the nasal and oral cavities to the larynx and conducts food from the mouth to the esophagus.

The three anatomic divisions are the nasopharynx, oropharynx, and laryngopharynx, lined with mucous membrane (Figure 1-15) and formed by three pairs of muscles: the superior, middle, and inferior constrictors.

NASOPHARYNX

The nasopharynx, the superior portion of the pharynx, lies behind the nasal cavities and extends from the posterior nares to the level of the uvula, a soft process attached to the posterior edge of the soft palate (see Figure 1-15). The eustachian tube opens into the nasopharynx approximately 1 cm behind the posterior end of the inferior turbinate. The posterior surface contains the pharyngeal tonsils (or adenoids), which help defend the body against infection. The nasopharyngeal space opens inferiorly into the oropharynx (see box below.)

OROPHARYNX

The oropharynx is located behind the oral cavity and extends from the uvula to the epiglottis (Figure 1-15). Located near the fauces, which is the opening of the oral cavity into the oropharynx, are the palatine tonsils and the lingual tonsil. The palatine tonsils are the ones most commonly removed by a tonsillectomy. The pharynx contains a large amount of lymphoid tissue, including the tonsils. The pharyngeal, palatine, and lingual tonsils form Waldeyer's lymphatic ring, which is the first line of immunologic defense.

LARYNGOPHARYNX

The laryngopharynx extends from the epiglottis to the openings of the larynx and the esophagus (see Figure 1-15). The oropharynx and laryngopharynx are spaces that form a passageway for the respiratory and diges-

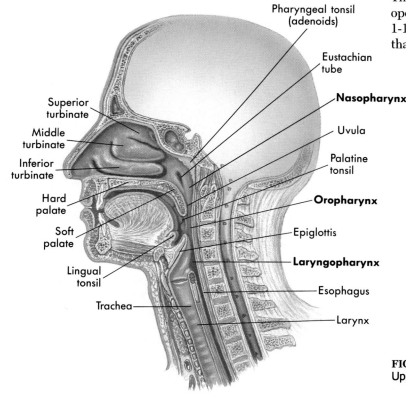

Pharyngeal tonsil (adenoids)

Eustachian tube

Nasopharynx

Uvula

Palatine tonsil

Oropharynx

Epiglottis

Laryngopharynx

Esophagus

Larynx

Superior turbinate

Middle turbinate

Inferior turbinate

Hard palate

Soft palate

Lingual tonsil

Trachea

SEVEN DIFFERENT OPENINGS ARE LOCATED IN THE PHARYNX:

Two posterior nares (into the nasopharynx)
Two eustachian tubes (into the nasopharynx)
The fauces (into the oropharynx)
The larynx (into the laryngopharynx)
The esophagus (into the laryngopharynx)

FIGURE 1-15
Upper respiratory structures. (From Thompson.[71])

tive tracts. The boundaries of the laryngopharynx are the superior constrictor muscle and vertebrae posteriorly; the larynx and pyriform sinuses inferiorly; and the hyoid bone, base of the tongue, and constrictor muscle superiorly.

Besides serving as a conduit for channeling air, food, and fluids to the appropriate areas, the pharynx affects vowel phonation by changing shape. The pharyngeal portion of swallowing, or deglutition, is accomplished by the action of the constrictor muscles in the pharynx and the suprahyoid and infrahyoid muscles. These muscles are also responsible for the gag reflex, which protects the air and food passages from any foreign material. The glossopharyngeal nerve (cranial nerve IX), the vagus nerve (cranial nerve X), and the hypoglossal nerve (cranial nerve XII) are responsible for the gag reflex and swallowing mechanism.

ORAL CAVITY

The oral cavity is surrounded by the lips anteriorly, the fauces posteriorly, the cheeks laterally, the palate superiorly, and the muscular floor inferiorly. The mouth can be divided into two regions, the oral cavity and the vestibule. The oral cavity lies inside the alveolar processes (which hold the teeth) and contains the tongue. The vestibule is the space between the lips and cheeks and the alveolar processes (Figure 1-16). The oral cavity is lined with moist, stratified epithelium, which protects against abrasion.

LIPS

The bulk of the lips is composed of the orbicularis oris, a sphincterlike muscle covered externally by skin and internally by a mucous membrane that is continuous with the lining of the vestibule and oral cavity. The lips are sharply separated from the surrounding facial skin by the vermilion cutaneous line. The red or pink coloring from the underlying blood vessels is seen through the transparent epithelium. The lips have a variety of sensory receptors that help judge the temperature and texture of food. The lips also keep food and saliva in the mouth during chewing (mastication), help form words during speech, and aid in facial expression.

BUCCAL MUCOSA

The buccal mucosa forms the lateral walls of the oral cavity and are composed of the buccinator muscles, fat, areolar tissue, nerves, vessels, and buccal glands. The small, numerous, mucus-secreting buccal glands

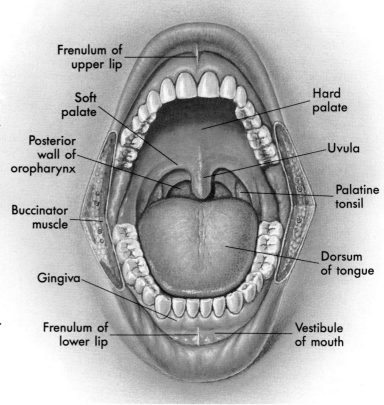

FIGURE 1-16
Anatomic structures of the oral cavity. (From Seidel.[58])

have ducts that open opposite the last molar teeth. The gums, or gingivae, are dense, fibrous tissue covered by a smooth mucous membrane.

Chewing (mastication) involves the stimulation of jaw muscles, many of which are innervated by the motor branch of cranial nerve V (the trigeminal nerve). When food is put in the mouth, a reflex inhibition of the muscles of mastication allows the lower jaw to drop. This drop initiates a stretch reflex in the jaw and causes a rebound contraction, raising the jaw and closing the teeth. The buccal mucosa also helps manipulate the food in the oral cavity or hold it in place while the teeth tear or crush it. The cheeks help form words during speech and help to produce facial expressions.

HARD AND SOFT PALATES

The roof of the mouth is formed by the hard and soft palates (see Figure 1-16). The anterior hard palate is formed by two palatine bones and parts of the superior maxillary bone. The mucous membrane of the hard palate is thick, pale, and corrugated and has a midline, called the linear raphe. Attached to the posterior portion of the hard palate is the soft palate, which forms a partition between the mouth and the nasopharynx. The soft palate is composed of muscle arranged in the shape of an arch. The opening in the arch, called the fauces, leads from the mouth into the oropharynx. The uvula is the conical, fingerlike projection on the posterior border of the arch. During swallowing, the soft palate moves upward, closing off the nasopharynx to prevent food and fluids from entering.

TONGUE

The tongue is a large, muscular organ that occupies most of the oral cavity when the mouth is closed. The posterior portion of the tongue is covered with mucous membrane and is anchored to the hyoid bone and the mandible. The anterior portion is relatively free but is attached to the floor of the mouth by the frenulum, a fold of mucous membrane. A mucous membrane also attaches the tongue to the epiglottis and the pharynx. The tip of the tongue is called the apex.

The muscles of the tongue are both intrinsic (origin and insertion are in the tongue) and extrinsic (muscle originates outside the tongue but is attached to it). The intrinsic muscles change the shape of the tongue and help position food during chewing or mastication. The extrinsic muscles assist in the protrusion, retraction, depression, and elevation of the tongue. Contraction of extrinsic muscles helps during swallowing (deglutition), and speech.

The anterior two thirds of the tongue's surface is covered by papillae, which contain most of the taste buds on their lateral surfaces. The posterior one third of the tongue has a large amount of lymphoid tissue (lingual tonsil), a few small glands, and a small number of taste buds, but no papillae.

Adults have approximately 10,000 taste buds, which begin to degenerate as the person ages, resulting in decreased taste acuity. The four primary sensations of taste are sweet, sour, salty, and bitter. Taste buds respond to these sensations with differing degrees of sensitivity. The brain actually determines the taste according to the degree of stimulation. The sense of smell also affects the sense of taste.

TEETH AND GUMS

An adult normally has 32 permanent teeth, which are set in sockets along the alveolar ridges of the maxilla and mandible. The alveolar ridges are covered by dense, fibrous connective tissue and stratified squamous epithelium, referred to as gums, or gingivae. The teeth are secured in the alveoli by periodontal ligaments, and the alveolar walls are lined with a periodontal membrane.

The teeth play an important role in the digestive process by cutting and mixing the food. Chewing increases the surface area exposed to the digestive enzymes and makes it easier to swallow the food.

SALIVARY GLANDS

The salivary glands secrete saliva (approximately 1 L a day), which moistens food particles, helps bind them together, and begins the digestion of carbohydrates. Saliva also acts as a solvent on various food chemicals so that the foods can be tasted.

There are three major pairs of salivary glands: the parotid glands, the submandibular glands, and the sublingual glands. In addition there are numerous small, coiled, tubular salivary glands, known as the lingual glands (in the tongue), the palatine glands (in the palate), the buccal glands (in the cheeks), and the labial glands (in the lips).

Two types of secretory cells, known as serous cells and mucous cells, occur in varying proportions in the different salivary glands. The serous cells produce amylase, which splits starch and glycogen molecules into disaccharides. The mucous cells produce a thick, stringy liquid, called mucus, that acts as a lubricant and binds food together during swallowing.

Parotid Glands

The parotid glands are the largest saliva glands. They are serous glands located anterior to the ear on each side of the head between the ramus of the mandible and the mastoid process. The parotid duct, or Stensen's duct, enters the oral cavity just adjacent to the upper second molar. The parotid gland is divided into a superficial lobe and a deep lobe. Along the anterior margin of the parotid gland are branches of cranial nerve VII (the facial nerve). The parotid gland produces ptyalin, which is salivary amylase.

Submandibular Glands

The submandibular (submaxillary) glands are found on the floor of the mouth on the mandible's inner surface They are smaller than the parotid glands and are predominantly serous glands. Each gland can be felt as a soft mass along the inferior border of the mandible's posterior half. The submandibular ducts, or Wharton's ducts, enter the oral cavity on either side of the frenulum.

Sublingual Glands

The sublingual glands are located under the tongue. They are the smallest of the three paired salivary glands and are predominantly mucous glands. Their primary purpose is lubrication. These glands enter into the floor of the mouth through 10 or 12 separate ducts.

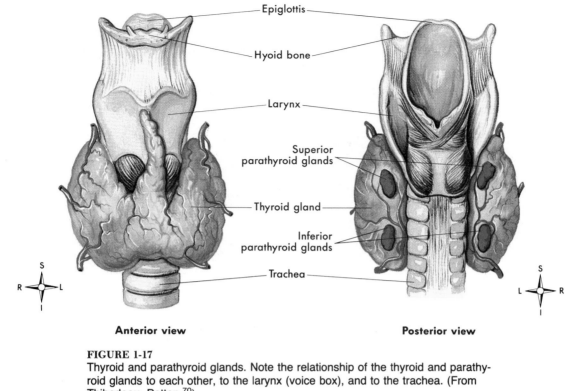

FIGURE 1-17
Thyroid and parathyroid glands. Note the relationship of the thyroid and parathyroid glands to each other, to the larynx (voice box), and to the trachea. (From Thibodeau, Patton.[70])

LARYNX

The larynx, or voice box, is a tubular vestibule between the trachea and pharynx. It is wider at the top, where it attaches to the laryngopharynx, and narrower below, where it attaches to the trachea. The larynx extends between the third and the sixth cervical vertebrae, although it is somewhat higher in females and during childhood. The lateral lobes of the thyroid gland and the carotid artery touch the sides of the larynx.

The larynx is composed of cartilage, ligaments, and muscles that prevent its wall from collapsing on inspiration. The cavity of the larynx extends from the triangular-shaped inlet at the epiglottis to the circular opening at the lower border of the cricoid cartilage (Figure 1-17). The larynx is lined with a ciliated mucous membrane. It has two pairs of folds that project inward from its lateral walls and divide it into three compartments: the vestibule, the false vocal cords, and the true vocal cords. The superior folds, or false vocal cords, play no part in vocalization. The lower folds are the true vocal cords. The slitlike space between the true vocal cords, which is the rima glottidis, is the narrowest part of the larynx. The true vocal cords are joined anteriorly and attach to the thyroid cartilage. The true vocal cords and the rima glottidis together form the glottis.

The compartment of the laryngeal cavity above the false vocal cords is called the vestibule. The middle compartment between the false and true vocal cords is the ventricle. Glands in the upper portion of the ventricle secrete mucus that lubricates the vocal cords. The lowest compartment of the laryngeal cavity, the area below the true vocal cords, is called the infraglottic larynx.

CARTILAGES OF THE LARYNX

The larynx is composed of nine cartilages. Three of these are paired structures (the arytenoid, corniculate, and cuneiform cartilages), and three are unpaired (the thyroid, epiglottis, and cricoid cartilages) (see Figure 1-18).

Paired Cartilages

The paired cartilages are stacked in two pillars between the cricoid cartilage and the thyroid cartilage.

The pyramid-shaped arytenoid cartilages are the largest and most important of the paired laryngeal cartilages. The base of each cartilage articulates with the superior border of the cricoid cartilage. The anterior edges serve as points of attachment for the vocal cords. The arytenoid cartilage swings in and out. This action opens or closes the space between the vocal cords.

The middle pair of cartilages is the conical-shaped corniculate cartilages. They rest on the apex of the arytenoid cartilages and serve as attachments for mus-

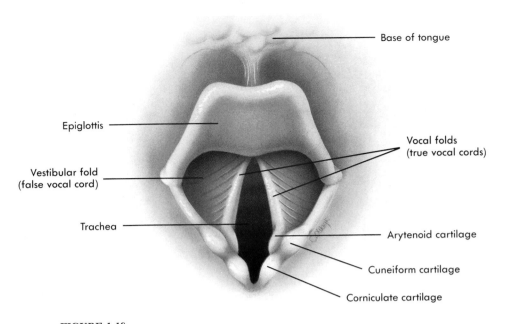

FIGURE 1-18
Vocal cords viewed from above, showing their relationship to the paired cartilages of the larynx and epiglottis. (From Seeley, Stephens, Tate.[57])

cles that help regulate the tension of the vocal cords during speech and help close the larynx during swallowing.

The uppermost cartilages, the wedge-shaped cuneiform cartilages, are the smallest of the paired laryngeal cartilages. Located near the base of the epiglottis, they stiffen the soft tissues in this region.

Unpaired Cartilages

The thyroid cartilage, named for the gland it partly covers, is the largest cartilage of the larynx. It is shaped like a shield and is commonly called the Adam's apple. This cartilage is the uppermost of the unpaired cartilages and often is larger in men than in women as a result of the effects of male sex hormones.

The second unpaired cartilage is the epiglottis, a small, leaf-shaped cartilage that projects upward behind the tongue and hyoid bone. It differs from the other cartilages in that it is elastic rather than hyaline cartilage. The inferior margin of the epiglottis is attached to the superior margin of the thyroid cartilage, but its free superior border can move up and down during swallowing to prevent food or liquids from entering the trachea.

The lowest unpaired cartilage is the cricoid cartilage. It forms the base of the larynx, on which the other cartilages rest. The cricoid cartilage is shaped somewhat like a signet ring and is the only complete cartilaginous ring in the respiratory tract. The cricoid cartilage can be palpated in a person with a normal neck and can be seen in a person with a thin neck.

MUSCLES OF THE LARYNX

The muscles of the larynx are divided into extrinsic and intrinsic groups. The extrinsic muscles connect the larynx to adjacent structures of the neck, such as the sternum and the hyoid bone. Contraction of the extrinsic muscles moves the larynx as a whole. The five intrinsic muscles connect the laryngeal cartilages and alter the shape of the laryngeal cavity. A branch of the vagus nerve, the recurrent laryngeal nerve, supplies each intrinsic muscle except the cricothyroid muscle, which is supplied by the superior laryngeal nerve. This innervation becomes particularly significant during endotracheal intubation, because mechanical manipulation of the vocal cords and musculature can result in bradycardia caused by vagal stimulation. Muscles in both groups play important roles in respiration, vocalization, and swallowing.

FUNCTIONS OF THE LARYNX

The most important function of the larynx is to act as a passage for air between the pharynx and the trachea. The larynx's inner mucous membrane warms and humidifies incoming air and continues to filter it by entrapping particles. The larynx helps prevent aspiration and assists in coughing, an important protective mechanism triggered whenever the highly sensitive laryngeal mucosa is touched by a foreign substance.

The larynx also serves as the organ of voice production as a result of vocal cord vibration. Air is expired through the glottis, which is narrowed by partial adduction of the true vocal cords; this causes the cords to vibrate (Figure 1-18). Words are formed when the vibrating column of air passes from the larynx to the tongue, lips, palate, and teeth. The greater the amplitude or force of the vibration, the louder or more intense the sound. Pitch is controlled by changes in the tension on the cords. Men usually have lower pitched voices than women because males usually have longer vocal cords. The size and shape of the nose, mouth, pharynx, and paranasal sinuses also help determine the quality of the voice.

TRACHEA

The trachea, or windpipe, is a flexible, cylindric tube about 2.5 cm in diameter and 11 cm long that extends downward in front of the esophagus from the cricoid cartilage to the left and right mainstem bronchi in the thoracic cavity. The trachea is composed of C-shaped pieces of hyaline cartilage, called tracheal rings, that are arranged one above the other to reinforce, protect, and maintain an airway. The open ends of these incomplete rings are directed posteriorly. The posterior wall of the trachea is composed of smooth muscle and connective tissue, which complete the rings and can alter the diameter. These soft tissues permit the esophagus (immediately behind the trachea) to expand as it carries a bolus of food to the stomach.

The trachea is lined with a ciliated mucous membrane that contains many goblet cells. This lining, which is typical of the entire respiratory tract, also filters incoming air and moves entrapped particles upward to the larynx, where they can enter the esophagus and be swallowed.

The trachea acts as a passageway for air to enter the lungs. Obstruction of this airway for just a few minutes causes asphyxiation, which may lead to death.

THYROID GLAND

The thyroid gland is the largest endocrine gland, weighing approximately 30 g. It is located in the anterior aspect of the neck just below the cricoid cartilage. The gland has two large, butterfly-shaped lobes, connected by a broad isthmus, that lie lateral to the upper portion of the trachea. The isthmus extends across the anterior aspect of the trachea (see Figure 1-17). The recurrent laryngeal nerve runs beside the trachea and behind the lobes of the thyroid gland. Blood is supplied by the superior and inferior thyroid arteries.

The thyroid gland is covered by a capsule of connective tissue and composed of tiny structural units called follicles. Each follicle is filled with a clear, viscous fluid called thyroid colloid. The follicle cells produce and secrete hormones (protein-iodine complexes, known as thyroglobulins) that can be stored in the colloid or released into the blood of nearby capillaries.

Between the follicular cells is a delicate network of loose, capillary-rich connective tissue. Parafollicular cells are found between the follicles and among the cells that make up the follicle wall.

THYROID HORMONE

The major secretory products of the thyroid gland are tetraiodothyronine, or thyroxine (T_4) (90%) and triiodothyronine (T_3) (10%). Although T_4 is the most abundant secretory product, once it enters the bloodstream it is converted to T_3. Therefore T_3 is the principal thyroid hormone.

T_3 helps regulate the metabolic rate of all cells, as well as the processes of cell growth and tissue differentiation. Because T_3 can interact with any cell in the body, it is said to have a "general" target.

CALCITONIN

The thyroid gland also secretes calcitonin, which is produced by the parafollicular cells. The primary target tissue for calcitonin is bone. Calcitonin controls calcium content of the blood by increasing bone formation by osteoblasts and inhibiting bone breakdown by osteoclasts. Calcitonin tends to decrease the blood calcium level and promote conservation of calcium in the bones.

PARATHYROID GLANDS

The parathyroid glands are embedded in the posterior portion of each lobe of the thyroid gland (see Figure 1-17). Normally four parathyroid glands are present, two associated with each lateral lobe. Each parathyroid gland is a small, round, yellowish brown structure covered by a thin capsule of connective tissue. Its numerous cells are organized in tightly packed, secretory masses, or cords, that are closely associated with capillary networks.

PARATHORMONE

The only hormone known to be secreted by the parathyroid glands is parathormone, an antagonist to calcitonin that helps maintain calcium homeostasis. The target tissues for parathormone are the bones, kidneys, and intestines. Without functional parathyroid glands, the body cannot maintain an adequate level of calcium in the blood. Normal neuromuscular excitability, blood clotting, cell membrane permeability, and the functioning of certain enzymes all depend on an adequate blood level of calcium.

CHAPTER 2

Assessment

Every nurse, regardless of education or focus of care, should be prepared to perform a complete nursing history and physical examination on a patient with an ear, nose, throat, head, or neck disorder. Nurses are involved in every aspect of the care of these patients, including prevention, detection, and treatment. Ear, nose, and throat disorders are common, can occur at any age, and often require immediate attention.

The nurse must be able to look at a patient with a disorder of the ear, nose, throat, head, or neck holistically. In other words, does the problem interfere with the patient's activities of daily living (ADLs)? Nurses can also participate in case findings involving these patients, as well as in rehabilitation and referral to appropriate agencies for assistance. Often the nurse is the first member of the health team whom the patient approaches about these problems.

HISTORY

Evaluation of a patient with a disorder of the ear, nose, throat, head, or neck begins with the patient's history, which can be the most important assessment tool. Both the patient and the nurse should be relaxed during this interview.

The nursing history should accomplish four goals: (1) establish a rapport with the patient, (2) determine the patient's chief complaints, (3) relate other health history problems to the current problem, and (4) deter-

COMPONENTS OF A GOOD HEALTH HISTORY

1. Identifying data (age, sex, race)
2. Chief complaint (put briefly in patient's own words)
3. Current illness (a chronologic, narrative account)
4. Past medical history
5. Family history
6. Psychosocial-cultural history (life-style, typical ADLs, religious beliefs)
7. Review of body systems (patient's responses, not physical findings)

mine the patient's emotional state regarding the current problem or other health problems.

PHYSICAL EXAMINATION

To perform a thorough, accurate physical examination, the nurse requires adequate lighting and the appropriate instruments.

EAR

Hearing is recognized as one of the five senses of the human body. Hearing and balance are very important in our activities of daily living. Sound helps us to be in touch with our environment, adding aesthetic pleasure as well as warnings of danger. The sense of hearing is essential for normal development and maintenance of speech, and the ability to communicate with others through speech depends on the ability to hear. The ear also contains the organs of balance, which relay information to the brain about the body's position and the direction of body motions.

Assessment of the External Ear

Inspect the external ear for size, configuration, symmetry, color, and angle of attachment to the head. To de-

HEALTH HISTORY

Body systems
Ears

Sense of hearing: degree of hearing loss, inability to discriminate words, unilateral or bilateral loss, sudden or gradual onset, fluctuating or stable hearing loss, events leading to loss of hearing

Tinnitus: onset, intensity, and frequency of tinnitus, intermittent or constant, unilateral or bilateral

Infection: consistency and amount of drainage, unilateral or bilateral, acute or chronic, swelling of ear canal, erythema or lesions of pinna

Otalgia: Intensity, type, unilateral or bilateral, constant or intermittent, location

Nose and paranasal sinuses

Drainage: consistency, frequency, unilateral or bilateral, postnasal drip, bleeding or blood-tinged mucus

Nasal breathing: obstruction to nasal breathing, continuous or intermittent obstruction, unilateral or bilateral obstruction

Sense of smell: altered sense of smell, anosmia (total loss of sense of smell), partial loss of sense of smell, events leading to loss of sense of smell

Sneezing

Oral cavity and oropharynx

Dental condition: edentulous, broken teeth, missing teeth, loose teeth, gingivitis, periodontitis

Excessive dryness of oral cavity, alterations in taste, difficulty moving tongue, altered sensations, swelling in mouth, halitosis, pain, ulcerations, raised lesions, change in articulation

Larynx

Voice changes, aspiration when swallowing, cough, shortness of breath, dyspnea

Neck

Discomfort, range of motion, swelling, or lumps

Pain

Local, referred (otalgia); instruct patient to pinpoint pain

Cranial nerves
See Table 2-3

Past medical history

Hypertension, diabetes mellitus, liver disease, bleeding disorders, allergy, emphysema or other pulmonary disorders, weight loss, use of medication

Social history

Smoking: method of smoking, amount of smoking, number of years

Use of smokeless tobacco

Alcohol use: beer, wine, liquor

Drug use: prescription medications, intranasal cocaine, IV drug use

Exposure to noxious fumes/chemicals: type, frequency, duration

Family history

Family history of otolaryngology–head and neck disorders, family history of cancer

termine the angle of attachment, draw an imaginary line between the greatest protuberance on the occiput to the outer canthus of the eye; the top of the auricle should touch or extend above the eye-occipital line. Draw another imaginary line perpendicular to the eye-occipital line just anterior to the auricle; the position of the auricle should be almost vertical, with a lateroposterior angle of no more than 10 degrees (Figure 2-1). An auricle set below the eye-occipital line or at a lateroposterior angle of more than 10 degrees can indicate chromosomal aberrations such as mongolism or renal disorders.

PHYSICAL EXAMINATION EQUIPMENT

Gloves
Light source (penlight, flashlight, indirect light with head mirror)
Suction
Otoscope
Tuning fork
Nasal speculum
Tongue blades
Laryngeal/nasopharyngeal mirrors
Gauze sponges

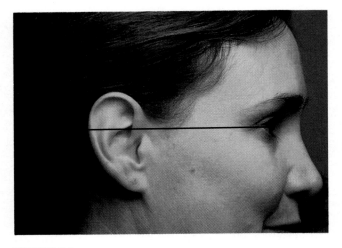

FIGURE 2-1
Auricle alignment assessment shows expected position.

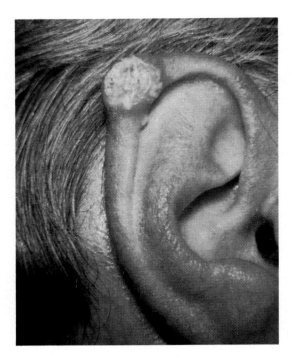

FIGURE 2-2
Tophus of the pinna.

Next, check the pinna for size, configuration, deformities, and protrusion. An unusual shape or size can be a familial trait or may indicate a pathologic condition. Darwin's tubercle, a thickening along the upper ridge of the helix, is a normal variation.

The auricle should be the same color as facial skin, and it should be smooth and without breaks or inflammation, especially behind the ear. Note the size and location of any skin tags, moles, cysts, nodules, or le-

sions. There should be no openings or discharge in the preauricular area.

Palpating and manipulating the pinna can produce information about tenderness, nodules, or tophi (Figure 2-2). *Tophi* are small, hard nodules in the helix that are deposits of uric acid crystals, characteristic of gout. In palpation, move the pinna, feel the mastoid area, and press on the tragus. Note whether any of the manipulations cause pain or discomfort that could indicate inflammation or infection. Also, fold the pinna forward; it should readily return to its usual position.

Inspection of the ear canal is by direct observation, otoscopy, or microscopic examination. For direct observation in an *adult*, ask the patient to tip his head slightly to the opposite side while you pull the pinna up, back, and out. Use a penlight to inspect the ear canal for any abnormalities such as extreme narrowing of the ear canal, excessive wax, redness, scaliness, swelling, drainage, cysts, or foreign objects. Normally none of these signs are present. Visualization of the eardrum with this method is unlikely.

Assessment of the Mastoid

To assess the mastoid bone and process, palpate the bone behind the pinna. A normal mastoid bone is smooth, hard, and not tender. In comparing the mastoid bones on either side, remember that the mastoid processes are not always equal in size. The patient sometimes mentions this discrepancy, but the condition is not pathologic. The skin of the mastoid area should look normal.

Assessment of the Eardrum

The eardrum is located in the head at the end of the only skin-lined canal in the body, the ear canal. Thus visualization is difficult and requires illumination; adding magnification allows a more accurate assessment of the ear. These aids can be provided by an otoscope, a device consisting of a handle, a light source, a magnifying lens, and an attachment for visualizing the ear canal and eardrum. Some otoscopes have a pneumatic device for injecting air into the ear canal to test the mobility and integrity of the eardrum.

Specula for the otoscope come in a variety of sizes. Because the diameter of the meatus and the length of the ear canal vary, use the speculum with the largest diameter that fits comfortably into the ear canal. Check the light source for brightness; if the light appears yellowish or dim (like a flashlight with weak batteries), the batteries must be recharged or replaced.

Hold the otoscope in your dominant hand, with the hand resting against the patient's head. Then, if the patient should move suddenly, the otoscope will move also, and the external canal is less likely to be damaged. With your other hand, pull the pinna up, back, and out, straightening the ear canal. While doing this, gently tilt the patient's head away from you, and insert the speculum slowly and carefully into the ear canal (Figure 2-3). Bring your eye close to the magnifying lens to view the ear canal and eardrum. Advance the otoscope far enough to make a good seal, to facilitate use of the pneumatic bulb.

Observe the ear canal while the speculum is entering and leaving. Move the otoscope in a circular fashion to allow inspection of the entire ear canal; note any abnormalities such as extreme narrowing of the ear canal, nodules, redness, scaliness, swelling, drainage, cysts, foreign objects, or excessive wax. Some of these abnormalities impair visualization of the eardrum. Sometimes the ear canal must be cleaned of wax, dead skin, and other debris. Wax and debris can be removed with a cerumen spoon, suction aspirator, or irrigation, or a combination of all three.

The presence of a small amount of cerumen should not interfere with the examination. Cerumen normally is present in the external ear and varies in color from light yellow to black. Because cerumen that is impacted in the ear canal can cause loss of hearing, assessing the amount of cerumen is important.

A normal eardrum is slightly conical, quite shiny and smooth, and pearly gray (Figure 2-4). The position of the drumhead is oblique with respect to the ear canal. When disease is present, not only does the color of the eardrum change, but other abnormalities appear as well, such as retraction, bulging, or perforation of the eardrum, or the development of a white plaque in the eardrum.

Carefully inspect the entire eardrum, including the border of the annulus, again rotating the otoscope in a circular fashion. The umbo and the long and short processes of the malleus should be easily visible through the eardrum (see Figure 2-4).

Test the mobility of the eardrum by using the pneumatic device of the otoscope to inject a small amount of air into the ear canal. Observe the eardrum for movement, which normally accompanies this procedure.

Assessment of the Middle Ear

Assessment of the middle ear involves both measuring hearing and inspecting the middle ear through the tympanic membrane. Measuring the hearing of the middle ear is discussed in the next section. Table 2-1 lists tympanic membrane signs and the associated pathologic condition of the middle ear. Common pathologic conditions of the middle ear are shown in Figure 2-5.

Assessment of the Inner Ear—Hearing

The inner ears cannot be examined directly. However, some inferences about their condition can be drawn by testing auditory and vestibular function. A gross assess-

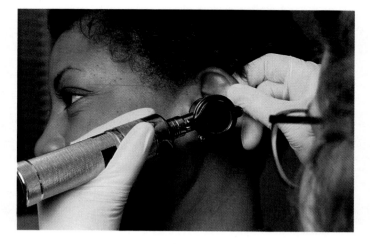

FIGURE 2-3
Otoscopic exam. Straighten the external auditory canal by pulling the auricle up and back to examine the ear with the otoscope.

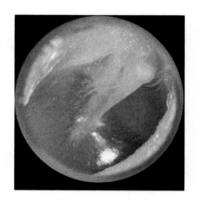

FIGURE 2-4
Normal tympanic membrane. (From Seidel.[58])

ment of the patient's hearing can be made simply through conversation and by evaluating the logical sequences of replies. A hearing questionnaire is helpful in assessment (see Appendix A).

Auditory Acuity
Whisper voice test

The ears must be tested separately to estimate the hearing in each. Occlude one of the patient's ears with a finger, and whisper two-syllable numbers softly toward the unoccluded ear; have the patient repeat the numbers. The intensity and volume of your voice can be decreased from a soft, medium, or loud voice to a soft, medium, or loud whisper. If you suspect that the patient is lipreading, turn your face away. Ask the patient if his hearing is better in one ear than in the other ear. If the auditory acuity is different, test the ear that hears better first. Then produce noise in the better-

Table 2-1

TYMPANIC MEMBRANE SIGNS AND ASSOCIATED CONDITIONS

Signs	Associated Conditions
Mobility	
Bulging with no mobility	Pus or fluid in middle ear
Retracted with no mobility	Obstruction of eustachian tube
Mobility with negative pressure only	Obstruction of eustachian tube
Excessive mobility on small areas	Healed perforation
Color	
Amber	Serous fluid in middle ear
Blue or deep red	Blood in middle ear
Chalky white	Infection in middle ear
Redness	Infection in middle ear, prolonged crying
Dullness	Fibrosis
White flecks, dense white plaques	Healed inflammation
Air bubbles	Serous fluid in middle ear

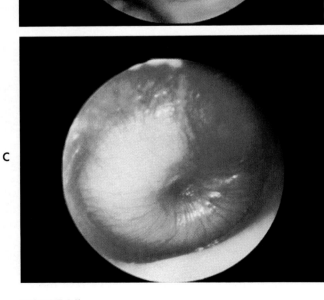

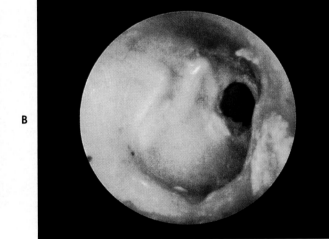

FIGURE 2-5
A, Cerumen in external ear canal. **B,** Perforation of tympanic membrane. **C,** Acute otitis media.

hearing ear by rapidly but gently moving the finger in the patient's ear canal while testing the other ear.

A watch tick can also be used to test hearing. However, a watch tick is a higher-pitched sound and less relevant to functional hearing than the voice test.

A tuning fork also provides a general estimate of hearing loss. The three major tuning fork tests date from the nineteenth century and are named after their originators: Rinne, Weber, and Schwabach (Table 2-2).

Rinne test

A vibrating tuning fork is shifted between two positions: against the mastoid bone (bone conduction) (Figure 2-6, **A**) and 2 inches from the opening of the ear canal (air conduction) (Figure 2-6, **B**). As the position is changed, the patient is asked to indicate which tone is

Table 2-2

INTERPRETING TUNING FORK TESTS

Site of problem	Rinne test	Weber test	Schwabach test
Normal hearing			
None	Air conduction is heard longer than bone conduction by 2:1 ratio (positive Rinne).	Tone is heard in center of head; no lateralization.	Examiner hears tone equally as long as patient.
Conductive loss			
External or middle ear	Bone conduction is heard longer than air conduction in poorer ear (negative Rinne).	Tone lateralizes to poorer ear.	Patient hears bone conduction longer than examiner.
Sensorineural loss			
Inner ear	Air conduction is heard longer than bone conduction (positive Rinne).	Tone is heard in better ear, because inner ear is less able to receive vibrations.	Examiner hears longer than patient.

louder (in front of the ear or behind the ear) or when one of the tones is no longer heard. The Rinne test is useful for distinguishing between *conductive* and *sensorineural* hearing loss.

With conductive hearing loss, the pathways of normal sound conduction are blocked. However, because vibrations against the mastoid bone can bypass the obstruction, bone conduction lasts longer than air conduction. With sensorineural hearing loss, the acoustic nerve is less able to perceive vibrations from either route; therefore the patient reports normal patterns.

Normally sound is heard twice as long or loud by air conduction (AC) as it is by bone conduction (BC). Therefore a normal response is one in which AC is heard louder or longer than BC (a positive Rinne test result). With conductive hearing loss, a person hears BC louder or longer than AC (a negative Rinne test result). With sensorineural hearing loss, a person hears better by AC, producing a positive Rinne test result.

Weber test

A tuning fork is set to vibrating by striking the tines on the examiner's knuckles or knee. The rounded tip of the handle is placed on the patient's forehead (Figure 2-7) or teeth (placement on the teeth generally is more reliable, even if the patient has false teeth). The patient is asked whether the tone is heard in the middle of the head, the right ear, or the left ear. The Weber test is useful in cases of *unilateral loss.*

A person with normal hearing hears the sound equally in both ears by bone conduction. If the person

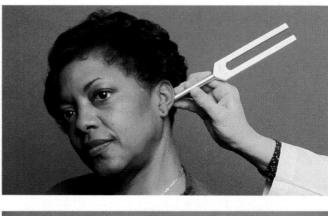

A

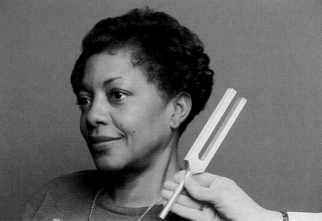

B

FIGURE 2-6
Rinne test. **A,** The tuning fork is placed on the mastoid bone for bone conduction. **B,** The tuning fork is placed in front of the ear for air conduction.

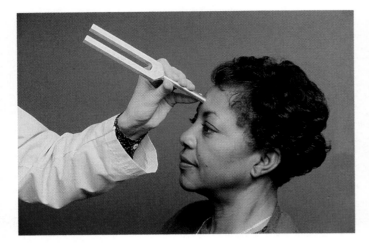

FIGURE 2-7
Weber test. The tuning fork is placed on the midline of the skull.

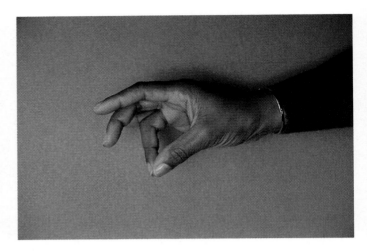

FIGURE 2-8
Examination of coordination with rapid alternating movements.

has a sensorineural hearing loss in one ear, the sound is heard in the better ear. If the person has a conductive hearing loss in one ear, the sound is heard better in that ear.

Schwabach test

This test is also used to distinguish between normal hearing and a hearing loss. The Schwabach test compares the hearing, both air and bone conduction, of the examiner (who must have normal hearing) with the patient by alternately placing a tuning fork on the mastoid process of the patient and the examiner.

Nurses can perform these tests at the bedside to obtain an indication of the amount of hearing the patient has. More elaborate and specific hearing tests, such as pure tone and speech tests, are performed in a soundproof room by an audiologist.

ASSESSMENT OF THE INNER EAR—BALANCE

Balance and equilibrium depend on *four systems* being intact: the *vestibular* system (the labyrinth of the ears), the *proprioceptive* system (somatosensors of joints and muscles), the *visual* system (the eyes), and the *cerebellar* system (coordination). The proprioceptive, vestibular, and visual sensations are integrated in the brainstem and cerebellum and perceived in the cerebral cortex. *Dizziness* is most likely to occur when *two* or *more systems* are *impaired simultaneously* or when they transmit sensory information that is contradictory.

Assessment of the inner ear for balance should include the same components as assessment of the inner ear for hearing: a complete health history, a dizziness questionnaire (see Appendix B), a review of systems, otoscopic examination, a whisper voice test, Rinne test, and Weber test. A neurologic screening examination focusing on the function of the cranial nerves and cere-

bellum should also be performed. The heart rate and rhythm should be determined, and the cardiovascular system should be checked for carotid bruits and orthostatic hypotension. Dizziness can have devastating effects on a patient's behavior. The disruption of the patient's routine, the severity of the attacks, and fear of the unknown can make the patient agitated, anxious, and depressed. Nurses must be aware of these feelings and demonstrate self-confidence, patience, courtesy, consideration, and gentleness.

Proprioception and Cerebellar Function
Coordination and fine motor skills

To test the patient's ability to do rhythmic, alternating movements quickly, have her touch the thumb to each finger on the same hand sequentially back and forth with increasing speed (Figure 2-8). Test each hand separately. The movements should be smooth and rhythmic.

Test movement accuracy by having the patient touch her nose with her index finger and then touch your index finger, which is held about 18 inches from the patient (Figure 2-9 **A** and **B**). Change the location of your finger several times. Repeat the test with the patient using the other hand. The movements during the finger-to-finger test should be rapid, smooth, and accurate.

The second test of movement accuracy is the finger-to-nose test. Have the patient close her eyes, then touch her nose with the index finger of each hand. The movements should be rapid, smooth, and accurate, even with increased speed.

The third test of movement accuracy is the heel-to-shin test. It can be done while the patient is sitting, standing, or lying down. Ask the patient to lightly run the heel of one foot up and down the opposite shin

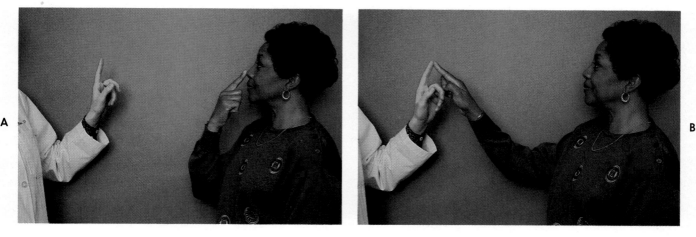

FIGURE 2-9
Examination of fine motor function. The patient touches **(A)** her nose, then **(B)** the examiner's finger.

(Figure 2-10). Repeat with the other heel. The patient should be able to do this in a smooth, straight line.

Finally, have the patient perform a series of facial movements to determine the functioning of the facial nerve. Ask her to clench her teeth, smile, purse her lips, pucker her lips, raise her eyebrows, and tightly close her eyes. Note any deviation from normal (See Figure 2-11).

CRANIAL NERVE FUNCTION

Cranial nerves are paired (12 pairs), and except for the first cranial nerve, all nerves originate in the brainstem. The involvement of cranial nerves in pathologic processes sometimes helps to localize the neurologic lesion. Thus certain tests have been developed to gauge the function of each cranial nerve. Table 2-3 can serve as a guide for the nurse in identifying each specific function and the corresponding test. Ordinarily taste and smell are not evaluated unless a problem is indicated. However, if any sensory loss is suspected, evaluation of the relevant cranial nerve is mandatory to determine the extent of the loss.

Cranial nerve function is expected to be intact as described in Table 2-3. Retrocochlear disorders, such as an acoustic neuroma, diminish the function of one or more of the cranial nerves on that side of the brain.

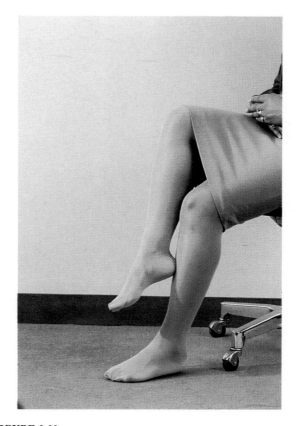

FIGURE 2-10
Examination of fine motor function. The patient runs the heel of one foot up and down the opposite shin.

A   B   C

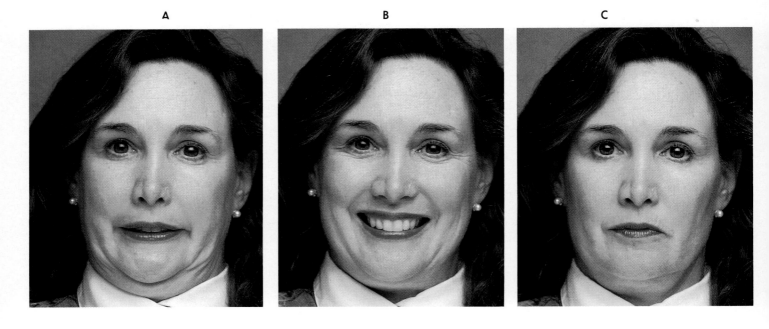

D   E   F

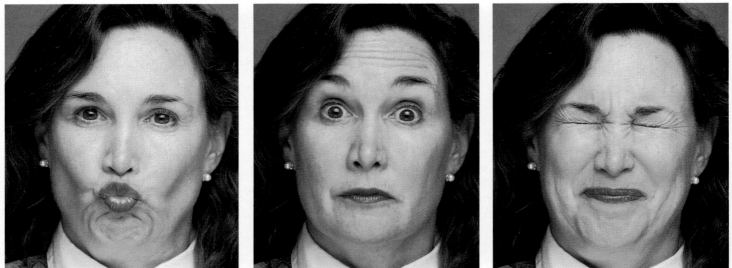

FIGURE 2-11
Patient performs facial movements in examination of facial nerve function. **A,**
Clenches teeth. **B,** Smiles, **C,** Purses lips. **D,** Puckers lips. **E,** Raises eyebrows.
F, Closes eyes tightly.

NYSTAGMUS

Nystagmus is the involuntary, rhythmic movement of the eyes. It is essentially an ocular disorder associated with vestibular dysfunction. Nystagmus occurs normally when a person watches a rapidly moving object. To check for *gaze nystagmus*, place your finger directly in front of the patient at eye level, and have the patient follow the finger without moving his head. Move your finger slowly from the midline toward the ear in each direction, and observe the patient's eyes for any jerking movements. For example, if the eyes jerk quickly to the left and drift slowly back to the right, the patient has a left nystagmus. Nystagmus can be horizontal, vertical, or rotary. Nystagmus is an abnormal condition that can be caused by a problem in the central or peripheral nervous system.

BALANCE—EQUILIBRIUM

Equilibrium is first tested with the Romberg test. Have the patient stand, feet together, arms at his sides, eyes open. Be prepared to steady or catch the patient if he begins to fall. Slight swaying is normal, but loss of balance (positive Romberg sign) is abnormal. Repeat the test with the eyes closed (Figure 2-12). If the positive Romberg sign recurs, additional balance tests may not be safe.

Balance may be tested in another way. Have the patient stand with his feet slightly apart; then push his shoulders to throw him off balance (being ready to catch him if necessary). The patient should recover his balance quickly.

Balance is also tested by having the patient stand on one foot, eyes closed, and arms held straight at his sides. Repeat on the opposite foot. Slight swaying is normal, but balance should be maintained for at least 5 seconds on each foot.

Table 2-3

PROCEDURES FOR CRANIAL NERVE EXAMINATION

Cranial nerve	Procedure
I (olfactory)	Test ability to identify familiar aromatic odors, one naris at a time with eyes closed.
II (optic)	Test vision with Snellen chart and Rosenbaum near vision chart.
	Perform ophthalmoscopic examination of fundi.
	Test visual fields.
III, IV, and VI (oculomotor, trochlear, and abducens)	Inspect eyelids for drooping.
	Inspect pupils' size for equality and direct and consensual response to light and accommodation.
V (trigeminal)	Inspect face for muscle atrophy and tremors.
	Palpate jaw muscles for tone and strength when patient clenches teeth.
	Test superficial pain and touch sensation in each branch. (Test temperature sensation if unexpected findings arise with pain or touch test.)
	Test corneal reflex.
VII (facial)	Inspect symmetry of facial features with various expressions (e.g., smile, frown, puffed cheeks, wrinkled forehead).
	Test ability to identify sweet and salty tastes on each side of tongue.
VIII (acoustic)	Test sense of hearing with whisper screening tests or by audiometry.
	Compare bone and air conduction of sound.
	Test for lateralization of sound.
IX (glossopharyngeal)	Test ability to identify sour and bitter tastes.
	Test gag reflex and ability to swallow.
X (vagus)	Inspect palate and uvula for symmetry with speech sounds and gag reflex.
	Observe for swallowing difficulty.
	Evaluate quality of guttural speech sounds (nasal or hoarse quality to voice).
XI (spinal accessory)	Test trapezius muscle strength (shrug shoulders against resistance).
	Test sternocleidomastoid muscle strength (turn head to each side against resistance).
XII (hypoglossal)	Inspect tongue in mouth and while protruded for symmetry, tremors, and atrophy.
	Inspect tongue movement toward nose and chin.
	Test tongue strength with index finger when tongue is pressed against cheek.
	Evaluate quality of lingual speech sounds (l, t, d, n).

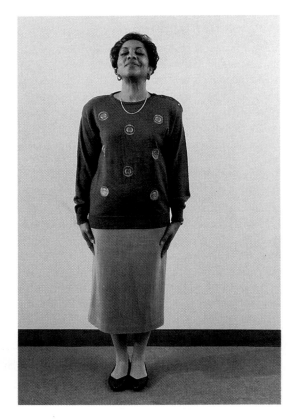

FIGURE 2-12
Evaluation of balance with the Romberg test.

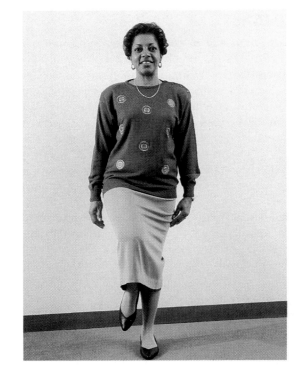

FIGURE 2-13
Evaluation of balance with the patient hopping in place on one foot.

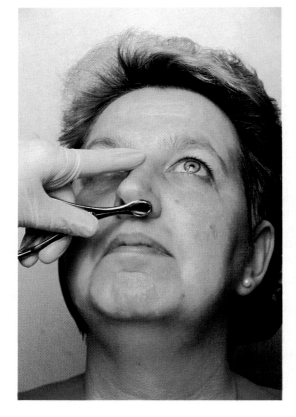

FIGURE 2-14
Use and placement of the nasal speculum.

Finally, have the patient open his eyes and hop in place, first on one foot and then on the other (Figure 2-13). The patient should be able to balance and hop on each foot for at least 5 seconds.

BALANCE—GAIT

Watch the patient walk down the hallway, first with her eyes open and then with them closed. Observe gait sequence, arm movements, and posture. Note any shuffling, toe walking, foot slapping, staggering, scissoring, widely placed feet, loss of arm swing, or hip hiking. The gait should be smooth and symmetric and have a regular rhythm. Posture should be a smooth sway with each step, and the arm swing should be smooth and symmetric.

Next, have the patient walk forward in a straight line, heel to toe, with her eyes open. Then have the patient reverse and walk heel to toe backwards. Some swaying is normal, but the patient should be able to consistently touch heel to toe.

CARDIOVASCULAR ASSESSMENT

Balance assessment includes taking the blood pressure in three positions: lying down, sitting, and standing up because orthostatic hypotension can mimic positional vertigo. The heart rate and rhythm should also be evaluated. Palpate the neck for masses, and auscultate for carotid bruits. All of these assessments can reveal hints for the cause of the patient's balance problem.

NOSE, NASOPHARYNX, AND SINUSES

First, evaluate the external nose and face. Examine the nose for edema and contour and the skin of the nose for color and any lesions. Is the columella in the midline? Notice any dryness or ulceration, or drainage from the nares. What is the shape of the nares? Are they equal in size? Is there flaring (which may indicate respiratory distress)? Are the nares narrow (which may indicate edema from an upper respiratory infection or nasal obstruction)? Can the patient breathe equally through both sides of the nose? Occlude one nasal passage, and instruct the patient to breathe. Repeat the procedure on the other nasal passage to determine whether there is equal passage of air. Gently insert the nasal speculum, placing the index finger on the tip of the nose for support (Figure 2-14). Do not overdilate the nares, because this will cause discomfort. Evaluate any nasal discharge according to character, amount, and color and whether the drainage is unilateral or bilateral. Gently suction the nasal cavity to visualize the structures. Examine the nasal turbinates on the lateral walls of the nose. Does the nasal cavity contain any crusting? Crusts may indicate excessive dryness of the nasal mucosa or denote an area of previous bleeding. Evaluate the nasal septum. Does it appear to be in the midline or is it deviated, making one side of the nasal cavity smaller than the other?

The sinuses can be examined with a nasopharyngoscope (Figure 2-15). A small telescope, available with various degrees of angularity, may be passed through or near the ostia to determine patency. The interior of the sinus cavities cannot be evaluated; however, the patient should be evaluated for asymmetry or edema over the sinuses. Does the patient have any tenderness to palpation when slight pressure is applied to the sinus areas, especially over the cheeks and forehead or at the bridge of the nose? Percussion with gentle tapping of the index finger over the sinuses may give an indication of fluid in the sinus cavity. Does the patient have equal sensation over the sinus areas? This can be determined by gently stroking the skin over the face and forehead.

Examine the nasopharynx with a small nasopharyngeal mirror. Gently depress the tongue with a tongue blade, and insert the warmed mirror behind the uvula,

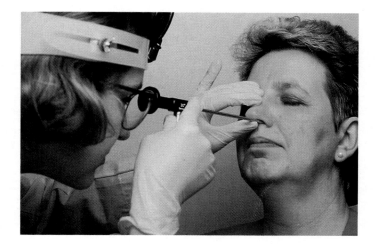

FIGURE 2-15
Use and placement of the nasopharyngoscope.

taking special care not to elicit a gag reflex or to touch the pharyngeal walls. Instruct the patient to say "aha" to elevate the palate. Evaluate the nasopharynx for lymphoid tissue, a mass, and any drainage. If drainage is present, note the color, consistency, and amount.

ORAL CAVITY

Evaluate the oral cavity systematically, beginning anteriorly with the lips. Inspect the external lips inside and outside. Note the color and symmetry, and any edema, excessive dryness, or lesions.

Evaluate the patient's bite. Examine the mouth for missing, jagged, or chipped teeth and for gingivitis or periodontitis. If the patient has dentures, partial or complete, instruct her to remove the dentures. Instruct her to open her mouth with the tongue remaining inside the oral cavity. Using two tongue blades as retractors, examine the buccal mucosa and the surface of the tongue (Figure 2-16, **A**); elevate the tongue to examine the floor of the mouth and the frenulum. Look at the hard and soft palates for ulceration or lesions. Evaluate the tonsils and tonsillar pillars; determine if there are crypts in the tonsils and whether the crypts contain any embedded food particles or purulent material. Apply slight pressure to the tongue, and instruct the patient to say "aha" in order to elevate the palate to determine movement (Figure 2-16, **B**). Instruct the patient to extend her tongue, noting any deviation, atrophy, fissures, ulcerations or lesions, and/or fasciculations. If the patient appears to have any plaques, red or white, attempt to remove them by gently scraping with the tongue blade.

Stensen's duct. Gently apply pressure to the parotid gland, and note the amount and color of saliva coming from the parotid gland through Stensen's duct. Repeat this procedure on the opposite side. Dry the floor of the mouth and apply slight pressure to the submandibular gland, noting the amount and consistency of saliva from Wharton's duct. Perform this test on both submandibular glands.

Using a gloved finger, gently palpate the floor of the mouth for any areas of induration. Then palpate the anterior tongue and the base of the tongue for any induration or ulceration.

LARYNX AND HYPOPHARYNX

To examine the larynx and hypopharynx, have the patient sit in an upright position, leaning slightly forward. Instruct him to extend his tongue while you hold the tongue firmly but gently with a piece of gauze. The laryngeal equipment should be warmed, or a defogging solution should be applied to it to prevent fogging of the lens, which distorts the findings of the examination.

Instruct the patient to breathe in and out through the mouth without holding his breath. Insert the laryngeal mirror over the base of the tongue, gently elevating the palate (Figure 2-17). Examine the area of the larynx and hypopharynx with the patient breathing in and out. Examine the area of the vocal cords with the cords in an open position and with the patient breathing; then have the patient say "a" and a high-pitched "e" to determine whether there is full movement of the vocal cords and to detect any lesions. If this procedure elicits a strong gag reflex, an adequate examination is not possible. An alternative examination may be performed with a flexible or rigid scope. Insert a rigid scope in the same manner as the laryngeal mirror, giving the patient the same instructions (Figure 2-18, **A**). Insert a flexible scope through the nose after applying a topical anesthetic (Figure 2-18, **B**). The pharynx may also be anesthetized with a topical anesthetic to decrease the gag reflex. If a topical anesthetic has been used in the oropharynx, instruct the patient to avoid drinking for 30 minutes to prevent aspiration.

NECK

Instruct the patient to unbutton or lower the collar of her clothing to inspect the neck area. First visually inspect the neck for symmetry or any lymph node enlargement. Then examine the area of the thyroid. You may choose to stand behind the patient, instructing her to swallow while you palpate the size of the thyroid gland and note any enlargement or nodules (see Figure 2-19). Next, examine the neck for enlarged lymph nodes, beginning with the jugulodigastric chain and moving both anterior and posterior (see Figure 2-20). Examine the area of the parotid gland and the submandibular gland for enlargement or masses.

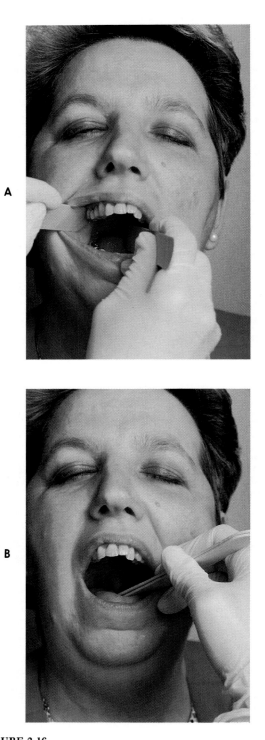

A

B

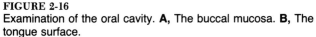

FIGURE 2-16
Examination of the oral cavity. **A,** The buccal mucosa. **B,** The tongue surface.

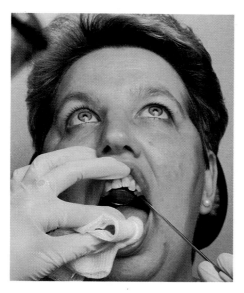

FIGURE 2-17
Laryngeal mirror in place for examination of the larynx and hypopharynx.

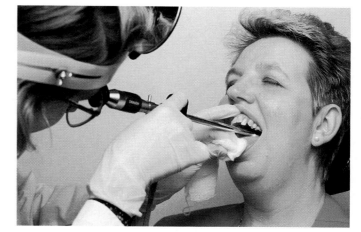

A

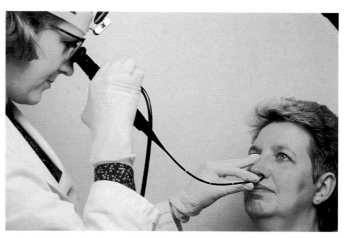

B

FIGURE 2-18
Laryngeal examination performed with **(A)** rigid scope and **(B)** flexible scope.

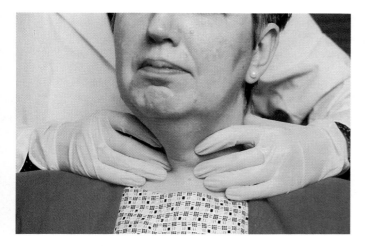

FIGURE 2-19
Palpation of the thyroid gland.

FIGURE 2-20
Palpation of the neck.

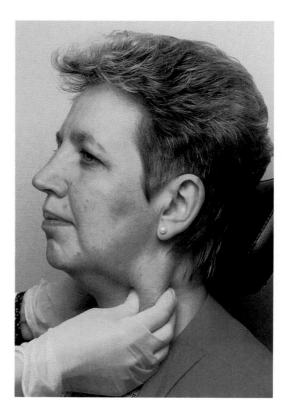

STAGING SYSTEM FOR TUMORS OF THE HEAD AND NECK

A general staging system, the TNM system, is used to stage cancers of the head and neck. This system was developed by the International Union Against Cancer (IUAC) and the American Joint Committee on Cancer (AJCC). The TNM staging system (see the box) evaluates the primary tumor (T), regional lymph nodes (N), and distant metastasis (M). It is used as a guide to plan treatment, to compare treatment results and prognoses among groups of patients, and to conduct and analyze cancer research.

Once the history and physical examination have been completed, any suspected tumor should be measured and documented according to the TNM system.

TUMOR STAGING SYSTEM

Classification	Characteristics
Tumor	
T_x	Primary tumor cannot be assessed
T_0	No evidence of primary tumor
T_{is}	Carcinoma in situ
T_1	Primary tumor ≤ 2 cm
T_2	Primary tumor 2-4 cm
T_3	Primary tumor >4 cm
T_4	Primary tumor involves adjacent structures
Regional lymph nodes	
N_x	Regional lymph nodes not assessed
N_0	No clinically palpable lymph node
N_1	Single ipsilateral lymph node <3 cm
N_{2a}	Single ipsilateral lymph node 3-6 cm
N_{2b}	Bilateral lymph nodes
N_{2c}	Contralateral lymph nodes
N_{3a}	Lymph nodes >6 cm
Distant metastasis	
M_x	Metastatic evaluation not performed
M_0	No clinical evidence of distant metastasis
M_1	Clinical evidence of metastasis

CHAPTER 3

Diagnostic Procedures

OTOSCOPY

Otoscopy is a magnified inspection of the external auditory canal and tympanic membrane using an otoscope. An otoscope consists of a handle, a light source, a magnifying lens, and an attachment for visualizing the inside of the ear. Specula for the otoscope are available in a variety of sizes. The largest speculum that will fit comfortably in the patient's ear is inserted to a depth of 1 to 1.5 cm, allowing examination of the auditory canal from the meatus to the tympanic membrane. If further evaluation is indicated, a microscopic examination is done, which allows a more detailed inspection (Figure 3-1).

INDICATIONS

To note any discharge, scaling, excessive redness, swelling, lesions, foreign bodies, or cerumen

To inspect the tympanic membrane for color, landmarks, contours, and perforations (the direction of the light can be varied to allow inspection of the entire tympanic membrane and annulus)

CONTRAINDICATIONS: None

NURSING CARE

No special nursing care is required.

PATIENT TEACHING

Explain the procedure to the patient.

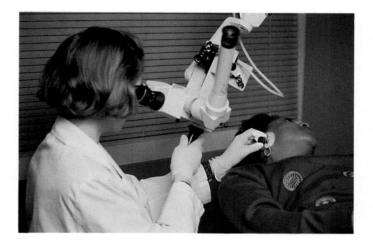

FIGURE 3-1
Examination of the tympanic membrane with an otoscope.

AUDIOMETRY

Audiometry is a hearing test performed in a soundproof booth by an audiologist. An electronic instrument, called an audiometer, produces sounds of varying tones and loudness, which are used to test the patient's hearing. Hearing is assessed by a special unit of measure, the decibel (db), which is a logarithmic function of sound intensity. For the test, the patient wears earphones and is asked to signal the audiologist by raising a hand or pressing a button when he hears a tone in each ear (Figure 3-2). The responses are plotted on a

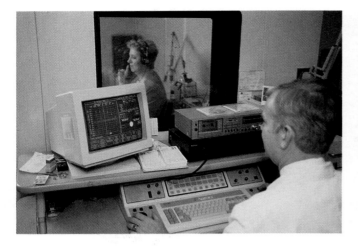

FIGURE 3-2
Patient undergoing an audiogram.

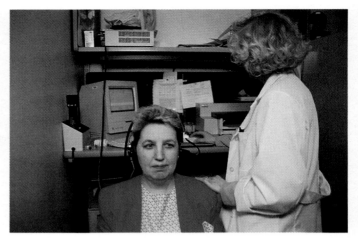

FIGURE 3-3
Tympanometry (middle ear pressure) and acoustic reflex thresholds are measured in a patient.

graph, the audiogram. The earphones are also used to measure the patient's level of speech hearing (speech reception threshold) and understanding of speech (speech discrimination).

AIR CONDUCTION

Air conduction is achieved by presenting tones through the earphones. By varying the loudness from 0 to 100 db and the frequency from 250 to 8,000 hertz (Hz), a hearing level can be established for air conduction. A normal hearing level is a pure tone average (derived by averaging the decibel level at 500, 1,000, and 2,000 Hz) of 20 db or less.

BONE CONDUCTION

Bone conduction is achieved by presenting the tones through a bone conduction oscillator placed on the mastoid bone. By varying the loudness (0 to 70 db) and the frequency (250 to 8,000 Hz), a hearing level can be established for bone conduction. The middle ear structures are bypassed during the bone conduction test, and the test result obtained is the nerve hearing level.

SPEECH TESTING

The speech reception threshold (SRT), which is determined through the earphones, is the lowest level at which a patient can hear correctly. The SRT test uses two-syllable words and serves as a check on the reliability of the air conduction result.

Speech discrimination is also tested through use of the earphones. This test determines the percentage of one-syllable words repeated correctly at a level 40 db above the speech reception threshold. A person with normal hearing usually repeats 88% or more of the words correctly.

IMPEDANCE AUDIOMETRY

Impedance audiometry includes assessment of middle ear pressure (tympanometry) and acoustic reflex thresholds.

Tympanometry

Tympanometry is the indirect measurement of the mobility (compliance) and impedance (resistance) of the tympanic membrane and ossicles of the middle ear. This automatic test is performed by placing a sealed probe in the external ear canal. By subjecting the external auditory canal and tympanic membrane to positive and negative air pressure, a distinctive tracing is formed on a graph called a tympanogram (Figure 3-3). Abnormalities on a tympanogram, categorized into types, point to the status of the tympanic membrane, middle ear space, eustachian tube, and ossicles; thus this test is useful for differentiating problems in the middle ear.

Acoustic Reflex Test

The acoustic reflex is the contraction of the stapedius muscle in response to an intense sound. In the acoustic reflex test, the stapedius muscle should show a bilateral response (stimulation to one ear causes a reaction in both ears) to loud acoustic stimulation from a probe. With pathologic conditions of the cochlea, acoustic reflex thresholds often are obtained at less intense stimulation levels (less than 60 db sensation level). With a retrocochlear lesion, the reflex thresholds often are elevated and may demonstrate abnormal decay or absence of the reflex. With conductive hearing loss, the reflexes may be elevated but usually are absent.

INDICATIONS

Chronic ear infection
Eustachian tube problems
Trauma
Otosclerosis
Tinnitus/hearing loss
Sensorineural hearing loss
Retrocochlear disorders

CONTRAINDICATIONS

Tympanic membrane perforation

NURSING CARE

No special nursing care is required.

PATIENT TEACHING

Explain to the patient the reason for the test, the procedure, and the results (when appropriate).

ELECTROCOCHLEOGRAPHY

Electrocochleography is the electrophysiologic measurement of electrical potentials of the eighth cranial nerve in response to acoustic stimuli applied by an electrode on the external auditory canal or tympanic membrane (noninvasive or extratympanic) or on the promontory (invasive or transtympanic). Other ground electrodes are placed on the head, mastoid process, and/or earlobe. Electrocochleography is used either to measure sensitivity or to determine whether a hearing loss stems from the level of the cochlea or from the eighth cranial nerve.

INDICATION

Hearing loss

CONTRAINDICATIONS: None

NURSING CARE

Because the electrodes for the test are applied with conductive paste, the patient should be instructed to wash after the procedure.

PATIENT TEACHING

Explain the purpose of the test, how long it will take (30 to 45 minutes), and the procedure. The patient will be seated in a comfortable chair and is permitted to fall asleep during the test. If the transtympanic approach is used, the electrode will be placed using a microscope. The pain is minimal because the electrode is very tiny.

ELECTRONYSTAGMOGRAPHY

Electronystagmography (ENG) is the measurement and graphic recording of the electrical potentials of eye movements during spontaneous, positional, or calorically evoked nystagmus. Electronystagmography is used to assess the oculomotor and vestibular systems and their corresponding interaction. The cornea of the eye carries a positive electrical charge, and the retina carries a negative electrical charge (corneoretinal potential). Electrodes are placed on the skin immediately lateral to each eye and on the skin above the bridge of the nose to detect horizontal eye movements; electrodes are also placed above and below the eye to detect vertical eye movements. The ENG test battery used in many vestibular clinics is: (1) spontaneous nystagmus, (2) gaze nystagmus, (3) positional test, (4) positioning test, (5) saccadic test, (6) pendular tracking test, (7) optokinetic test, and (8) caloric tests. These procedures are designed to test each function, investigate any pathologic nystagmus (spontaneous, gaze, positional, and positioning), and reflect the status of each labyrinth. Electronystagmography can also reflect disorders of the central nervous system.

The patient is seated for two thirds of the test and is lying supine with the head at a 30-degree angle for one third of the test (caloric stimulation). The skin is cleansed with alcohol to reduce the skin-electrode impedance, and the electrodes are applied (Figure 3-4). Most of the ENG is accomplished by having the patient look at lights or change head and body positions while seated. The caloric testing is the instillation of cool (30° C) and warm (44° C) water or air into the external auditory canal. If there is no response, then water at (20° C) can be introduced.

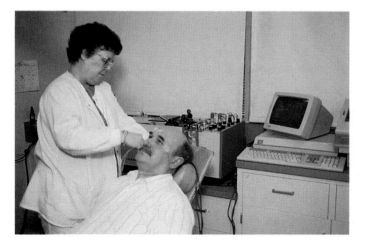

FIGURE 3-4
Electrodes are applied to a patient in preparation for electronystagmography.

INDICATIONS FOR VESTIBULAR TESTING

Indication	Possible diagnostic considerations
Unilateral or sensorineural hearing loss	Ménière's disease, lesion of the cerebellopontine angle, posterior fossa mass or deformity
Bilateral asymmetric sensorineural hearing loss	Ménière's disease, lesion of the cerebellopontine angle, posterior fossa mass or deformity, several other causes (e.g., presbycusis plus Ménière's disease)
Bilateral symmetric sensorineural hearing loss (profound)	Meningitis, head injury, developmental disorder
Bilateral symmetric sensorineural hearing loss with vertigo and ataxia	Bilateral Ménière's disease, ototoxicity
Conductive hearing loss, vertigo	Otosclerosis, circumscribed labyrinthitis
Persistent unilateral tinnitus with or without ipsilateral hearing loss	Small acoustic neuroma
Childhood failure of speech development with severe bilateral sensorineural hearing loss	Congenital malformation, acquired infection (e.g., meningitis)

INDICATIONS

See box on indications for vestibular testing.

CONTRAINDICATIONS: None

NURSING CARE

The nurse should obtain an adequate history of drug and alcohol use before ENG testing, because many drugs affect nystagmus. Patients should be instructed to stop taking vestibular sedatives, tranquilizers, and alcohol at least 24 hours before the tests. Patients prone to nausea or vomiting should not eat heavy meals before the tests.

PATIENT TEACHING

Advise the patient about the restriction on certain medications. Explain the reason for the tests, the different procedures, and what sensations to expect. The entire battery takes approximately 1 to 1½ hours to accomplish. Testing is painless, although vertigo and nausea may occur during the caloric irrigations. In rare cases vomiting is evoked. Reassure the patient of the benign nature of the test to reduce anxiety and obtain more accurate records.

ROTARY CHAIR

The rotary chair or rotational test is used as an adjunct to ENG. The physical forces applied by the rotary chair on the semicircular canal mechanism can be measured precisely. The subject is seated in a chair that can be rotated at a constant velocity and abruptly brought to rest or can be accelerated smoothly for a period of time (Figure 3-5). The patient is seated in darkness while viewing a light rotating with the chair. Rotational testing is useful for documenting recovery after a unilateral labyrinthine loss.

INDICATIONS

See the box on indications for vestibular testing.

CONTRAINDICATIONS: None

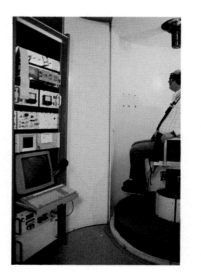

FIGURE 3-5
Patient undergoing rotary chair assessment.

NURSING CARE

As with ENG, the nurse should obtain an adequate history of drug and alcohol use before rotary chair testing, because many drugs affect nystagmus. Patients should be instructed to stop taking vestibular sedatives, tranquilizers, and alcohol at least 24 hours before the tests. Patients prone to nausea or vomiting should not eat heavy meals before the tests.

PATIENT TEACHING

Explain the procedure, expected sensations, and medication restriction to the patient. The procedure is painless, but nausea or vomiting may occur. Reassure the patient to reduce anxiety.

PLATFORM POSTUROGRAPHY

Platform posturography is a series of tests designed to detect the cause of problems with balance. The patient stands with each foot on a special sensor plate surrounded by a visual field wall. He is protected from falling by a safety harness (Figure 3-6). Sensors from each corner of the plate detect body sway and feed the data to a computer. The sensor plates on which the patient stands and the wall of the booth on which he fixates can be moved. The tests rely on the hypothesis that three sensory inputs are responsible for balance: the labyrinth, the proprioceptors, and vision. Six different tests are performed to determine which sensory input, or combination of them, is responsible for the balance problem. The procedures are: (1) eyes open, platform stable, visual field stable; (2) eyes shut, platform stable (Romberg test); (3) eyes open, platform stable, visual field swayed; (4) eyes open, platform swayed, visual field stable; (5) eyes shut, platform swayed; and (6) eyes open, platform swayed, visual field swayed.

Platform posturography can help distinguish among three types of vestibular dysfunction: (1) bilaterally or unilaterally reduced labyrinthine function; (2) fluctuations in vestibular function (e.g., as from a perilymphatic fistula); and (3) distortions of vestibular reflux function caused by benign paroxysmal positional nystagmus.

INDICATIONS

Same as for vestibular testing (see page 36).

CONTRAINDICATIONS: None

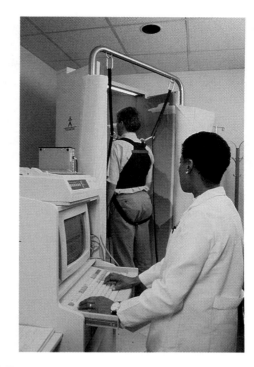

FIGURE 3-6
Patient wears a harness during the platform posturography exam to protect him from falling.

NURSING CARE

Advise the patient about the restriction on certain medications. Explain the reason for the tests, the different procedures, and what sensations to expect. Testing is painless, although vertigo and nausea may occur. Reassure the patient of the benign nature of the test to reduce anxiety and obtain more accurate records.

PATIENT TEACHING

Discuss the purpose of the test with the patient, and explain the procedure.

AUTOMATIC BRAINSTEM RESPONSE (ABR)

Brainstem auditory evoked potential testing is one approach to assessment of the auditory nervous system for evaluating dysfunction at the level of the eighth cranial nerve (acoustic nerve), pons, or midbrain. Evoked potentials measure and record changes in brain electrical activity that occur in response to auditory sensory stimulation; that is, the evoked potential measures and re-

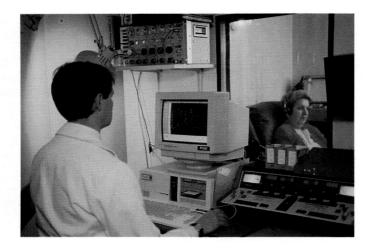

FIGURE 3-7
Patient undergoing test for auditory brainstem response (ABR).

cords brain electrical activity after auditory stimuli have been administered. Auditory evoked potentials measure electrical activity along the central auditory pathways of the brainstem in response to clicking sounds. The test involves placing electrodes on the vertex, mastoid process, and/or earlobes while the patient is seated in a comfortable chair (Figure 3-7). The data are fed into a computer. The abnormal findings suggest dysfunctions at the various levels in the auditory nervous system. For example, abnormal test results suggest a lesion of the acoustic nerve or brainstem.

INDICATIONS

Unilateral hearing loss
Unilateral tinnitus
Intracranial tumor
Acoustic tumor
Head injury

CONTRAINDICATIONS

None

NURSING CARE

Because the electrodes are applied with conductive paste, the patient's hair should be cleaned after the test.

PATIENT TEACHING

Explain the purpose of the test. Explain that the procedure takes 30 to 45 minutes and is done while the patient is seated in a comfortable chair. The patient will hear clicks but can fall asleep during the test.

PLAIN FILM X-RAYS

In diagnosing head and neck disorders, plain film x-rays may be taken of the chest, sinuses, and neck. A routine chest x-ray is taken to determine a baseline lung condition; to detect abnormalities that may require further investigation, such as nodules; and to monitor changes in the patient's pulmonary condition, such as pneumonia or atelectasis.

Plain film x-rays of the sinuses have been mostly replaced by computed tomography (CT) scans, but x-rays may be taken for an initial evaluation or to monitor the patient's response to therapy.

Plain film x-rays of the neck can be used to detect abscesses and to detect metal foreign bodies, especially before magnetic resonance imaging (MRI).

INDICATIONS

To establish baseline condition
To detect changes in baseline condition
To monitor response to therapy
To detect metallic foreign bodies
To determine need for more extensive procedures
To develop template for frontal sinus surgery

CONTRAINDICATIONS

Pregnancy

NURSING CARE

The patient should be instructed to remove jewelry and clothing above the waist and to put on a hospital gown.

PATIENT TEACHING

Explain the reason for the test, and emphasize that it is painless.

SIALOGRAPHY

Sialography is the x-ray examination of the salivary glands and ducts after introduction of a radiopaque material into the ducts. A sialogram may be recommended in patients with either parotid or submandibular gland swelling related to narrowing of the duct or calculus in the duct. Radiopaque dye is introduced through a small catheter placed in Stensen's duct to evaluate parotid swelling, or Wharton's duct to evaluate the submandibular gland. X-ray films are taken.

INDICATIONS

Ductal abnormality of Wharton's or Stensen's duct

CONTRAINDICATIONS

Complete stenosis of the duct
Allergy to radiopaque dye
Pregnancy

NURSING CARE

A local anesthetic is injected, and the patient will feel slight pressure or discomfort near the duct. The punctum of the duct should be observed for redness, edema, and drainage after the procedure.

PATIENT TEACHING

Instruct the patient to rinse her mouth with half-strength hydrogen peroxide and water after meals and at bedtime. She may apply heat to the gland after the procedure if it is causing her discomfort.

COMPUTED TOMOGRAPHY

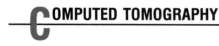

Computed tomography (CT scanning) involves sending an x-ray beam through the body at various angles (Figure 3-8). The images that are obtained by the x-ray beam are passed through a computer to produce cross-sectional images. The area being examined can be evaluated in thin sections, or slices, producing more and smaller components than a plain film x-ray. The CT scan may also be done with a contrast medium, an iodinated dye that is useful in imaging vascular lesions and in increasing the clarity of the images.

INDICATIONS

To diagnose and evaluate tumors
To detect abscesses
To evaluate the extent of sinus disease
To determine upper or lower airway obstruction

CONTRAINDICATIONS

Allergy to iodinated dye (manifested by allergy to shell-fish)
Pregnancy
Weight over 300 pounds

NURSING CARE

The patient should be questioned about allergies to iodinated dye; this is best accomplished by asking the patient if he has ever had an allergic reaction when eating shellfish. The patient is instructed to remove jewelry and clothing above the waist and to put on a hospital gown. If an intravenous contrast medium is to be used,

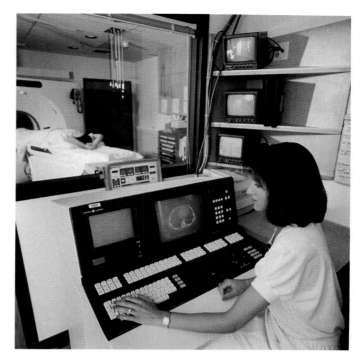

FIGURE 3-8
X-ray technician performs computed tomography.

an intravenous line should be placed. After the procedure the patient should be monitored for any allergic reactions to the dye.

PATIENT TEACHING

Explain the procedure to the patient, and provide information about use of a contrast medium. Inform the patient that the procedure will take approximately 30 to 60 minutes; during this time the patient will be asked to lie still, but he can communicate with the physician and technician performing the scan. The patient should be instructed to tell the physician if any untoward effects occur from use of the dye, such as itching, rash, rapid heartbeat, nausea, or vomiting.

MAGNETIC RESONANCE IMAGING

Magnetic resonance imaging (MRI) uses a large magnet rather than ionizing radiation to emit energy. The patient is placed in a tube or tunnel containing a large magnet equipped with radiofrequency coils, which transmit radio waves into the body part being imaged (Figure 3-9). The patient's own atoms (mainly hydrogen atoms) are given additional bursts of energy by these radiofrequency waves and in turn emit signals that are processed and displayed as computer-generated images of the body part.

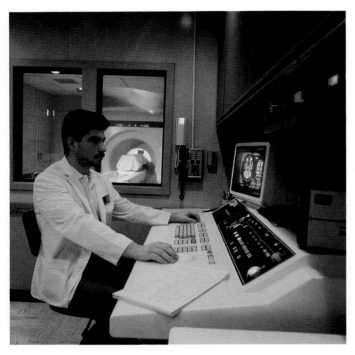

FIGURE 3-9
X-ray technician performs magnetic resonance imaging.

INDICATIONS

Tumors (to distinguish tumor mass from fibrosis)
Sinus disease (infection and tumors)

CONTRAINDICATIONS

Claustrophobia
Weight over 300 pounds
Pregnancy
Implanted metal devices

NURSING CARE

The patient is instructed to remove all jewelry, other metal items, credit cards, and clothing. Ear plugs or music may be provided in some units to help block the pounding sound emitted during the procedure. The nurse evaluates the patient's ability to complete the procedure and any complaints of claustrophobia. If severe claustrophobia is detected, a mild sedative (e.g., Valium) can be given 30 minutes before the procedure. In addition, a family member or friend may be allowed in the room during the procedure to offer reassurance if necessary.

The patient should be questioned about previous surgery that may have involved implantable devices such as aneurysm clips, pacemakers, or cochlear implants. If a metallic foreign body may be present, plain film x-rays must be taken to determine the actual location.

PATIENT TEACHING

Explain the procedure to the patient. Inform her that a mirror may be present to decrease anxiety from claustrophobia. Also tell her that she will not be exposed to radiation during the MRI. Tell the patient that the procedure usually takes 30 to 60 minutes, and during that time she must remain still on a hard table. Encourage the patient to talk to the x-ray technician performing the scan during the procedure if she needs to. Additional instructions are given to the patient during the procedure.

NUCLEAR MEDICINE SCANNING

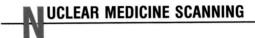

In nuclear medicine scanning, a radioactive isotope specific to the area being scanned is ingested or injected. The isotope is absorbed by the particular tissue, and the remainder is excreted through the kidneys. The patient is scanned to detect the uptake of the isotope in the body tissue.

Thyroid scans may be done to detect abnormalities in the thyroid gland, and bone scans may be performed to detect bony metastases. Additional scans such as liver-spleen scans may be ordered to detect liver metastases, but these scans generally have been replaced by CT scanning.

INDICATIONS

Thyroid abnormality (enlargement or mass)
To evaluate for metastasis

CONTRAINDICATIONS: Pregnancy

NURSING CARE

The radioactive isotope is either ingested or injected, depending on the isotope used. The injection site should be evaluated for redness, warmth, and irritation. The patient should be encouraged to drink plenty of fluids after the procedure to ensure excretion of the isotope.

PATIENT TEACHING

Explain the procedure to the patient. After the dye is injected, tell him to increase his fluid intake and to notify the physician if any changes occur at the injection site. Give the patient instructions to return for the completion of the scan at a specific time. Emphasize to the patient that the amount of radiation involved is minimal and that he poses no danger to other people.

BARIUM SWALLOW (ESOPHAGOGRAPHY)

With a barium swallow (barium esophagography), the patient is given a radiopaque drink, and videofluoroscopy is performed with the patient in a sitting position and lying down. A motion x-ray film is taken to detect any abnormality. A barium swallow (esophagogram) is done to evaluate a patient's swallowing ability if dysphagia (difficulty swallowing) is a presenting symptom, or to detect any abnormality in the esophagus if gastroesophageal reflux or a tumor of the upper aerodigestive tract is suspected. If solid food dysphagia is the complaint, a modified swallow is done using foods of various consistencies coated with barium. A modified swallow usually is done with the aid of the speech/swallowing therapist, who can help evaluate the patient's condition and recommend treatment, depending on test results.

INDICATIONS

Dysphagia
Gastroesophageal reflux
To rule out a tumor of the upper aerodigestive tract

CONTRAINDICATIONS: Pregnancy

NURSING CARE

The patient is instructed to avoid eating or drinking for 4 hours before the test. The chalky-tasting liquid she will drink will be taken in sips while a series of x-ray films is taken.

PATIENT TEACHING

After the procedure, instruct the patient to increase fluids and to use a laxative to prevent a barium impaction.

ANGIOGRAPHY

Angiography is the x-ray examination of vessels after injection of a radiopaque dye. The procedure is performed by a neuroradiologist in the radiology department. An angiogram may be performed to demonstrate a vascular tumor in the head and neck, to show the proximity of a tumor to the carotid artery, to determine the vascular supply to a tumor or area of bleeding, or to embolize a bleeding area.

The patient is instructed to have nothing by mouth for several hours before the procedure. Blood tests are done before testing to evaluate bleeding time, platelet counts, and kidney function. The patient is admitted to an outpatient radiology or same-day surgery unit the morning of the procedure. The patient is transported to radiology by stretcher and moved to a hard table (Fig-

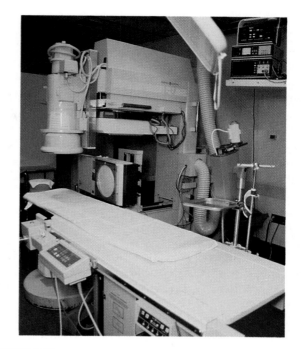

FIGURE 3-10
Equipment used for angiography.

ure 3-10). An intravenous line is started once the patient has been positioned. The patient's head and shoulders are immobilized, and the groin area is draped and prepared.

A local anesthetic is injected into the groin. Then a catheter is inserted into the femoral artery and threaded up to the carotid artery (or arteries) to be evaluated. An iodinated dye is periodically injected into the catheter, and a series of x-ray films taken. The procedure takes approximately 1 hour, and the patient must remain in bed for 8 hours before being discharged.

INDICATIONS

To identify vascular tumors
To demonstrate tumor involvement of the carotid artery
To determine the vascular supply to a tumor or area of bleeding
To embolize an area of bleeding or a vascular tumor

CONTRAINDICATIONS

Allergy to dye
Anticoagulant therapy
Recent embolic or thromboembolic event

COMPLICATIONS

Hematoma, bleeding

NURSING CARE

A nursing assessment should be completed before the procedure is scheduled. The patient is questioned about (1) possible allergy to the iodinated dye; (2) use of anticoagulants, including aspirin and nonsteroidal anti-inflammatory drugs; and (3) his general medical condition, especially renal function and any previous embolic or thromboembolic events. An informed consent form is signed, and blood tests are done. The patient is instructed to have nothing by mouth for 8 hours before the procedure. An intravenous line is started, and the groin area is prepared and draped. The patient's vital signs and neurologic status are monitored before and during the procedure.

After the procedure, the patient is kept in bed for 8 hours, with the affected leg kept straight. The catheter insertion site should be evaluated for bleeding, hematoma, or edema. A pressure dressing is kept over the insertion site.

Fluids are forced after the procedure to promote excretion of the dye. A general diet and normal activities can be resumed after 8 hours of bed rest.

PATIENT TEACHING

Explain the procedure to the patient and family member or friend. Inform the patient that he will be asked questions and his vital signs will be monitored frequently. Explain to the patient that he may experience a warm feeling, flushing, or pressure sensations during the procedure.

Explain the reasons for bed rest after the procedure and the need for increasing his fluid intake.

BALLOON OCCLUSION TESTING

If the carotid artery is at risk during surgery (involved with tumor), it is necessary to determine the patient's ability to withstand ligation of the blood supply. A balloon occlusion test is performed after the angiogram. A catheter with a balloon at the tip is inserted through the catheter used for the angiogram. Once the catheter is in place in the carotid artery, the balloon is inflated to occlude the blood flow. The patient is monitored closely during this procedure to ensure adequate cerebral blood flow by way of the other carotid artery and collateral circulation. The patient is asked to respond to simple questions, to squeeze the examiner's hands, and to push his feet against the examiner's hands to ensure adequate circulation. If the patient's response changes in any way, the procedure is immediately discontinued.

After the catheter and balloon are removed, a pressure dressing is put on the catheter insertion site, and the patient is instructed to remain in bed for 8 hours before discharge.

EMBOLIZATION PROCEDURE

If the angiogram demonstrates a vascular tumor or an area of bleeding, embolization may be performed. The same procedure as was described for the angiogram is performed. Embolization material is passed through the catheter to the major vessel supplying the mass or bleeding area in order to occlude the blood flow. This results in a decrease of the blood supply, shrinking of the tumor mass, and a decrease in bleeding during the surgical procedure.

LABORATORY TESTS

Four laboratory tests are useful for assessment of head and neck disorders: (1) blood tests, (2) cultures, (3) cerebrospinal fluid (CSF) identification, and (4) pathologic tissue examination.

Blood tests that are diagnostic for systemic abnormalities are only secondarily significant for specific disease. For example, an elevated white blood count points to an infection but is not diagnostic of ear disease. However, with an ear infection and in the absence of other infection, blood tests for infection are necessary to assess the ear infection.

Drainage from abscesses or a surgical incision usually is *cultured* to identify the causative organism. This is especially necessary with acute infections to choose the appropriate antibiotics. When long-term drainage is present (such as in chronic otitis media), cultures are less helpful because gram-negative bacilli cover up the original pathogen. In these cases many surgeons do not culture the drainage but begin treatment with broad-spectrum antibiotics.

Drainage found in the ear presents a dilemma. Is this clear fluid *cerebrospinal (CSF) fluid?* A fistula from the inner ear to the middle ear and external ear can produce CSF fluid. Because this pathway also can lead to meningitis by retrograde contamination, analysis of clear fluid often is helpful in diagnosing a problem.

Pathologic examination of abnormal tissue harvested during surgery is necessary both to rule out a malignancy and to identify unusual disorders. If the surgeon is in doubt as to the findings, then a tissue sample (biopsy) is taken for examination.

CHAPTER 4

Disorders of the Ear—Hearing

Impaired hearing is the most common disability in the United States and the third most prevalent chronic condition among people 65 years of age or older. Hearing impairment is a state of diminished auditory acuity that ranges from partial to complete loss of hearing. More than 28 million people in the United States have a hearing impairment. By the year 2050 about one out of every five people in the United States, or almost 58 million individuals, will be 55 years of age or older. Of these almost half (26 million) are expected to have a hearing impairment.

Because of the expected scope of this problem, nurses face two major responsibilities: identifying individuals with a hearing impairment and developing effective techniques for communicating with these patients. Nursing care is impossible if the nurse and patient cannot communicate. Also, a hearing disability may be alleviated if the nurse detects the problem and refers the patient for appropriate treatment.

Each person's economic and social well-being depends on the ability to communicate. Impaired hearing can hinder communication with others, limit social activities, and reduce constructive use of leisure time. It can jeopardize career options, job opportunities, and financial security. Hearing problems can also influence a person's ability to remain independent or to feel that he or she is a contributing member of society. People with impaired hearing are less able to enjoy the beauty of life that stems from sound, and their ability to share the human experience is temporarily or permanently curtailed. Hearing impairment diminishes the quality of life for one third of U.S. adults between 65 and 75 years of age.

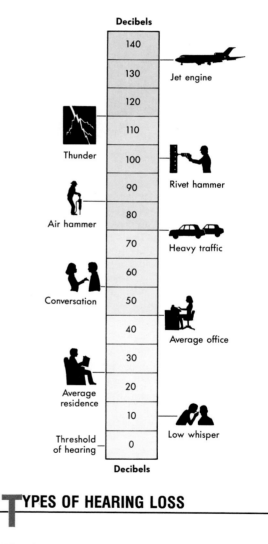

TYPES OF HEARING LOSS

CONDUCTIVE HEARING LOSS

Any interference with the conduction of sound waves through the external auditory canal, the eardrum, or the middle ear results in *conductive hearing loss*, or transmission deafness. The inner ear is not involved in

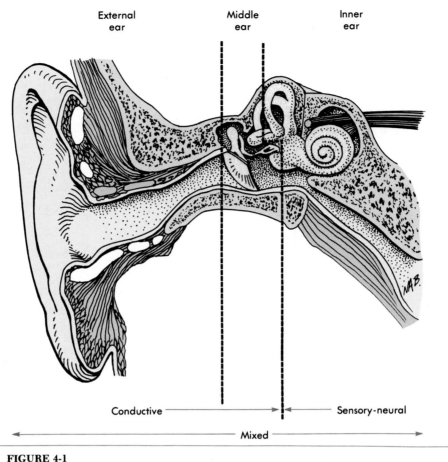

External
ear

Middle
ear

Inner
ear

Conductive ————————————►|◄——— Sensory-neural

◄——————————————— Mixed ———————————————►

FIGURE 4-1
Three types of hearing loss. Conductive loss results from interference with conduction in external and middle ears; sensorineural loss from interference with conduction in the inner ear; and mixed hearing loss results from interference with conduction in all three areas. (From Phipps, Long, Woods, Cassmeyer.[48a])

pure conductive loss, and amplified sound waves will reach the inner ear.

Conductive hearing loss may be caused by anything that blocks the external ear (e.g., wax, a foreign body, or edema or drainage from an infection); by thickening, retraction, scarring, or perforation of the tympanic membrane; or by any pathophysiologic changes in the middle ear that affect or fix one or more of the ossicles (Figure 4-1).

SENSORINEURAL HEARING LOSS

Sensorineural hearing loss is caused by a disease or injury that affects the inner ear, neural structures, or nerve pathways leading to the brainstem (Figure 4-1). Some of the causes of "nerve" deafness are infectious diseases (measles, mumps, meningitis); arteriosclerosis; ototoxic drugs (see the box on page 68); neuromas of cranial nerve VIII (the acoustic nerve); otospongiosis (a form of progressive deafness caused by the formation of new, abnormal spongy bone in the labyrinth); injury to the head or ear; or degeneration of the organ of Corti,

which occurs most often as a result of advancing age (in such cases the condition is known as presbycusis).

CENTRAL DEAFNESS

Central deafness is also known as central auditory dysfunction. It is a condition in which the central nervous system (CNS) cannot interpret normal auditory signals. Thus the ability to hear tests as normal, although the patient is "deaf." Diseases that alter the central nervous system, such as cerebrovascular accidents and tumors, cause this rare form of sensorineural hearing loss.

OTHER TYPES OF HEARING LOSS

Different types of hearing loss are listed in the box on page 45. A person is considered to have a *mixed* loss when conductive and sensorineural hearing loss are present simultaneously. A *functional* loss is a hearing loss for which no organic lesion can be found. A hearing loss may also be congenital or acquired. *Most people with ear problems have some degree of hearing loss.*

TYPES OF HEARING LOSS

Air conduction hearing loss: loss of hearing through the external and middle ears

Bone conduction hearing loss: loss of hearing through the inner ear

Central hearing loss: loss of hearing from damage to the brain's auditory pathways or auditory center

Conductive hearing loss: loss of hearing in which air conduction is worse than bone conduction

Fluctuating hearing loss: a sensorineural hearing loss that varies with time

Functional hearing loss: loss of hearing for which no organic lesion can be found

Mixed hearing loss: both air and bone conduction hearing loss occur

Neural hearing loss: a sensorineural hearing loss originating in the nerve or brainstem

Sensorineural hearing loss: loss of hearing involving the cochlea and hearing nerve; bone and air conduction are equal but diminished

Sensory hearing loss: a sensorineural hearing loss originating in the cochlea and involving the hair cells and nerve endings

Sudden hearing loss: a sensorineural hearing loss of sudden onset

External Ear Disorders

PATHOPHYSIOLOGY

Congenital Ear Disorders

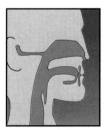

In the embryo the auricle and external ear canal develop separately, a process that results in two types of congenital disorders of the external ear. The pinna may be deformed or absent while the external ear canal is normal (see Figure 4-2), or the pinna and ear canal may both show congenital changes. Abnormalities of the external ear canal cause different degrees of incomplete development, or *canal atresia.* Congenital findings of the external ear do not necessarily mean that the middle or inner ear is involved. One minor congenital finding is protruding ears, in which the auricle is set at a larger than normal angle to the head. Cysts and skin tracts that develop from incomplete formation of the pinna are quite common.

Depending on their severity, congenital disorders of the external ear usually require cosmetic surgery. Postoperative nursing care for such procedures is discussed in Chapter 6, Therapeutic Interventions for Ear Disorders.

Masses/Tumors

Benign masses of the external ear canal usually are cysts that arise from a sebaceous gland (in rare cases the cyst may develop from the cerumen, or earwax,

glands). *Sebaceous cysts* are glands that have become obstructed with sebum, a soft, cheesy material (see Figure 4-2). Cysts can also be congenital. The small, hard, bony protrusions sometimes seen in the lower posterior bony portion of the ear canal are called *exostoses.* The skin covering exostosis is normal; if the skin is red, the mass usually is an abscess. Exostoses most often occur bilaterally, are rare in children, and are more common in men than in women. *Infectious polyps* found in the ear canal arise from the tympanic membrane or, more commonly, from the middle ear through a hole in the tympanic membrane. Malignant tumors also may be found in the external ear. The most common *cutaneous carcinomas* are *basal cell carcinoma* on the pinna and *squamous cell carcinoma* in the ear canal. If left untreated, these carcinomas can invade the underlying tissue, and squamous cell carcinoma may spread throughout the temporal bone. Rare tumors of the cerumen glands are of the *adenoma* cell type.

Benign or malignant masses and tumors require surgery. Postoperative nursing care for these procedures is discussed in Chapter 6 and Chapter 11.

Keloids

Keloids are an overgrowth of hypertrophied scar tissue that may result from surgery, trauma, or ear piercing. Keloids are more common in blacks than in whites. Treatment of keloids involves excision followed by re-

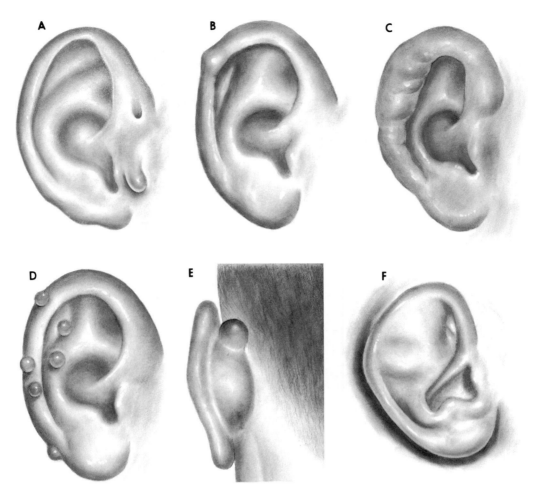

FIGURE 4-2
Congenital external ear problems. **A**, Preauricular skin tag and sinus. **B**, Darwin's tubercle. **C**, Cauliflower ear. **D**, Tophi. **E**, Sebaceous cysts. **F**, Malformation of the auricle. (From Seidel.[58])

peated injections of steroids. Postoperative nursing care for this procedure is discussed in Chapter 6.

Impacted Cerumen

On inspection of the external ear canal, the most common problematic finding is impacted cerumen (earwax). Although the ear canal cleans itself, cerumen may become impacted as a result of disease or improper cleaning. The cerumen must be removed carefully, and this may need to be done before the tympanic membrane can be examined.

Trauma, either sharp or blunt, is becoming a more common finding. Repeated blunt trauma produces a residual finding of hypertrophic scar formation, known as *cauliflower ears* (see Figure 4-2), an occupational hazard for boxers. With prompt treatment traumatic injuries can be corrected successfully.

Foreign Bodies

Surprisingly, a wide array of items, or *foreign bodies*, fit into the ear canal. In adults the foreign bodies most commonly found are a piece of cotton or (also the most

annoying) an insect. In children the most common foreign body is a small toy. Equally surprising is the difficulty that can be encountered in removing a foreign body. The least traumatic method is to use an *operating microscope*. To remove a live insect, the ear canal is filled with mineral oil, **not water.** Water causes the insect to swell, making it difficult to remove.

External Otitis

The most common problems in the external ear are infections, primarily bacterial or fungal. The most common infection, called *external otitis*, involves the external ear canal. External otitis is a term used to describe inflammatory diseases of the auricle and the external auditory canal. This infection begins in the skin lining of the ear canal and can occlude the canal (see Color Plate 2 on page x). External otitis occurs more often in the summer than in the winter. A localized form of this infection is seen as an ear canal furuncle or abscess. If the individual has a systemic disease such as diabetes mellitus, the external otitis can spread wildly through cartilage and bone; it is then referred to as *malignant external otitis* caused by *Pseudomonas* organisms. The most common form of external otitis is called *swimmer's ear,* because it is prevalent when water remains in the ear canal. Opportunistic fungal infections are also common, as are contact and seborrheic dermatitis. See Nursing Care Plan on pages 50-53.

Perichondritis

Occasionally an infection can involve the cartilage of the auricle, a condition known as perichondritis. Perichondritis may be caused by trauma, ear piercing, insect bites, or a skin infection, all of which allow bacteria to enter. The bacteria cause pus to form between the cartilage and the perichondrium. Perichondritis can diminish the blood supply to the cartilage and surrounding tissue, causing breakdown and necrosis of the cartilage and loss of the auricle's distinctive shape. Early, aggressive treatment (usually with parenteral antibiotics) is needed to prevent this disorder from following a lengthy and destructive course.

Frostbite of the auricle has similar findings. See Nursing Care Plan on pages 53-55.

CLINICAL MANIFESTATIONS

Pain is the most common symptom of problems in the external ear. The pain can range from mild to severe, and painful sites also cause tenderness because of the close proximity of bone (a hard surface) when palpating the ear. A clue to external otitis is tenderness when gently pulling on the pinna. A forerunner of pain in external otitis is pruritus in the ear canal. Inflammation (redness) can be easily identified with an otoscope, but an otoscopic examination may not be possible because of pain and swelling, and the inflammation may prevent visualization of the tympanic membrane. At different stages of infection, *drainage* is found exiting the ear canal. Early in an infection the drainage may be clear and not discolored by pus.

Patients with an occluded ear canal commonly complain of loss of hearing. Both infection and cerumen can cause a sudden hearing loss. The patient may also complain of a *blocked* ear, or a feeling of fullness in the ear. In some forms of external otitis, the patient may have a low-grade temperature. With perichondritis or frostbite, the pinna may be edematous, inflamed, and/or shiny.

COMPLICATIONS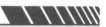

Abscess	Keloid
Cellulitis	Lymphadenopathy
Discoloration	Metastasis
Disfigurement of pinna	Osteitis
Hearing loss	Septicemia
Infection of middle ear	Stenosis
Ischemia/necrosis of pinna	

DIAGNOSTIC STUDIES AND FINDINGS

Diagnostic test	Findings
Culture of discharge	To identify specific microbe (bacteria, fungus, virus)
Otoscopic/microscopic examination	To diagnose specific external ear disorder or infection, remove cerumen and/or foreign body
Audiometric testing	To identify hearing loss
Biopsy	To rule out malignancies and to identify tissue
Complete blood count	To detect a systemic infection
Imaging studies	To diagnose tumors, osteitis, or exostoses

MEDICAL MANAGEMENT

GENERAL MANAGEMENT

Infections of the external ear are treated with antibiotics, either as drops or ointment or in oral and parenteral forms. If the ear canal is swollen shut, a wick can be inserted to allow drops to penetrate the canal. If the infection is both systemic and localized, systemic antibiotics are the standard treatment.

Debris from the infection and cerumen can be cleaned out with medicinal irrigations. External ear infections are very painful, and the patient usually needs analgesics. Perichondritis must be treated aggressively to prevent complications.

MEDICAL MANAGEMENT—cont'd

The treatment for an external ear infection is determined by the stage of the infection. The four principles of treatment are:
1. Frequent and thorough cleansing of the external auditory canal.
2. Use the appropriate topical antibiotics (add systemic antibiotics if the infection extends beyond the ear canal into other tissues).
3. Treat associated symptoms such as pain and inflammation.
4. Teach the patient the basics of ear care and how to prevent problems in the external ear.

DRUG THERAPY

Analgesic agents (aspirin, acetaminophen, codeine): 30 mg PO q 4 h.

Corticosteroids (with or without wick): 1% hydrocortisone with antibiotics in drops.

Antiinfective agents: Antibiotic or antifungal ear drops may be prescribed (usually 0.5% neomycin or 10,000 U/ml of polymyxin). Systemic antibiotics may be prescribed if the infection is severe; the specific drug depends on the causative organism. The systemic parenteral antibiotics depend on the cultured organism. Local irrigations with antibiotic solutions (usually polymyxin B [10,000 U/ml], bacitracin, neomycin 0.5%, or a combination of these) can be prescribed.

SURGERY

Surgical treatment of infections involves incision and drainage in the acute phase for abscesses and, at times, for perichondritis. Chronic infection can also require surgical treatment. The most common surgical treatment is excision of cysts and cutaneous carcinomas. For the most part, the surgery involved is minimal. For conditions that occlude the ear canal such as congenital atresia or exostoses, more extensive surgery involving skin grafting (canalplasty) is performed. Extensive surgery of the external ear usually is needed to repair congenital defects of the pinna. The correction of protruding ears is called otoplasty.

IMPACTED CERUMEN/FOREIGN BODIES

1 ASSESS

ASSESSMENT	OBSERVATIONS
Hearing loss	Varies from no hearing loss to moderate hearing loss according to amount of occlusion
Aural pressure/ fullness	Cerumen may be pressing on ear canal
Aural itching	Varies from no itching to mild itching according to degree of irritation
Aural discomfort/ pain	Varies from no pain to dull ache according to consistency of cerumen

ASSESSMENT	OBSERVATIONS
Drainage	Varies from no drainage to mild drainage according to consistency of cerumen
Altered communica-tion pattern	Does not respond to oral communication because hearing is impaired

2   DIAGNOSE

NURSING DIAGNOSIS	SUBJECTIVE FINDINGS	OBJECTIVE FINDINGS
Altered auditory sensory perception related to occlusion of external ear canal by cerumen or foreign body	Complains of decreased ability to hear or understand and aural fullness	Decreased hearing on audiogram; responds inappropriately or not at all to spoken word; asks that words or phrases be repeated
Impaired skin integrity related to pressure necrosis	Complains of itching, discomfort, and/or drainage in the ear canal	Cerumen causing pressure and/or excoriation; damage to skin's surface from scratching of ear canal due to itching or attempts to remove cerumen or foreign body

3   PLAN

Patient goals

1. The patient will have a patent ear canal.
2. The patient will have good skin integrity.

4   IMPLEMENT

NURSING DIAGNOSIS	NURSING INTERVENTIONS	RATIONALE
Altered auditory sensory perception related to occlusion of external ear canal by cerumen or foreign body	Assess for recent changes in hearing acuity; assess audiogram/tympanogram for hearing impairment.	Hearing may be decreased as a result of occlusion of ear canal.
	Speak distinctly and without shouting.	Shouting distorts words.
	Carefully remove earwax as indicated (see Chapter 6).	To improve hearing.
Impaired skin integrity related to pressure necrosis	Teach patient how to use prescribed ear drops and ear wash (see Patient Teaching Guide, Chapter 12).	To remove debris and/or infection from ear canal so that topical antibiotics are effective.
	Discourage itching or scratching of ear canal.	To prevent further skin irritation.

5 EVALUATE

PATIENT OUTCOME	DATA INDICATING THAT OUTCOME IS REACHED
Patient has a patent external ear canal.	Hearing loss has resolved or stabilized.
Patient has good skin integrity.	Patient feels no aural pressure or fullness; has no itching, discomfort, or tenderness and does not scratch the ear canal.

PATIENT TEACHING

1. Teach the patient how to administer ear drops and/or ear wash.
2. Teach the patient how to prevent the buildup of cerumen.
3. Reassure the patient that the hearing loss from occlusion of the ear canal is temporary.

EXTERNAL OTITIS

1 ASSESS

ASSESSMENT	OBSERVATIONS
Otorrhea	Varies from mild to moderate drainage according to amount of infection
Erythema of pinna and/or external auditory canal	Varies according to severity of infection
Edema or protrusion of pinna	Varies according to severity of inflammation
Excoriation of skin of external ear	Varies according to severity of inflammation
Pruritus	Varies from no itching to intense itching
Otalgia	Varies from no pain to intense pain related to degree of swelling in external ear canal
Aural tenderness	Upon gentle palpation of pinna, ranges from slight to intense; differential diagnosis for external and middle ear infection
Hearing loss	Varies from no hearing loss to moderate hearing loss according to amount of occlusion
Aural fullness	Drainage, infection, and swelling that may exert pressure on ear canal
Altered communication	Does not respond to oral communication

2 DIAGNOSE

NURSING DIAGNOSIS	SUBJECTIVE FINDINGS	OBJECTIVE FINDINGS
High risk for infection related to broken skin	Complains of drainage	Drainage from ear canal, edema of pinna and erythema of ear canal on otoscopic examination; elevated temperature
Impaired skin integrity related to pressure necrosis	Complains of itching, pain, tenderness, and prickling or burning in ear canal	Excoriation and discoloration of skin, skin lesion, edema, crusting
Pain (acute) related to physical factors	Complains of tenderness, pain, discomfort, itching skin, and fullness in ear	Pain on gentle palpation of external auditory canal; patient requests medication for pain
Impaired verbal communication related to hearing deficit	Complains of decreased ability to understand and fullness in ear	Hearing deficit caused by partial or total occlusion of external auditory canal
Altered auditory sensory perception related to drainage and/or swelling of external ear canal	Complains of decreased ability to hear or understand and fullness in ear	Decreased hearing on audiogram; responds inappropriately or not at all to communication; asks for words or phrases to be repeated

3 PLAN

1. The patient will have no infection.
2. The patient will have good skin integrity.
3. The patient will have no pain.
4. The patient will be able to communicate appropriately.
5. The patient will have resolution or stabilization of hearing loss.

4 IMPLEMENT

NURSING DIAGNOSIS	NURSING INTERVENTIONS	RATIONALE
High risk for infection related to broken skin	Obtain and document otologic history. Pertinent history may include exposure to water, ear trauma, allergic responses, cerumen impaction, use of earphones or hearing aid, diabetes. Pertinent symptoms include otalgia, otorrhea, pruritus, hearing loss, and aural fullness.	To document outcome and evaluation of treatment.
	Perform and document otoscopic examination, including edema of pinna, inflammation of ear canal, auricular or tragal tenderness, presence of drainage or debris in ear canal, color and appearance of tympanic membrane, middle ear fluid.	To compare pretreatment condition with posttreatment evaluation.

→ > >

NURSING DIAGNOSIS	NURSING INTERVENTIONS	RATIONALE
	Administer antibiotic or topical otologic preparations as ordered.	To reduce infections.
	Teach instillation of ear drops and irrigation of ear if ordered; instruct patient in administration of medications and the drugs' side effects.	Mechanical cleansing and topical antibiotics may be necessary to reduce infection.
	Evaluate and document response to medications.	To evaluate treatment.
	Inform patient of water restrictions (not getting water in the ear).	Water in the ear canal intensifies and perpetuates infection.
Impaired skin integrity related to pressure necrosis	Assess ear canal and auricle for edema, erythema, crusting, scabs, pustules, and discharge, and document.	To evaluate pretreatment condition with posttreatment outcome.
	Discourage itching or scratching of the ear canal.	To prevent further skin irritation.
Pain (acute) related to physical factors	Assess and document location, intensity, and frequency of otalgia.	To compare pretreatment condition with posttreatment outcome.
	Gently palpate pinna and tragus, and document findings.	To distinguish between external and middle ear disorder.
	Observe ear canal for inflammation and swelling, and document findings.	To evaluate cause of pain.
	Administer analgesics as ordered.	To relieve pain.
	Instruct patient in administration of analgesics and the drugs' side effects.	To ensure that patient takes medication safely.
	Evaluate and document response to analgesics.	To evaluate response to kind, amount, and frequency of analgesics.
Impaired verbal communication related to hearing deficit	Assess degree of hearing impairment.	Lack of ability to understand speech may be due to decreased hearing caused by occlusion of ear canal.
	Use an alternate means of communication (e.g., louder voice, writing).	To help patient communicate comfortably.
	Speak distinctly without shouting.	Shouting distorts words.
Altered auditory sensory perception related to drainage and/or swelling of external ear canal	Assess for and document recent change in hearing acuity; assess audiogram and/or tympanogram for hearing impairment.	Hearing may be reduced because of occlusion of ear canal.
	Speak distinctly without shouting.	Shouting distorts words.

5 EVALUATE

PATIENT OUTCOME	DATA INDICATING THAT OUTCOME IS REACHED
Patient has no infection.	Patient's temperature is normal, and there is no otorrhea, itching, erythema, or edema of the ear canal.
Patient demonstrates good skin integrity.	Patient has no discolored, excoriated, or edematous skin in the ear canal and no itching.
Patient has no discomfort or pain.	Patient does not complain of pain and has no pain on palpation of the ear canal; facial grimacing is reduced.
Patient is able to hear as well as before the infection.	Patient does not complain of hearing loss or aural fullness caused by occlusion of the ear canal by infection and debris.
Patient can communicate normally.	Patient can hear and understand spoken word.

PATIENT TEACHING

1. Instruct the patient how to avoid getting water in the ears by using ear plugs or cotton smeared with petroleum jelly.
2. Teach the patient how to prevent future external ear infections or swimmer's ear.
3. Teach the patient how to administer drops, ointment, and/or ear wash.
4. Teach the patient about the purpose of wicks when the external auditory canal is occluded.
5. Reassure the patient that hearing loss from an external ear infection is temporary.

PERICHONDRITIS

1 ASSESS

ASSESSMENT	OBSERVATIONS
Erythema	Characteristic initial finding; lobule typically is not involved, since this part of auricle has no cartilage
Drainage	Varies greatly according to pathogen and extent of infection
Edema of auricle	Varies according to stage of infection that treatment is initiated
Temperature	Varies from normal to high according to stage of infection that treatment is initiated
Abscess	Infection has spread beneath perichondrium, producing a subperichondrial abscess
Skin excoriation/ necrosis	Abscess and untreated perichondritis have caused necrosis of underlying cartilage

ASSESSMENT	OBSERVATIONS
Pain/tenderness	Varies according to stage and severity of infection
Lymphadenopathy	Acute infection can cause enlargement of lymph nodes in the neck

2 DIAGNOSE

NURSING DIAGNOSIS	SUBJECTIVE FINDINGS	OBJECTIVE FINDINGS
High risk for infection related to broken skin, traumatized tissue, and tissue destruction	Complains of drainage; reports recent injury, surgery, or ear piercing	Elevated temperature, drainage from auricle, edema and erythema of auricle, lymphadenopathy
High risk for impaired skin integrity related to altered circulation and alterations in skin turgor	Complains of pain, tenderness, itching, and/or tingling or burning sensation	Excoriation, abscess, and/or necrosis of skin and cartilage
Pain (acute) related to physical factors	Complains of discomfort, tenderness, and pain	Grimacing, restlessness, moaning; requests pain medicine

3 PLAN

Patient goals

1. The patient will have no infection.
2. The patient will have good skin integrity and no disfigurement of the auricle.

3. The patient will have no pain.

4 IMPLEMENT

NURSING DIAGNOSIS	NURSING INTERVENTIONS	RATIONALE
High risk for infection related to broken skin, traumatized tissue, and tissue destruction	Administer oral, parenteral, and/or topical antibiotics as ordered.	High doses of antibiotics are used promptly and aggressively to prevent complications.
	Evaluate and document response to medication.	To evaluate treatment.
	Inform patient of possibility of incision and drainage.	A fluctuant subperichondrial abscess requires incision and drainage.
	Take vital signs q 4 h, especially temperature.	Elevated temperature indicates infection.

NURSING DIAGNOSIS	NURSING INTERVENTIONS	RATIONALE
High risk for impaired skin integrity related to altered circulation and alterations in skin turgor	Supplement antibiotic treatment with wet compresses.	To soothe skin and provide cleansing.
	Inform patient of possibility of debridement.	Evidence of necrosis requires debridement of tissue.
	Assess auricular cartilage for erythema, edema, excoriation, and pus.	To compare pretreatment condition to post-treatment outcome.
Pain (acute) related to physical factors	Assess and document location, intensity, and frequency of pain.	To compare pretreatment condition with posttreatment outcome.
	Administer analgesics as ordered.	To relieve pain.
	Instruct patient in administration of analgesics and the drugs' side effects.	To ensure patient takes medications safely.
	Evaluate and document response to analgesics.	To evaluate response to kind, amount, and frequency of analgesics.

5 EVALUATE

PATIENT OUTCOME	DATA INDICATING THAT OUTCOME IS REACHED
Patient has no infection.	Patient's temperature is within normal range and there is no drainage, erythema, or edema.
Patient has good skin integrity and no disfigurement of the auricle.	Patient's skin has no discoloration, excoriation, abscess, or necrosis.
Patient has no pain.	The patient does not grimace, moan, appear restless, or complain of pain.

PATIENT TEACHING

1. Teach the patient how to administer oral or topical antibiotics and antiinflammatory drugs (i.e., type, amount, frequency, and side effects).
2. Teach the patient the signs and symptoms of an abscess and of tissue necrosis.
3. Teach the patient how to monitor her temperature and how to take antipyretic drugs (i.e., type, amount, frequency, and side effects).
4. Inform the patient and family that minor surgery such as incision and drainage or debridement may have to be done if infection cannot be controlled medically.

Tympanic Membrane Disorders

PATHOPHYSIOLOGY

Infection

Infections of the external ear canal can involve the surface of the tympanic membrane, making the membrane a "window" for infection of the middle ear. Infection can cause hard deposits in the tympanic membrane, a condition called *tympanosclerosis*, as shown in Color Plate 4 on page x (discussed later in this chapter under Middle Ear Disorders). One particular infection of the tympanic membrane, either viral or bacterial, is known as *bullous myringitis*. In this inflammatory disease, blisters or bullae form on the tympanic membrane. Infection or trauma can also cause holes, or perforations, in the tympanic membrane.

Tumors

Both benign and malignant tumors can involve the tympanic membrane, but they seldom arise from it. However, an infectious glandular polyp can be isolated to the tympanic membrane.

Perforations

The most common finding in tympanic membrane disorders is a *perforation*. A perforation may be either *acute*, as seen in trauma and acute infection, or *chronic*, as seen in repeated infection. An acute perforation has a better chance of healing spontaneously than does a chronic perforation. A perforation located away from the annulus of the tympanic membrane is a cen-

tral perforation; a perforation involving the annulus is a marginal perforation. A marginal perforation has less chance of spontaneous closure and a greater chance of invasion of skin from the external ear, resulting in a cholesteatoma (see page 58). A perforation causes hearing loss, the extent of which depends on the size and location of the hole. The largest hearing loss found with a perforation was approximately 35 dB, or one third of normal hearing. If a perforation is present, damage to the ossicles should be suspected, which causes even greater hearing loss.

CLINICAL MANIFESTATIONS

Because the tympanic membrane is semitransparent, it can reflect what lies beneath it, as well as showing discoloration and displacement of the membrane. Therefore both fluid in the middle ear and infection can be seen. The tympanic membrane may be dull or red instead of its normal pearl grey. The membrane may bulge because of pressure in the middle ear caused by infection. In some cases this pressure is strong enough to "burst" the eardrum and produce drainage. A ruptured eardrum is more common in children than adults and usually heals spontaneously. Disorders of the tympanic membrane (such as bullous myringitis) are painful, perhaps the most painful of all ear disorders. Negative pressure in the ear causes retraction of the tympanic membrane, outlining the ossicles. Fluid is also found in these cases. Any change in the tympanic membrane can cause hearing loss.

NURSING CARE

See pages 60 to 65.

Middle Ear Disorders

PATHOPHYSIOLOGY

Infection (Otitis Media)

The most prevalent diseases of the middle ear are infections, collectively known as *otitis media*. Otitis media is caused by various types of bacteria, depending on the patient's age and the type of infection. When the infection appears suddenly and lasts only a short time, the diagnosis is *acute otitis media* (see Color Plate 1 on page x).

When the infection recurs, usually causing drainage and perforation, the diagnosis is *chronic otitis media*. Between bouts of otitis media, fluid may form in the middle ear *(serous otitis media)*. This fluid results from a vacuum in the middle ear caused by a blocked eustachian tube. Infection causes swelling of the mucosa throughout the middle ear and eustachian tube. When the swelling subsides, the remaining fluid can be too thick to drain. At times serous otitis media is found in conjunction with upper respiratory infections or allergies. If the fluid remains over a period of years, causing the tympanic membrane to retract, *adhesive otitis media* becomes the diagnosis. Infection that persists for a long period can cause necrosis of the tympanic membrane (perforations) or of the ossicles. Both problems cause conductive hearing loss. Necrosis of the bony covering of the facial nerve may cause facial paralysis. Because of the extraordinary anatomy of the temporal bone, middle ear infection can also lead to a brain abscess that is life threatening if not treated properly.

Tympanosclerosis is a result of repeated infection and deserves special emphasis. It is a deposit of collagen and calcium within the middle ear that can harden around the ossicles, causing conductive hearing loss. Tympanosclerosis can also be found mounded up in the middle ear or as plaque on the tympanic membrane (see Color Plate 4, page x).

Cholesteatoma is a complication of otitis media but is primarily a problem of the mastoid and mastoid disorders.

Otosclerosis

Otosclerosis, or "hardening of the ear," which involves the stapes, is important in middle ear disorders. This bony disease of the otic capsule causes excess bone to form, impeding normal movement of the stapes. The conductive hearing loss that results is the second most common correctable middle ear disorder, after infection of the ear (see Stapedectomy in Chapter 6). Another form of otosclerosis that does not involve the stapes is *cochlear otospongiosis,* which can cause a toxic sensorineural hearing loss.

Tumors

The most common benign growth in the middle ear is an *infectious polyp.* Next in frequency is a *cholesteatoma.* The rarest forms of benign middle ear tumors involve either the blood vessels or the facial nerve. A tumor that arises from the jugular vein is a *glomus jugulare,* known as a *glomus tympanicum* when limited to the middle ear (see Color Plate 6, page x). A *facial nerve neuroma* is a tumor found along the course of the facial nerve. Malignant tumors involving the middle ear can be primary or secondary.

Trauma

Trauma to the tympanic membrane from a blast or blunt injury can involve the middle ear, fracturing or dislocating the ossicles and tearing the tympanic membrane. The facial nerve is also vulnerable to trauma. A *basal skull fracture* involves the temporal bone and, depending on the fracture site, can damage the ossicles and cause facial nerve paralysis.

Eustachian Tube Disorders

The eustachian tube is part of the middle ear but presents separate problems. Because the eustachian tube connects the middle ear to the nasopharynx, pharyngeal disorders cause eustachian tube dysfunction and secondary middle ear problems. For example, the most common disorder is blockage of the eustachian tube by enlarged adenoidal tissue in children. The most common blockage in adults is swelling of the mucosa in the eustachian tube during an upper respiratory infection, which can lead to serous otitis media. If only one tube is blocked, a malignant tumor must be ruled out as the cause. Acute blockage from *barotrauma* (altitude changes) during flying or underwater diving also can cause middle ear problems. Any long-term blockage of the eustachian tube leads to serous otitis media and hearing loss.

CLINICAL MANIFESTATIONS

Because the middle ear is the transformer for hearing (i.e., it transmits the sound vibrations from the tympanic membrane to the inner ear), hearing loss is the most common middle ear finding. Fortunately, 95% of problems involve conductive hearing loss that can be corrected either medically or surgically. Pain is also a common finding, because fluid or swelling from infection exerts pressure on the tympanic membrane. Once an infection has caused a perforation, drainage of pus, blood, and other material often is seen. In chronic middle ear and mastoid disorders, a thick, yellow, purulent discharge is common. With acute otitis media, all three findings (hearing loss, pain, and discharge) may be present.

NURSING CARE

See pages 60 to 67.

Mastoid Disorders

PATHOPHYSIOLOGY

Infection (Mastoiditis)

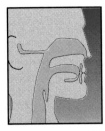

Before the discovery of antibiotics, a mastoid infection was a life-threatening event. Now, those drugs have made *acute mastoiditis* a rare condition. *Chronic mastoiditis*, on the other hand, is not as uncommon. With repeated middle ear infections, the mastoid cavity becomes part of the problem, increasing the amount of drainage. A chronic infection also leads to formation of a *cholesteatoma*, a skin-lined sac that sheds debris into its center, thus enlarging the sac. Infection often is present in the mass of the cholesteatoma. These chronic infectious changes produce cholesterol granules, which give the condition its name. Although they are benign growths, cholesteatomas have prompted stories of brain abscesses, dizziness, and facial paralysis. These conditions are still seen, but like acute mastoiditis, they are much less common.

Tumors

The same tumors that arise in the middle ear can be found in the mastoid cavity. Because the mastoid cavity is connected to other air cells throughout the temporal bone, malignant tumors in the mastoid carry a poor prognosis. (Tumors are discussed in Chapter 11.)

CLINICAL MANIFESTATIONS

Drainage from the mastoid cavity is the most common sign of mastoiditis. The drainage courses through the middle ear and out of the tympanic membrane through a perforation. Tenderness over the mastoid cavity behind the ear points to an infection but usually is caused by a sudden exacerbation of chronic mastoiditis rather than an episode of acute mastoiditis. The pinna may protrude because of swelling over the mastoid, especially in children.

COMPLICATIONS

Central nervous system abscess
Complete loss of balance
Cerebrospinal fluid (CSF) leak
Facial nerve paralysis
Complete hearing loss
Infection of surrounding structures
Leukocytosis
Lymphadenopathy
Meningitis
Metastasis
Septicemia
Sigmoid sinus thrombosis
Subperiosteal abscess
Vertigo

NURSING CARE

See pages 62 to 65.

DIAGNOSTIC STUDIES AND FINDINGS

Diagnostic test	Findings
Otoscopic/microscopic examination	To diagnose middle ear or mastoid disorder, to remove debris of infection, and to perform minor surgery
Culture	To identify specific infecting microbe
Biopsy	To identify tissue and rule out malignancy
Audiometric testing	To determine amount of hearing loss and middle ear impedance
Imaging	To diagnose tumors, masses, infection, fluid osteitis, and metastasis
Complete blood count	To detect a systemic infection
Facial nerve testing	To determine extent of damage to facial nerve and prognosis for paralysis
Electronystagmography	To determine extent of damage to labyrinth

MEDICAL MANAGEMENT

GENERAL MANAGEMENT

Antibiotics are the most common treatment of tympanic membrane, middle ear, and mastoid problems, and they are given in both local and systemic forms. If drainage is present, a culture and sensitivity should be performed. However, most episodes of acute otitis media do not produce drainage, and the most probable bacterial cause must be identified. In chronic ear drainage and mastoiditis, the normal contaminants of the ear abound and unfortunately do not respond to the common antibiotics; thus local treatment is used (e.g., irrigation, drops, and powders).

Blood in the ear canal usually points to a minor problem, such as a scratch, and not to a major disease. Persistent bleeding must be checked by an otologist.

Because the eustachian tube plays a pivotal role in middle ear disorders, decongestants and antihistamines are used to decrease the swelling and open the eustachian tube. Pain medication is used when necessary.

DRUG THERAPY

Antiinfective agents

Amoxicillin (Amoxil, Larotid): 500 mg PO tid for 10 days.

Sulfamethoxazole (Septra or Bactrim): 1 tab PO bid or qid (if allergic to penicillin).

Penicillin G or V: 250-500 mg PO q 6 h for 10 days for patients older than 8 years.

Ampicillin (Amcil, others): 50-100 mg/kg/day for 10 days for children under 8 years because of frequency of *Haemophilus influenzae* infections in this age group

If patient is allergic to penicillin, erythromycin (E-Mycin, others): 250 mg PO for adults and older children; combination of erythromycin and sulfisoxazole for children younger than 8 years.

Ear wash for cleansing, such as supersaturated solution of boric acid in alcohol.

Analgesic/antipyretic or narcotic analgesics

Codeine: 30 mg PO q 4 h (for severe pain); sedatives are sometimes given to small children.

Antihistamines/decongestants

Chlorpheniramine (Chlor-Trimeton): 4 mg PO q 4-6 h for 7-10 days for adults.

Pseudoephedrine (Sudafed): 60 mg PO q 6-8 h for adults.

SURGERY

Surgical treatment involves using a surgical microscope to enlarge the tympanic membrane; the power of magnification most commonly used is 6 to 25 times normal. The major surgical procedure performed is closure of a perforation. This procedure is called a *myringoplasty* if only the perforation is in the surgical field, and a *tympanoplasty* if more of the middle ear is involved. Sometimes the ossicles must also be reconstructed, altering the type of tympanoplasty performed (types I through IV). A tympanoplasty may also be performed in conjunction with surgery involving the mastoid. A stapedectomy is performed for otosclerosis. (A detailed description of these surgical procedures is found in Chapter 6.)

SEROUS OTITIS MEDIA/ACUTE OTITIS MEDIA WITHOUT PERFORATION

1 ASSESS

ASSESSMENT	OBSERVATIONS
Upper respiratory infection	May be contributory cause of fluid in middle ear
Temperature	May be elevated (a sign of generalized infection)
Earache	Varies from mild to moderate according to amount of fluid in middle ear
Allergy	May be contributory cause of fluid in middle ear
Fullness/blocked sensation in ear	May be present because of fluid in middle ear and hearing loss
Decreased or fluctuating hearing	Varies according to amount of fluid in middle ear
Lack of response or inattention to spoken word	Varies according to amount of fluid in the middle ear and whether problem involves one or both ears
Unilateral versus bilateral problem	Chronic unilateral fluid in an adult may indicate carcinoma of nasopharynx

2 DIAGNOSE

NURSING DIAGNOSIS	SUBJECTIVE FINDINGS	OBJECTIVE FINDINGS
High risk for infection related to tissue destruction	Complains of fullness or blockage in ear, frequent colds, and/or allergies	Fluid in middle ear, redness and/or bulging of tympanic membrane, chronic ear disease, elevated temperature
Altered auditory sensory perception related to fluid in middle ear	Complains of fullness or pressure in ear and decreased or fluctuating hearing	Fluid in middle ear
Pain (acute) related to physical factors	Complains of earaches	Decreased hearing on audiogram, abnormal tympanogram, asks that words or phrases be repeated, holds affected ear or ears, uses cotton or protective covering over ear, shows grimacing and restlessness, requests pain-relief medication

3 PLAN

Patient goals
1. The patient will have no infection.
2. The patient will have resolution or stabilization of hearing loss.

3. The patient will have no earaches or ear discomfort.

4 IMPLEMENT

NURSING DIAGNOSIS	NURSING INTERVENTIONS	RATIONALE
High risk for infection related to tissue destruction	Obtain and document otologic history (recent upper respiratory infection, exposure to water, ear trauma, allergy, ear infections); pertinent symptoms include otalgia, otorrhea, pruritus, hearing loss, and aural fullness.	To compare pretreatment symptoms with posttreatment outcome.
	Perform and document otoscopic examination; check for drainage or debris in ear canal, color and appearance of tympanic membrane, and fluid in middle ear.	To compare pretreatment symptoms with posttreatment outcome.
	Administer antibiotic and antipyretic preparations as ordered.	To reduce infection and fever.
	Teach patient instillation of ear drops or irrigation of ear if ordered; instruct patient in administration of medications and the drugs' side effects.	Mechanical cleansing, topical antibiotics, and antiinflammatory drugs may be needed to reduce infection.
	Monitor and document response to drugs.	To evaluate effectiveness of treatment.
	Instruct patient about water restrictions.	Water in ear canal creates an environment conducive to bacterial or fungal growth.
Altered auditory sensory perception related to fluid in middle ear	Assess and document recent change in hearing acuity; assess audiogram and/or tympanogram for hearing impairment.	Hearing may be decreased because of fluid in middle ear.
	Speak distinctly without shouting.	Shouting distorts speech.
Pain (acute) related to physical factors	Assess and document location, intensity, and frequency of pain.	To compare pretreatment symptoms to posttreatment outcome.
	Observe ear canal for inflammation and swelling and tympanic membrane for redness, bulging, and/or bubbles.	To compare pretreatment symptoms with posttreatment outcome.
	Administer analgesics as ordered, and instruct patient in administration and side effects of drugs.	To relieve pain and to teach patient how to take medications safely.
	Monitor and document response to analgesics.	To evaluate response to kind, amount, and scheduling of analgesics.

→ > >

5 EVALUATE

PATIENT OUTCOME	DATA INDICATING THAT OUTCOME IS REACHED
Patient has no infection.	Temperature is normal; there is no blocked sensation, redness, or bulging of eardrum, or bubbles of fluid in middle ear.
Patient has resolution or stabilization of hearing loss.	Patient does not complain of hearing loss or fullness in ear; audiogram shows no hearing loss from recent infection.
Patient has no earaches or ear discomfort.	Patient does not complain of earaches, does not protect his ear in any way, and does not grimace or seem restless.

PATIENT TEACHING

1. Teach the patient the causes, signs, and symptoms of serous otitis media.
2. Stress that the patient should see his physician about any significant earache; teach him how to carry out medical treatment of serous otitis media (antihistamines, decongestants, and/or the Valsalva maneuver).
3. Inform the patient that minor surgery may be needed to remove fluid from or to ventilate the middle ear.
4. Reassure the patient that hearing loss caused by serous otitis media is temporary.

CHRONIC OTITIS MEDIA/CHRONIC MASTOIDITIS/ACUTE OTITIS MEDIA WITH PERFORATION

1 ASSESS

ASSESSMENT	OBSERVATIONS
Otorrhea with or without foul odor	Varies from mild to severe drainage, with or without odor, according to type of bacteria, amount of infection, and stage of disease
Erythema of tympanic drum	Varies according to stage of infection
Perforation of tympanic drum	May be present as a result of increased pressure in middle ear cavity caused by infection
Cholesteatoma of middle ear and/or mastoid	May be present; can enlarge as disease progresses
Tympanosclerosis of tympanic drum	Small, chalk white plaques on tympanic membrane

ASSESSMENT	OBSERVATIONS
Otalgia	Varies from no pain to moderate discomfort
Hearing loss	Varies from mild to severe according to chronicity and severity of infection
History of chronic ear disease with acute exacerbations	Chronic ear disease usually means that ear surgery is indicated to remove infection and restore hearing
Vertigo	Present if there is erosion of the labyrinth

2 DIAGNOSE

NURSING DIAGNOSIS	SUBJECTIVE FINDINGS	OBJECTIVE FINDINGS
High risk for infection caused by tissue destruction and chronic disease	Complains of drainage from ear and chronic ear problems	Erythema, otorrhea with or without pus, perforation, and/or tympanosclerosis of the tympanic membrane with or without cholesteatoma
Pain (chronic) related to physical factors	Complains of pain, usually a dull ache deep in the ear canal; requests medication for pain	Grimacing, fatigue, withdrawal
Altered auditory sensory perception related to partial or total perforation and/or destruction of middle ear ossicles	Complains of decreased ability to hear and understand spoken word and a sense of fullness in the ear	Decreased hearing on audiogram, abnormal tympanogram, asks that words or phrases be repeated, responds inappropriately or not at all to spoken word
Impaired verbal communication related to hearing deficit	Complains of decreased hearing and decreased ability to understand spoken word	Answers inappropriately or not at all to verbal communication; asks that words be repeated
High risk for trauma related to balance difficulties	Complains of spinning sensation or hallucination of movement; complains of some loss of hearing	Nystagmus, unsteady gait: positive result on Romberg test (see page 27).

3 PLAN

Patient goals
1. The patient will have no infection.
2. The patient will have no pain.
3. The patient's hearing loss will resolve or stabilize.
4. The patient will be able to communicate adequately.
5. The patient will not experience vertigo.

4 IMPLEMENT

NURSING DIAGNOSIS	NURSING INTERVENTIONS	RATIONALE
High risk for infection caused by tissue destruction and chronic disease	Obtain otologic history (previous ear infections, exposure to water, allergies, use of earphones or hearing aids); pertinent symptoms include otorrhea, otalgia, pruritus, hearing loss, and vertigo.	To compare pretreatment symptoms with posttreatment outcome.
	Perform otoscopic examination; check for drainage or debris in ear canal, color and appearance of tympanic membrane, perforation, tympanosclerosis, and/or cholesteatoma.	To compare pretreatment symptoms with posttreatment outcome.
	Administer antibiotic and antiinflammatory preparations as ordered.	To reduce infection.
	Teach instillation of ointment, drops, and ear wash as ordered.	Mechanical cleansing and topical antibiotics may be needed to eliminate infection.
	Monitor response to all medication.	To evaluate effectiveness of treatment.
	Instruct patient about water restrictions.	Water in ear canal and middle ear provides an environment conducive to bacterial or fungal growth.
Pain (chronic) related to physical factors	Assess location, intensity, and frequency of pain.	To document effectiveness of treatment.
	Use otoscope to check the tympanic membrane for redness, perforation, or drainage.	To compare pretreatment symptoms with posttreatment outcome.
	Administer analgesics as ordered.	To relieve pain.
	Instruct patient in administration of analgesics and the drugs' common side effects.	To teach patient how to take medications safely.
	Monitor response to analgesics.	To evaluate response to kind, amount, and frequency of analgesics.
Altered auditory sensory perception related to partial or total perforation of tympanic membrane and/or destruction of middle ear ossicles	Assess changes in hearing acuity; assess audiogram or tympanogram for hearing impairment.	Hearing may be decreased because of secondary changes from chronic infection.
	Speak distinctly without shouting.	Shouting distorts words.
Impaired verbal communication related to hearing deficit	Assess degree of hearing impairment.	Lack of ability to understand speech may be due to decreased hearing caused by occlusion of the ear canal.

NURSING DIAGNOSIS	NURSING INTERVENTIONS	RATIONALE
	Use an adequate alternative method of communication (e.g., raise the voice, write notes).	To help patient cope with hearing impairment.
	Speak distinctly without shouting.	Shouting distorts words.
High risk for trauma related to balance difficulties	Assess for vertigo by observing for nystagmus, abnormal gait, positive Romberg's sign, and inability to perform tandem Romberg test.	Secondary changes arising from chronic infection can cause erosion of the labyrinth, resulting in vertigo, dizziness, and balance problems.
	Assist with ambulation when indicated.	Abnormal gait may predispose patient to unsteadiness and falls.

5 EVALUATE

PATIENT OUTCOME	DATA INDICATING THAT OUTCOME IS REACHED
Patient has no infection.	The tympanic membrane, middle ear, and mastoid show no drainage, erythema, or edema.
Patient has no pain.	Patient does not complain of pain and shows no fatigue or facial grimacing.
Patient's hearing loss has resolved or stabilized.	Patient will have continued loss of hearing with chronic ear infections, but controlling infection prevents a rapid loss.
Patient can communicate adequately.	Patient can hear and understand spoken word with or without amplification.
Patient has no trauma secondary to falls.	Patient does not complain of vertigo or dizziness and has a normal gait.

PATIENT TEACHING

1. Instruct the patient to avoid getting water in the ears by using earplugs or cotton with petroleum jelly on it.
2. Teach the patient how to use drops, ointment, or ear wash.
3. Teach the patient the causes, signs, symptoms, and treatment of chronic otitis media.
4. Inform the patient that surgery may be needed to remove the infection and restore some degree of hearing.

OTOSCLEROSIS

1 ASSESS

ASSESSMENT	OBSERVATIONS
Hearing	Loss of hearing and/or decreased comprehension of spoken word (unilateral or bilateral)
Tympanic membrane	Normal (tympanic membrane is not affected by otosclerosis)
Tinnitus	May be present in varying degrees or may be absent
Vertigo	May be present (20% to 25% of patients experience vertigo, especially after bending over)
Voice	Quiet, well modulated (patient can hear own voice because sound is conducted through bones in the head)
Hereditary predisposition	May have family history of disease
Inappropriate conversation	May be present because of inability to hear

2 DIAGNOSE

NURSING DIAGNOSIS	SUBJECTIVE FINDINGS	OBJECTIVE FINDINGS
Altered auditory sensory perception related to gradual fixation of stapes footplate in oval window	Complains of gradual loss of hearing and understanding; reports ringing, whistling, or other strange noises in ears	Partial or total loss of hearing on audiogram; no reflexes shown on impedance audiometry; history of otosclerosis in patient's family; normal tympanic membrane.
Impaired verbal communication related to hearing deficit	Complains of inability to hear or understand what is being said	Frequently asks that words or phrases be repeated; responds inappropriately or not at all to communication; audiogram shows partial or total loss of hearing unilaterally or bilaterally
High risk for trauma related to balance difficulties	Reports intermittent feeling of giddiness or spinning	Nystagmus, abnormal gait, and/or positive result on Romberg's test

3 PLAN

Patient goals

1. The patient will understand that progressive loss of hearing is caused by the disease.
2. The patient will be able to communicate.

3. The patient will understand the intermittent vertigo that is experienced is caused by the disease.

4   IMPLEMENT

NURSING DIAGNOSIS	NURSING INTERVENTIONS	RATIONALE
Altered auditory sensory perception related to gradual fixation of stapes footplate in oval window	Assess hearing acuity level; assess audiogram and tympanogram for hearing impairment.	Hearing is decreased due to unilateral or bilateral otosclerosis.
	Speak distinctly without shouting. Assess tympanic reflex.	Shouting distorts words. Reflex usually is absent with otosclerosis.
Impaired verbal communication related to hearing deficit	Assess degree of hearing impairment.	Lack of ability to understand speech may be due to decreased hearing caused by occlusion of ear canal.
	Use an adequate alternate method of communication (e.g., raise voice, write).	To help patient cope with disability.
	Speak distinctly without shouting.	Shouting distorts words.
High risk for trauma related to balance difficulties	Assess for vertigo by observing for nystagmus, abnormal gait, positive Romberg's sign, and inability to perform a tandem Romberg test.	Secondary change resulting from chronic infection can cause erosion of the labyrinth, resulting in vertigo, dizziness, and balance problems.
	Assist with ambulation when indicated.	Abnormal gait can predispose patient to unsteadiness and falls.

5   EVALUATE

PATIENT OUTCOME	DATA INDICATING THAT OUTCOME IS REACHED
Patient understands that her progressive loss of hearing is caused by the disease process.	Patient understands the course of otosclerosis and the medical and surgical options for maintaining or regaining hearing.
Patient can communicate.	Patient is aware that the spoken word may not always be heard correctly, and asks others to repeat or speak more distinctly.
Patient understands that the intermittent vertigo she experiences is caused by the disease process.	Patient understands that the intermittent vertigo is caused by otosclerosis and that surgical treatment of the condition can eliminate or lessen the vertigo.

PATIENT TEACHING

1. Teach the patient the signs, symptoms, and causes of otosclerosis.
2. Inform the patient that hearing loss can be helped by surgery (called a stapedectomy) or by a hearing aid.
3. Explain the procedure for a stapedectomy.
4. Teach the patient the dosage, administration, and side effects of any medications prescribed.

Inner Ear Disorders

PATHOPHYSIOLOGY

Congenital Disorders

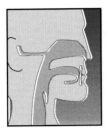 Incomplete development of the cochlea is the most common congenital disorder of the inner ear; it results in sensorineural hearing loss. In contrast, congenital disorders of the vestibular system do not usually cause dizziness or equilibrium problems.

Infection (Labyrinthitis)

An infection of the inner ear, called *labyrinthitis*, can be either viral or bacterial in origin. Viral labyrinthitis usually is isolated to the inner ear, whereas the rarer bacterial labyrinthitis is associated with infection in the middle ear and mastoid (see Chapter 5).

Tumors

Both benign and malignant tumors of the temporal bone can involve the inner ear (see Chapter 11 for malignant tumors). The most common benign tumor is an *acoustic neuroma* of cranial nerve VIII (the acoustic nerve) that arises in the internal ear canal. Spread of this tumor out of the internal ear canal toward the brainstem produces neurologic problems that can be life threatening. Other tumors in the cerebellopontine angle can involve cranial nerves VII (the facial nerve) and VIII as they enter the internal acoustic meatus. Acoustic neuromas are discussed in greater detail in Chapter 6.

Hearing Disorders

Sensorineural hearing loss is the most common disorder of the inner ear. This type of hearing loss may occur in conjunction with a known disorder, but it usually is an isolated finding. Factors influencing the type and amount of hearing loss are heredity, disease, aging, toxic substances, and noise-induced hearing loss. The hearing loss may fluctuate, but it usually proceeds to progressive loss.

Noise-induced hearing loss can be caused by trauma, as in a blast injury from a sudden explosion. More commonly, the hearing loss occurs over time as a consequence of repeated injury from noise. The major cause of such injury is industrial noise; the use of firearms is a distant second. Whatever the cause, this type of hearing loss is characterized by greater loss of hearing in the higher frequencies. There is no treatment for noise-induced hearing loss; the best course is to pre-

vent the injury by avoiding noise or by wearing ear protection.

Sudden or *fluctuating hearing loss* is recognized as a separate hearing disorder because of the isolated findings and dramatic outcome. Although the exact cause of this disorder is unknown, it is thought to be vascular in nature. Because of this, treatment attempts focus on altering the vascular system in some way. Autoimmune disease should also be ruled out by a blood test. Sudden or fluctuating hearing loss is treated primarily with steroids.

Occasionally the patient's hearing may return to normal without apparent reason. Unfortunately, most patients do not regain normal hearing. One cause that is becoming better recognized is a fistula from the inner ear to the middle ear via the oval or round windows. If this condition is suspected, the fistulas are closed by a tissue graft (see Chapter 6).

Presbycusis is a hearing loss found in the elderly. Changes in the delicate labyrinthine structures over the decades cause a hearing loss predominantly in the higher frequencies. The amount of hearing loss will have familial differences and can start in middle age. Tinnitus usually accompanies presbycusis. Most people eventually develop presbycusis as they age. In some of these people, the amount of hearing loss warrants the use of a hearing aid. Presbycusis cannot be cured (Table 4-1).

OTOTOXIC DRUGS AND OTHER SUBSTANCES

Aminoglycoside antibiotics

Amikacin
Gentamicin
Kanamycin
Netilmicin
Neomycin
Streptomycin
Tobramycin

Other antibiotics

Capreomycin
Erythromycin
Minocycline
Polymyxin B
Polymyxin E
Vancomycin
Viomycin

Chemotherapeutic drugs

Cisplatin
Nitrogen mustard

Diuretics

Acetazolamide
Ethacrynic acid
Furosemide

Other drugs

Bleomycin
Quinidine
Quinine drugs
Salicylates

Chemicals

Alcohol
Arsenic

Metals

Gold
Mercury
Lead

Table 4-1

CHANGES IN HEARING CAUSED BY AGING

Change in structure	Change in function
Cochlear hair cell degeneration	Inability to hear high-frequency sounds (sensorineural loss)
Loss of auditory neurons in spiral ganglia of organ of Corti	Inability to hear high-frequency sounds (sensorineural loss)
Degeneration of basilar conductive membrane of cochlea	Inability to hear at all frequencies but more pronounced at higher frequencies (cochlear conductive loss)
Decreased vascularity of cochlea	Equal loss of hearing at all frequencies (strial loss)
Loss of cortical auditory neurons	Diminished hearing and speech comprehension

(From McCance/Huether.)

Some medicines, called ototoxic drugs, can affect the cochlea, vestibular labyrinth, or cranial nerve VIII (see the box on page 68). Patients taking ototoxic drugs need to know the signs and symptoms of the side effects of these drugs to prevent loss of hearing or balance. If symptoms such as dizziness, decreasing hearing acuity, and tinnitus occur, the patient should not take the next dose of the drug and should consult the physician. Audiometric and vestibular testing may be necessary.

CLINICAL MANIFESTATIONS

Hearing Loss

Sensorineural hearing loss is found with almost any inner ear disorder. The hearing loss usually is incomplete but can be progressive in some illnesses. A characteristic of a severe hearing loss is the loss of discrimination (understanding of words).

Tinnitus

Ringing or any other noises in the ear are called tinnitus. Tinnitus accompanies most types of sensorineural hearing loss and is very annoying. In some patients the tinnitus becomes the problem, and the underlying cause may be forgotten.

Tinnitus is not a disease but a very distressing symptom and often a warning of hearing loss or other more serious disorder. Ear noise that cannot be heard by an observer is classified as subjective tinnitus (the most common kind). Any ear noise that can be heard by someone other than the patient is called objective tinnitus. In some cases the tinnitus is so severe or disruptive that these persons have attempted suicide.

People may have tinnitus without hearing problems. The pathophysiology of tinnitus is still in the realm of speculation, and a number of theories have been proposed to explain this common symptom. Some of those theories involve vascular disorders, nerve inhibition, and trigger mechanisms.

The major nursing responsibility with tinnitus is to perform a thorough history and assessment about the onset, frequency, constancy, and level of intensity of the tinnitus. Unilateral tinnitus merits a complete neurotologic evaluation with the goal of ruling out a tumor (most likely an acoustic neuroma). The nurse should keep in mind that tinnitus is a symptom of an underlying pathologic condition that warrants referral to an otologist.

Many approaches to alleviating tinnitus have been tried, including biofeedback, electrostimulation, hypnosis, medication, hearing aids, and tinnitus maskers. Tinnitus maskers are quite similar to hearing aids except that they generate filtered bands of noise. The tinnitus masker can cause a phenomenon known as *residual inhibition*, which is the absence of the tinnitus for a period of 1 minute to a few weeks after treatment. However, every approach has proved only moderately successful at best.

COMPLICATIONS

Central nervous system abscess
Complete loss of balance
Loss of cerebrospinal fluid
Dehydration
Falling
Complete hearing loss
Inability to ambulate
Septicemia
Meningitis

DIAGNOSTIC STUDIES AND FINDINGS

Diagnostic test	Findings
Audiometric testing	To determine amount and kind of hearing loss
Automatic brainstem response test	To determine site of lesion and extent of involvement
Imaging studies	To identify tumors, masses, retrocochlear disorders, and necrosis
Electronystagmography	To determine extent of damage to labyrinth

MEDICAL MANAGEMENT

GENERAL MANAGEMENT

For hearing loss, general treatment approaches include vasodilators and steroids, but there is no specific therapy. The patient is offered some form of aural rehabilitation, hearing aids, or implantable hearing devices. With tinnitus, psychologic counseling, biofeedback, drugs, self-hypnosis, and tinnitus maskers sometimes are useful.

DRUG THERAPY

Hypocholesterolemic agents

Nicotinic acid (niacin): 50-200 mg/bid or tid PO to vasodilate blood vessels that supply inner ear (efficacy is questionable).

Antianxiety agents (used for sedative effect)

Diazepam (Valium): 5 mg PO q 4-6 h.

Anticonvulsants (used for sedative effect)

Carbamazepine (Tegretol): 200 mg PO bid for 1 day, then maintenance dosage of 800 mg—1.2 g qd.

Phenytoin (Dilantin): 100 mg PO tid.

Primidone (Mysoline): 100-125 mg/day at bedtime for 3 days, then 250 mg tid or qid, and carbamazepine in combination; has helped in some cases, but exact mechanism is unknown.

SURGERY

Implantable hearing devices such as cochlear implants are available and are discussed on page 78. Other devices such as bone conduction devices and semiimplantable hearing aids are under investigation.

HEARING LOSS

1 ASSESS

ASSESSMENT	OBSERVATIONS
Failure to respond to oral communication	Unable to hear, therefore does not respond
Inappropriate response to oral communication	Unable to hear, therefore responds incorrectly or inappropriately
Excessively loud speech	Unable to hear own voice, therefore raises voice to audible level
Abnormal awareness of sounds	Recruitment (an abnormally rapid increase in loudness)
Strained facial expressions	Often accompanies difficulty in hearing
Tilted head when listening	Better-hearing ear often is directed toward speaker
Constant need of clarification of conversation	Discrimination (the ability to understand communication) often decreases with hearing
Irritability, hostility, hypersensitivity in interpersonal relations	Behavior accompanies increased frustration with communication problems
Constantly complains that people mumble	Complaints of hearing impaired often are misdirected to family or friends
Volume turned up on TV or radio	Volume is increased so that the TV or radio is amplified, like a hearing aid
Tinnitus	Noises, such as ringing, often accompany hearing loss
Poor eye contact	Can be caused by embarrassment, denial, or insecurity
Expresses insecurity in large or small groups	Background noise of any kind, including groups of people who are talking, makes hearing more difficult
Tension or stress	Hearing impairment, especially a nerve hearing loss for which there is no cure, can produce stress
Loss of hearing and/or inability to understand oral communication	Varies from mild to total loss; gradual loss of hearing may go undetected

→ > > >

2 DIAGNOSE

NURSING DIAGNOSIS	SUBJECTIVE FINDINGS	OBJECTIVE FINDINGS
Altered auditory sensory perception related to sensorineural hearing loss	Reports abnormal awareness of sounds; constantly complains that people mumble; expresses insecurity in groups; complains of a hearing loss and of inability to understand spoken word	Hearing deficit on audiogram; fails to respond or inappropriate response to oral communication; loud speech, strained facial expressions, tilted head when listening, constant need of clarification; turns volume up on TV or radio
Anxiety related to threat of change or change in interaction patterns	Expresses insecurity in small or large groups; reports increased tension or stress	Irritability, poor eye contact, hostility, strained facial expressions
	Expresses feeling of regret or anticipated change in life situation	Shows hypersensitivity in interpersonal relationships
Impaired verbal communication related to decreased hearing	Complains of not being able to hear or understand oral communication; complains that people mumble	Responds inappropriately to oral communication or fails to respond at all; constantly requests clarification of conversations
Diversional activity deficit related to environmental lack of such activity	Complains of boredom and of not being able to interact with others because of hearing deficit	Decrease in recreational and leisure activities; displays anger because of inability to hear human speech; withdrawn behavior

3 PLAN

Patient goals
1. The patient's hearing loss will resolve or stabilize.
2. The patient will be less anxious.
3. The patient will be able to communicate adequately.
4. The patient will take more interest in recreational and leisure activities.

4 IMPLEMENT

NURSING DIAGNOSIS	NURSING INTERVENTIONS	RATIONALE
Altered auditory sensory perception related to sensorineural hearing loss	Assess hearing acuity level; assess audiogram or tympanogram for extent of hearing impairment.	Hearing loss varies from mild to total.
	Speak distinctly without shouting.	Shouting distorts words.
Anxiety related to threat of change or change in interaction patterns	Assess level of anxiety (mild, moderate, severe, panic).	To guide therapeutic interventions.
	Assess patient's perception of needs and expectations.	To facilitate problem solving.

NURSING DIAGNOSIS	NURSING INTERVENTIONS	RATIONALE
	Help patient recall coping skills used successfully in the past.	Past coping skill may relieve anxiety.
	Provide information about hearing loss and medical and surgical treatments.	Knowledge can decrease anxiety; fear and stress increase anxiety.
Impaired verbal communication related to decreased hearing	Assess degree of hearing impairment.	Failure to respond or inappropriate response to oral communication can be caused by decreased hearing.
	Use an adequate alternative method of communication (e.g., raising voice, writing).	To help patient cope with disability.
	Check hearing aid for power level, battery, and other problems (see Care of a Hearing Aid and What To Do if Hearing Aid Fails to Work, page 79).	Hearing aid may not be turned on; batteries may need to be replaced.
	Get patient's attention by raising an arm or hand.	Patient may be unaware that nurse is speaking.
	Shine a light on your face; face and talk directly to the patient; speak clearly but do not overaccentuate words.	To help patient lip read.
	Speak in a normal tone without shouting.	Shouting distorts words.
	If patient does not seem to understand what is said, express it differently.	To avoid long explanations.
	Move closer to patient and toward better ear.	To facilitate hearing.
	Write out proper names or any statement patient may not have understood.	To reinforce what was discussed.
	Do not smile, chew gum, or cover your mouth when talking.	May confuse lip readers.
	Do not show annoyance by careless facial expression.	Patients with hearing loss depend on visual cues for understanding.
	Encourage patient to use a hearing aid if one is available; allow the patient to adjust it before speaking.	Alternate methods of communication may be necessary.
	Do not use the intercommunication system.	This may distort sound and cause poor communication.
	Do not avoid conversation with a person who has impaired hearing.	May indicate nonacceptance.

NURSING DIAGNOSIS	NURSING INTERVENTIONS	RATIONALE
Diversional activity deficit related to environmental lack of such activity	Encourage patient to participate in group social events.	To alleviate boredom.
	Encourage patient to talk about anger over disability.	Anger is a normal reaction; expressing it can help control it.
	Inform patient of treatment options to increase or maximize hearing and to increase effective communication with others.	If hearing is increased, communication is more effective and socialization is enriched.

5 EVALUATE

PATIENT OUTCOME	DATA INDICATING THAT OUTCOME IS REACHED
Patient's hearing loss has resolved or stabilized.	Patient is knowledgeable about the cause of hearing loss and the options for medical or surgical treatment.
Patient is less anxious.	Patient acknowledges anxiety and can identify actions to cope with it.
Patient can communicate adequately.	Patient can hear and understand the spoken word with or without amplification, or uses an alternative means of communication.
Patient has taken more interest in recreational and leisure activities.	Patient can express anger, has overcome withdrawn behavior, and can identify appropriate treatment plan for loss of hearing.

PATIENT TEACHING

1. Teach the patient how to use and maintain a hearing aid if required.
2. Explain the cause of the patient's hearing loss and the medical or surgical treatment options.
3. Make appropriate referrals for aural rehabilitation, hearing aids, or appointments with an otologist.
4. Encourage the patient to ask questions about anything that is not understood.

TINNITUS

1 ASSESS

ASSESSMENT	OBSERVATIONS
Noises in one or both ears	May be minimal or extremely loud, intermittent or continuous; may vary from ringing to whistling to humming to crackling
Hearing loss	Commonly associated with tinnitus
History of exposure to loud noise, family history of deafness, tinnitus, or previous ear disease	Factors that contribute to likelihood of tinnitus
Ototoxic drugs	Certain drugs are toxic to the labyrinth and should be discontinued
Vertigo	Vestibular problems such as labyrinthitis and Ménière's disease cause tinnitus
Unilateral tinnitus	May be first symptom of acoustic neuroma or other retrocochlear problem
Vascular changes in central nervous system	Tinnitus may fluctuate with blood pressure or heart beat (pulsatile tinnitus)
Life-style	Psychosocial parameters and quality of life vary
Anxiety, stress, tension, or depression	Vary from mild adaptation problems to threat of suicide
Dietary habits and alcohol ingestion	Certain dietary factors or alcohol provoke tinnitus
Irritability and distress	Poor adaptation to tinnitus
Sleep disturbance	Tinnitus usually is louder in quiet environment
Lack of control	Constant noise may produce high levels of stress
Unsteady gait	Tinnitus often a symptom that occurs with vertigo

→ > >

2 DIAGNOSE

NURSING DIAGNOSIS	SUBJECTIVE FINDINGS	OBJECTIVE FINDINGS
Altered auditory sensory perception related to sensorineural hearing loss	Complains of hearing loss, decreased understanding, and tinnitus, history of exposure to loud noise, family history of ear disease, family history of deafness or tinnitus	Hearing loss on audiogram; tinnitus-matching audiometry; asks that words and phrases be repeated; takes ototoxic drugs
Anxiety related to threat of change or change in interaction patterns	Complains of anxiety, depression, increased stress and tension; complains of sleep disturbances; reports lack of control because of tinnitus or of being overwhelmed by life events	Irritability, distress
High risk for trauma related to balance difficulties	Complains of dizziness, vertigo, abnormal gait, tendency to fall	Abnormal gait, gaze nystagmus, positive Romberg's test

3 PLAN

Patient goals

1. The patient's tinnitus will resolve or stabilize.
2. The patient will understand the problem of tinnitus and will be less anxious.

3. The patient's vertigo will be resolved or controlled.

4 IMPLEMENT

NURSING DIAGNOSIS	NURSING INTERVENTIONS	RATIONALE
Altered auditory sensory perception related to sensorineural hearing loss	Obtain otologic history, including pertinent questions about tinnitus (subjective loudness; sound steady or fluctuating, continuous or intermittent; pitch or frequency; affects one or both ears).	Can help establish cause and pathologic considerations.
	Assess family history, history of ear disease, and any exposure to loud noises.	Can help establish cause and pathologic considerations.
	Perform a review of systems with special attention to central nervous system and cardiovascular system.	Can help establish cause and pathologic considerations.
	Assess dietary habits, alcohol ingestion, and current prescribed medications.	Can help establish cause and pathologic considerations.
	Assess auditory acuity level.	Hearing loss may vary from mild to total.
	Speak distinctly without shouting.	Shouting distorts words.

NURSING DIAGNOSIS	NURSING INTERVENTIONS	RATIONALE
Anxiety related to threat of change or change in interaction patterns	Assess level of anxiety (mild, moderate, severe, panic).	To guide therapeutic interventions.
	Assess patient's perception of needs and expectations.	To facilitate problem solving.
	Help patient recall coping skills used successfully in the past.	Past coping skills may alleviate anxiety.
	Provide information about tinnitus and its treatment.	Knowledge can decrease anxiety.
	Administer antidepressants as ordered.	To reduce anxiety and depression.
	Suggest psychologic evaluation.	Psychotherapy, biofeedback, and self-hypnosis have been effective in the treatment of some patients with tinnitus.
	Encourage patient to express her feelings and concerns.	Open discussion is necessary to alleviate distress, fear, and anxiety.
High risk for trauma related to balance difficulties	Assess for vertigo by observing for nystagmus, abnormal gait, positive Romberg's sign, and inability to perform a tandem Romberg test.	Tinnitus can occur with vestibular problems such as labyrinthitis and Ménière's disease.
	Help with ambulation when indicated.	Abnormal gait can predispose patient to unsteadiness and falls.

5 EVALUATE

PATIENT OUTCOME	DATA INDICATING THAT OUTCOME IS REACHED
Patient's tinnitus has resolved or stabilized.	Patient demonstrates knowledge and acceptance of tinnitus and of treatment options.
Patient understands the problem of tinnitus and is less anxious.	Patient acknowledges anxiety and can identify ways to cope with it.
Patient's vertigo has resolved or is controlled.	Patient understands that vertigo often accompanies tinnitus in vestibular disorders.

PATIENT TEACHING

1. Explain the signs and symptoms related to the cause of the patient's tinnitus.
2. Explain how the patient's hearing loss is related to tinnitus.
3. Explain the reason for retrocochlear testing and imaging studies for unilateral tinnitus and hearing loss.
4. Refer the patient for psychologic evaluation when appropriate.

TREATMENT OF HEARING DISORDERS

Because most hearing losses are permanent, use of a hearing aid should always be considered. A patient should undergo a trial period to establish the hearing aid's benefit before purchasing the device. Bilateral or binaural aids are desirable when applicable.

The technology of aided hearing is part of the current electronic explosion (see Aural Rehabilitation, page 79). The evolution in hearing aid development has led to smaller and more effective aids (see Figure 4-3). Small hearing aids that in general fit into the ear canal are currently available; however, the greater the hearing loss, the larger the hearing aid must be. Hearing aids also are available for placement within the ear concha or behind the ear. Special hearing aids can transmit sound by radio waves to the opposite ear or by vibration to the inner ear through the skull. In the future, hearing aids will be semiimplantable and eventually totally implantable in the middle ear and mastoid.

IMPLANTABLE HEARING DEVICES

Three types of implanted hearing devices are either available for use or in the investigational stage. They are *cochlear implants*, *bone conduction devices*, and *semi-implantable hearing devices*.

Cochlear implants are for patients with little to no hearing. A cochlear implant incorporates a small computer that changes the spoken word to electrical impulses. The impulses are transmitted across the skin to an implanted receiver, which carries the impulse to the hearing nerve endings in the cochlea by means of an electrode introduced through the round windows. The best of the cochlear implants use multichannels and can return about half of the patient's hearing and understanding.

In some cases of hearing loss sound can be transmitted through the skull to the inner ear by *bone conduction devices*. Patients with conductive hearing loss can use a device in which an orthopedic screw is implanted under the skin into the skull. An external device transmits the sound through the skin. This device is worn above the ear and not in the ear canal.

Patients who already use a hearing aid gain the most from an implantable device. Clinical research has shown that a magnet implanted in the middle ear can be stimulated by an ear canal driver, which changes sound to a magnetic force. This system eliminates several bothersome problems of hearing aids such as feedback and difficulties with hearing in noisy environments. A *semi-implantable hearing device* is the first step to a totally implantable device that would eliminate any external device. However, many challenges must be met before a workable device is available.

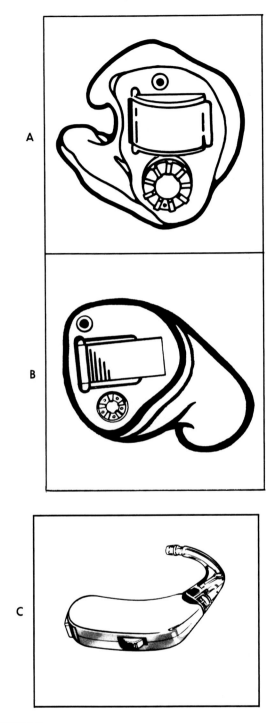

FIGURE 4-3
Types of commonly used hearing aids. **A,** Canal aid. **B,** In-the-ear aid. **C,** Behind-the-ear aid.

AURAL REHABILITATION

If hearing loss is irreversible or not amenable to surgical intervention or if the person elects not to have surgery, aural rehabilitation may be beneficial. The purpose of aural rehabilitation is to maximize the hearing-impaired person's communication skills.

The auditory sense is our primary mode of communication, and rehabilitation is directed toward teaching the person more effective use of the senses of vision, touch, and vibration plus maximizing the use of any remaining hearing ability. Rehabilitation is affected by the person's background and by the severity of impairment. As with other forms of rehabilitation, its success depends on the degree of the patient's motivation.

Aural rehabilitation includes auditory training, speech reading, speech training, and the use of hearing aids. The use of instruments and training is involved. *Auditory training* enhances listening skills. The hearing-impaired person initially is exposed to gross differences in sound and then gradually "fine tuned" so that subtle differences in discrimination of two similar sounds can be made. The primary purpose of auditory training exercises is to help the person concentrate on the speaker. For some people, only gross differences between sounds may be recognized.

Speech reading, the current term for lip reading, is an important means of communication. Speech reading is the process of understanding vocal communication by the integration of lip movements with facial expressions, gestures, environmental clues, and conversation contexts. Speech reading is very difficult, however, without auditory cues. Many movements for speech are very rapid, many sounds look very similar (b, m, p), and certain sounds of any language are invisible (the h in English). A high percentage of the words have to be guessed at by the hearing-impaired person. Recognizing this fact alone will help the nurse be more understanding of the person who is speech (lip) reading.

Because of reduced auditory feedback (the inability of hearing-impaired individuals to monitor their own speech), the clearness, pitch quality, or rate of their speech may deteriorate. These abnormal effects alter the efficiency of communication and reduce the intelligibility of speech. The goal of *speech training* is to conserve, develop, or prevent deterioration of speech skills.

HEARING AIDS

Hearing aids are instruments made up of miniature parts working together as a system to amplify sound in a controlled manner. They are used by people who are hard of hearing (slight or moderate hearing loss) and by deaf people (severe or profound hearing loss). Hearing aids make sound louder but do not improve the ability to understand. Therefore people with decreased discrimination (the ability to understand what is spoken) benefit less from a hearing aid. Appropriate aural rehabilitation ensures successful adjustment of most problems. The hearing aid amplifies many background noises (e.g., hospital machinery, footsteps, department store noises) as well as speech. These noises may mask conversation or confuse the hearing-impaired person, especially the elderly.

A person with a hearing aid should know how to care for the device and know what to do if the aid does not work (see the following boxes). The nurse must also have a basic knowledge of the hearing aid to assist a person who is unable or unwilling to do this when ill. The patient is encouraged to use the hearing aid and to store it safely in its case when it is not in use.

CARE OF A HEARING AID

1. Turn the hearing aid off when not in use.
2. Open the battery compartment at night to avoid accidental drainage of the battery.
3. Keep an extra battery available at all times.
4. Wash the earmold frequently (daily if necessary) with mild soap and warm water, using a pipe cleaner to cleanse the cannula.
5. Dry the earmold completely before reconnecting it to the receiver.
6. Do not wear the hearing aid during an ear infection.

WHAT TO DO IF HEARING AID FAILS TO WORK

1. Check the on-off switch.
2. Inspect the earmold for cleanliness.
3. Examine the battery for correct insertion.
4. Examine the cord plug for correct insertion.
5. Examine the cord for breaks.
6. Replace the battery, cord, or both, if necessary. The life of batteries varies according to the amount of use and the power requirements of the aid. Batteries last from 2 to 14 days.
7. Check the position of the earmold in the ear. If the hearing aid "whistles," the earmold is probably not inserted properly into the ear canal, or the person needs to have a new earmold made.

CHAPTER 5

Disorders of the Ear — Balance

Disorders of balance and the vestibular system afflict a large number of Americans, particularly the elderly. More than 90 million people age 17 or older have experienced dizziness or difficulty with balance. Balance-related falls account for more than half of accidental deaths in the elderly. Few symptoms are more personal or private than those involving an individual's sense of balance. Balance problems can be debilitating and embarrassing; they can create handicaps and impair the quality of life by causing anxiety, uncertainty, and depression.

Unlike with vision and hearing, no single organ is responsible for balance problems. The vestibular system (ear) must work in concert with other body systems to maintain balance. The brain integrates information from the visual system, the proprioceptive system (the position and movement sensors of the muscles and joints), and the vestibular system to execute precise motor commands that maintain the body's equilibrium, posture, and stability of gaze.

Vestibular disorders can produce symptoms of imbalance, vertigo, disorientation, instability, falling, blurred vision, and gait disturbances. Autonomic reactions of the digestive system (diarrhea, nausea, vomiting) and the circulatory system (pallor, slow heart rate, low blood pressure) frequently accompany a severe episode of *vertigo* because of the connections between the vestibular and autonomic centers.

Vestibular Neuronitis

Vestibular neuronitis is a disorder of the vestibular nerve characterized by severe vertigo with normal hearing.

The condition is common and has a number of causes such as viruses, vascular and demyelinating disorders, and toxins. Many patients with vestibular neuronitis have had previous ear, nose, and throat infections. Most probably a number of factors are involved in the pathogenesis of the disorder.

PATHOPHYSIOLOGY

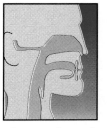

Vestibular neuronitis is characterized by a sudden onset of severe vertigo even though the person's hearing remains normal. The first episode usually is the worst, with subsequent attacks manifesting less and less vertigo. Recovery can occur without treatment over a period of several weeks to months. A less common chronic form can persist for many months to years. The reason for this extension is not understood.

COMPLICATIONS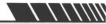

Trauma from falling
Permanent balance disability
Decreased quality of life

DIAGNOSTIC STUDIES AND FINDINGS

Diagnostic test	Findings
Audiometry	Normal hearing or no additional loss for patient with previous hearing impairment
Tympanometry	Compliance and impedance within normal limits
Electronystagmography	Reduced vestibular response on affected side

---

MEDICAL MANAGEMENT

GENERAL MANAGEMENT

Vestibular suppressants are used to treat acute attacks; labyrinthine exercises are done to hasten compensation and recovery.

DRUG THERAPY

Vestibular suppressants such as dimenhydrinate (Dramamine), meclizine (Bonine, Antivert), and buclizine (Bucladin-S) are prescribed (see the box on page 83 for dosage and administration of these and other vestibular suppressants).

SURGERY

If symptoms persist for several years, the condition can be treated with vestibular nerve section in some patients.

NURSING CARE

See pages 87 to 94.

Labyrinthitis

Labyrinthitis is an inflammation of the inner ear (labyrinth) caused by a viral or bacterial infection.

Viral labyrinthitis is a common medical diagnosis, but remarkably little is known about this disorder, which affects both hearing and balance. The causes of viral labyrinthitis can include sequelae of measles, mumps, rubella, and encephalitis; viral illnesses of the upper respiratory tract; and herpetiform disorders of cranial nerves VII (the facial nerve) and VIII (the acoustic nerve) (Ramsey Hunt's syndrome). However, dizziness or vertigo with decreased hearing on the affected side may be the only symptoms of the infection.

Bacterial labyrinthitis owes its source of infection to otitis media. Infection may enter the labyrinth by penetrating the oval or round window. A cholesteatoma (benign skin growth) causes erosion of the lateral semicircular canal, the nearest vulnerable point to the middle ear. If inflammation or a cholesteatoma damages this canal bone, a fistula forms between the middle ear and the labyrinth. Another source of infection is bacterial meningitis, which is conveyed to the labyrinth by two tracts, the cochlear aqueduct and the internal auditory canal.

Viral labyrinthitis is by far the most prevalent form.

PATHOPHYSIOLOGY

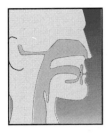

Labyrinthitis is characterized by sudden onset of severe vertigo with varying degrees of hearing loss; tinnitus may or may not be present. Most patients recover their balance function, but the hearing loss usually is permanent. Persistent balance dysfunction is rare, and spontaneous recovery of balance is expected in most patients. Recurrent acute episodes can continue for 5 to 6 weeks. Nausea and vomiting can also occur.

COMPLICATIONS

Partial to total loss of hearing on affected side
Trauma from falling
Permanent balance disability
Meningitis
Decreased quality of life

NURSING CARE

See pages 87 to 94.

DIAGNOSTIC STUDIES AND FINDINGS

Diagnostic Test	Findings
Audiometry	Varying degrees of sensorineural hearing loss on affected side
Tympanometry	*Viral disease:* compliance and impedance within normal limits; *bacterial disease:* compliance and impedance abnormal if labyrinthitis is accompanied by middle ear disease
Electronystagmography	Reduced vestibular response on affected side

MEDICAL MANAGEMENT

GENERAL MANAGEMENT

Vestibular suppressants are used to treat acute attacks; labyrinthine exercises are done to hasten compensation and recovery. Bacterial labyrinthitis is treated with antibiotics.

DRUG THERAPY

Vestibular suppressants such as dimenhydrinate (Dramamine), meclizine (Bonine, Antivert), and buclizine (Bucladin-S) are prescribed (see the box on page 83 for dosage and administration of these and other vestibular suppressants). Antibiotics that cross the blood-brain barrier should be given intravenously to treat bacterial labyrinthitis.

SURGERY

If symptoms do not respond to medical treatment and persist for several years, the condition can be treated with a labyrinthectomy or vestibular nerve section in some patients.

DOSAGE AND ADMINISTRATION OF VESTIBULAR SUPPRESSANTS

Drug (adult dose)	Nursing considerations
Buclizine (Bucladin-S) 50 mg tid	Used sublingually or orally for nausea.
Cyclizine (Marezine) 50 mg q 4-6 h	Drowsiness, dry mouth common.
Diazepam (Valium) 2-5 mg q 4-6 h	May be addictive.
Dimenhydrinate (Dramamine) 50 mg q 4-6 h	Drowsiness common with continued use.
Haloperidol (Haldol) 0.5 mg PO qid	Drowsiness, dry mouth common.
Meclizine* (Antivert, Bonine) 25 mg tid-qid prn	Dose is titrated to just below side effect level. Compensation of balance system may not occur with continued use.
Prochlorperazine (Compazine) 25 mg PO or suppositories q 4-6 h	Has strong antiemetic properties.
Promethazine (Phenergan) 12.5-50 mg q 4-6 h oral or suppositories	Drowsiness common; has strong antiemetic properties.
Scopolamine (Transderm Scop) 0.5 mg patch q 3 days	Diminished short-term memory and dry mouth common; hallucinations reported.
Trimethobenzamide (Tigan) 250 mg tid-qid	More effective for moderate to severe nausea.

*Drug of choice.

Benign Paroxysmal Positional Vertigo

Benign paroxysmal positional vertigo (BPPV) is a brief period of incapacitating vertigo that occurs when the position of the patient's head is changed with respect to gravity (typically by placing the head back with the affected ear turned downward).

Four factors predispose a patient to this disorder: advanced age, trauma, inactivity, and other ear disease. BPPV has been explained by two different theories, cupulolithiasis and canalithiasis. The cupulolithiasis theory proposes that the posterior semicircular canal is rendered sensitive to gravitation by degenerative debris (fragments of otoconia) acting upon the cupula. The canalithiasis theory suggests that this degenerative debris does not adhere to the cupula of the posterior canal, but is free floating in the endolymph. When the head is moved into the provoking position, the debris sinks into the canal. This theory appears more consistent with clinical observations.

The causes of BPPV are not all benign. The condition can be caused by labyrinthine ischemia, vertebrobasilar insufficiency, central nervous system (CNS) neoplasms, and other CNS diseases. However, typical cases are idiopathic or develop secondary to an inner ear disorder. The condition often resolves spontaneously without any need for intervention.

PATHOPHYSIOLOGY

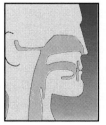

Benign paroxysmal positional vertigo typically is sudden in onset and is followed by a continuous propensity for positional vertigo, usually for hours to weeks but occasionally for months or years. Many patients experience periodic remissions and exacerbations. Severe cases involve vertigo induced by almost any head movement, accompanied by continuous nausea and sometimes vomiting. The symptoms typically are worse in the morning and improve during the day, with fatigue being the prevailing symptom by day's end.

The essential feature of BPPV is nystagmus, which

is evoked by the Dix-Hallpike maneuver. This test is performed by positioning the patient quickly from sitting to head hanging right, head hanging left, and head hanging straight back for 30 seconds in each position. This nystagmus in its classic form is rotary; is directed toward the undermost ear; has a latency of onset of 5 to 10 seconds; usually lasts less than 20 seconds; reverses when the head is returned upright; and is fatigable (response declines with repetition of maneuver).

COMPLICATIONS

Trauma from falling
Permanent balance disability
Decreased quality of life

NURSING CARE

See pages 87 to 94.

DIAGNOSTIC STUDIES AND FINDINGS

Diagnostic Test	Findings
Audiometry	Hearing loss is not expected, but BPPV and hearing loss may have a common cause; thus varying degrees of hearing loss may be found on affected side
Auditory brainstem response test	Should be within normal limits for BPPV (done to screen for retrocochlear problems)
Electronystagmography	Vestibular response may or may not be reduced on affected side
Dix-Hallpike maneuver	Positive for critical provocative position (performed with or without electronystagmography)

MEDICAL MANAGEMENT

GENERAL MANAGEMENT

A common treatment strategy with BPPV is to wait it out. Antivertiginous drugs generally do not prevent the paroxysmal attacks. Vestibular habituation therapy is used, as is a canalith repositioning procedure, which involves manuevers designed to transpose the canaliths out of the posterior semicircular canal and into the utricle.

DRUG THERAPY

None

SURGERY

When conservative treatment fails and incapacitation is significant, a singular neurectomy or occlusion of the posterior semicircular canal is recommended.

Presbyastasis (Presbyvertigo)

Presbyastasis, also known as **presbyvertigo,** is the balance disorder of aging. It is the result of generalized degenerative changes in the labyrinth.

PATHOPHYSIOLOGY

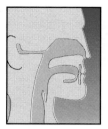

Presbycusis is well-recognized and has been defined as the *hearing* disorder of aging, which involves aging of the cochlear end organ. Presbyastasis, or presbyvertigo, is the *balance* disorder of aging, which involves aging of the vestibular end organ. Decreased visual acuity and compromised proprioception, in addition to vestibular dysfunction, contribute to balance problems. With all three systems involved, the elderly have difficulty with gait, resulting in falls and subsequent injury. As with all age-related disorders, the symptoms can be controlled in some patients but cannot be cured.

COMPLICATIONS

Permanent balance disability
Trauma from age-related falls
Decreased quality of life

NURSING CARE

See pages 87 to 94.

DIAGNOSTIC STUDIES AND FINDINGS

Diagnostic Test	Findings
Audiometry	Sensorineural hearing loss with decreased discrimination in affected ear or ears
Electronystagmography	May have reduced vestibular response in affected ear or ears
Imaging studies with enhancement	To evaluate cardiovascular status and to rule out labyrinthine ischemia caused by spasm, occlusion, or hemorrhage

MEDICAL MANAGEMENT

Management of an elderly patient may include physical therapy, the use of canes or walkers, vasodilators, and neurologic referrals. Control of symptoms is the overall goal.

DRUG THERAPY

Vasodilators such as niacin (nicotinic acid) and papaverine (Pavabid) are prescribed.

Ménière's Disease

Ménière's disease is characterized by a triad of symptoms: attacks of incapacitating vertigo, usually with nausea and vomiting; sensorineural hearing loss; and tinnitus.

Ménière's disease is a common disorder of both auditory and vestibular function that affects an estimated 545,000 people in the United States. Ménière's disease of the inner ear has been likened to glaucoma of the eye. The cause of Ménière's disease is still unknown, but the condition is thought to affect the vestibular system by metabolically altering the labyrinthine fluid, causing the membranous labyrinth to dilate with endolymph. Recurring disabling attacks of vertigo with nausea and vomiting can last several hours and typically subside to a sense of unsteadiness or dizziness. Although the disease is never fatal, its violent symptoms make it a dreaded diagnosis. Although cure is not available, control is possible. Circulatory, metabolic, toxic, allergic, and/or emotional factors may influence the intensity of the attacks or may precipitate an attack.

PATHOPHYSIOLOGY

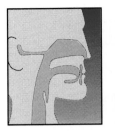

Prodromal symptoms of aural fullness or pressure and/or tinnitus can occur before an episode. Incapacitating vertigo occurs, along with other autonomic symptoms (e.g., nausea, vomiting, diarrhea, and diaphoresis), as well as hearing loss on the affected side. Initially, the hearing loss usually fluctuates. Attacks can last 20 minutes or several hours and can occur many times a week. After a severe attack, the individual is exhausted and sleeps for several hours. Between the attacks the person is completely free of vertigo.

COMPLICATIONS

Partial to total loss of hearing on affected side
Permanent balance disability
Trauma from falling
Dehydration
Decreased quality of life

DIAGNOSTIC STUDIES AND FINDINGS

Diagnostic Test	Findings
Audiometry	Fluctuating hearing loss, normal hearing, but as disease progresses, sensorineural hearing loss develops; low-pitched, peaked, or high-frequency hearing loss to profound sensorineural hearing loss in "burned out" ear
Laboratory evaluation	To rule out other metabolic problems (hypoglycemia, fluorescent treponema antibody [FTA], and thyroid, lipid, and autoimmune disorders)
Electronystagmography	Normal to decreased vestibular response on affected side
Electrocochleography	Negative-summating potential relative to action potential is larger than in normal hearing
Auditory brainstem response	To screen for a retrocochlear problem (normal in Ménière's disease)
Imaging studies with enhancement	To rule out acoustic neuroma

MEDICAL MANAGEMENT

GENERAL MANAGEMENT

Medical management is the mainstay of Ménière's disease, but treatment varies widely among physicians. The overall goals are to preserve hearing and to control vertiginous attacks.

Treatment usually consists of a low-sodium diet; use of diuretics, vestibular suppressants, and vasodilators; and labyrinthine exercises.

Avoiding tobacco, alcohol, and caffeine can sometimes be recommended. Psychologic evaluation may be indicated if the patient is anxious, uncertain, fearful, or depressed.

MEDICAL MANAGEMENT—cont'd

DRUG THERAPY

Vestibular depressants: AMT 25 mg qid prn; diazepam (Valium): 5 mg tid prn; Ativan: 1 mg qid prn.

Diuretic: Hydrochlorothiazide and triamterene (Dyazide): one capsule PO daily.

Vasodilators: Niacin: tid; papaverine (Pavabid): tid.

Cholinergic drugs: Atropine; scopolamine (Transderm Scop): 0.5 mg patch q 3 days.

Anticholinergic drugs: Glycopyrrolate (Robinul): 2 mg PO bid.

Antiemetic: Prochlorperazine (Compazine) 10 mg or Phenergan 25 mg PO or suppository q 4-6 h.

SURGERY

Ototoxic ablation therapy: Streptomycin injected for bilateral Ménière's disease; vestibular nerve section for uncontrollable unilateral Ménière's disease.

CHRONIC VERTIGO

1 ASSESS

ASSESSMENT	OBSERVATIONS
Vestibular signs/ symptoms	Vertigo, spinning, imbalance, inability to stand with legs and feet together without falling, unsteady or abnormal gait, veering in either direction, altered mobility due to imbalance, history of falls and trauma, change in ability to estimate spatial relationships of body to environment
Cerebellar signs/ symptoms	Inability to perform rapid alternating movements, inability to maintain an upright posture, inability to walk heel to toe, balancing difficulties
Cranial nerve signs/ symptoms	Blurred vision, diplopia, pupillary abnormalities, visual field deficits, ocular palsies, facial palsies, deafness, vertigo, alteration in taste or smell
Auditory signs/ symptoms	Decreased sensorineural hearing (unilateral or bilateral), tinnitus, auditory distortions, change in sensory acuity, inattention to communication on affected side, altered pattern of communication
Cardiovascular signs/symptoms	Increased heart rate and/or blood pressure, altered respiratory rhythm, orthostatic hypotension, carotid bruits
Fluid-electrolyte status	Change in gastrointestinal activity, vomiting, diarrhea, altered intake, use of medications such as diuretics
Psychosocial factors	Dependency, disability requiring life-style change, change in social involvement, verbalizes changes in life-style, verbalizes inability to cope, complains of frustration in not being able to continue usual activities, boredom, increase in daytime sleep period, nonparticipation, withdrawal, depression

→ ❯ ❯

ASSESSMENT	OBSERVATIONS
Mental/behavioral factors	Increased tension, fear, apprehension, phobias, panic, increased concentration on vertigo, anger, verbalizes lack of control over disease and vertigo, helplessness, hopelessness, chronic anxiety, irritability, fatigue, powerlessness, uncertainty, distress, chronic worry, facial tension, concern about health, withdrawn behavior, crying

2 DIAGNOSE

NURSING DIAGNOSIS	SUBJECTIVE FINDINGS	OBJECTIVE FINDINGS
Impaired adjustment related to disability requiring change in life-style due to unpredictability of vertigo	Reports feeling powerless, expresses lack of confidence in ability to be fully independent	Lack of movement toward independence, inability to problem solve or set goals
Anxiety related to threat of or change in health status and/or role functioning	Reports feeling increased tension, apprehension, helplessness, lack of control, uncertainty, and fear; feels scared or distressed and under stress because of decreased hearing	Irritability, crying, facial tension, increased perspiration
Body image disturbance related to biophysical factors of vertigo	Reports feeling helpless, hopeless, and powerless; complains of changes in life-style and/or social involvement	Change in ability to estimate spatial relationship of body to environment; change in balance function (abnormal gait); change in social involvement
Ineffective individual coping related to personal vulnerability and unmet expectations stemming from vertigo	Reports inability to cope or to meet role expectations, inability to problem solve, and emotional tension	Change in usual communication patterns, chronic worry and anxiety, general irritability, chronic depression
Diversional activity deficit related to environmental lack of such activity	Complains of boredom, expresses anger, complains of not being able to initiate or continue with usual activity and of not being able to interact with others because of hearing and/or balance problems	Anger, increase in daytime sleep periods, withdrawn behavior
Fear related to sensory impairment or phobia	Reports increased tension and apprehension and feeling scared or panicky	Increased blood pressure, pulse, and respiration; diaphoresis; change in gastrointestinal activity; increased concentration on vertigo, crying
High risk for fluid volume deficit related to increased fluid output, altered intake, and medications	Complains of fatigue, thirst, and/or dizziness	Vomiting, diarrhea, diaphoresis, diuretics, inability to eat or drink due to vertigo, nausea, and vomiting

NURSING DIAGNOSIS	SUBJECTIVE FINDINGS	OBJECTIVE FINDINGS
High risk for injury related to altered mobility because of gait disturbance and vertigo	Complains of vertigo	Abnormal gait, imbalance, history of injuries related to falls
Powerlessness related to illness regimen and being helpless in certain situations due to vertigo	Reports lack of control over or unpredictability of vertigo, expresses frustration over inability to perform previous tasks or activities, feels depressed	Increased dependence on others leading to anger, nonparticipation, and withdrawal
Altered auditory sensory perception related to altered state of the ear	Reports change in sensory acuity, anxiety; complains of decreased hearing and understanding and of tinnitus	Abnormal results on audiogram, inappropriate response to communication, inattention to stimulus on affected side, altered communication pattern
High risk for trauma related to balancing difficulties	Complains of vertigo and hearing deficit; has history of falls and/or injuries	Unsteady, abnormal gait; balancing difficulties; poor vision

3 PLAN

Patient goals

1. The patient will adjust to or modify life-style to decrease disability and exert maximum control and independence within limits posed by chronic vertigo.
2. The patient will have less or no anxiety.
3. The patient will have a positive body image.
4. The patient will develop coping skills necessary to decrease vulnerability and unmet needs and demonstrate effective coping.
5. The patient will engage in diversional activities.
6. The patient will have decreased fear through increased knowledge of vertigo.
7. The patient will maintain a normal fluid-electrolyte balance.
8. The patient will remain free of any injuries associated with imbalance and/or falls.
9. The patient will feel an increased sense of control over life and activities despite vertigo.
10. The patient's hearing loss will stabilize.
11. The patient will reduce the risk of trauma by adapting the home environment and by using rehabilitative devices if necessary.

4 IMPLEMENT

NURSING DIAGNOSIS	NURSING INTERVENTIONS	RATIONALE
Impaired adjustment related to disability requiring change in life-style due to unpredictability of vertigo	Encourage patient to identify personal strengths and roles that can still be fulfilled.	To maximize sense of regaining control and independence.
	Provide information about chronic vertigo and what to expect.	To reduce fear and anxiety.
	Assist in selection of self-care practices (e.g., increased aerobic activity and balance exercises).	Such practices enhance adjustment to disability and compensation of balance system.

➔ ➤ ➤ ➤

NURSING DIAGNOSIS	NURSING INTERVENTIONS	RATIONALE
	Include family and significant others in rehabilitative process.	Perceived beliefs of significant others are important for patient's adherence to medical regimen.
	Encourage patient to maintain sense of control by making decisions and assuming more responsibility for care.	To reinforce positive psychologic and social outcomes.
Anxiety related to threat of or change in health status and/or role functioning	Assess level of anxiety.	To guide therapeutic interventions and participation in self-care.
	Help patient identify coping skills used successfully in the past.	Past coping skills can relieve anxiety.
	Provide information about vertigo and its treatment.	To decrease anxiety through increased knowledge.
	Encourage patient to discuss anxieties and explore concerns about vertigo attacks and/or decreased hearing.	To help patient gain awareness and understanding of relationship between anxiety level and behavior.
	Teach patient stress management techniques.	Improved stress management can reduce the frequency and severity of some vertiginous attacks.
	Suggest psychotherapy for patient who is anxious and depressed.	To reduce anxiety and depression.
Body image disturbance related to biophysical factors of vertigo	Encourage patient to discuss feelings and concerns about vertigo.	Articulation of feelings reduces anxiety.
	Assess patient's current perceptions and feelings.	To identify distortions and misconceptions.
	Help patient identify, label, and express feelings about diagnosis, treatments, and anticipated prognosis.	Patient can then accept body change and incorporate it into self-concept.
	Promote acceptance of a positive, realistic body image.	To improve patient's self-image.
Ineffective individual coping related to personal vulnerability and unmet expectations stemming from vertigo	Assess patient's cognitive appraisal of illness and factors that may be contributing to patient's inability to cope.	To enhance coping process.
	Provide factual information about treatment and future health status.	To clarify any misinformation or confusion.
	Encourage and help patient participate in decision making about adjustments in lifestyle.	To help patient regain sense of power and control in self-care with activities of daily living.

NURSING DIAGNOSIS	NURSING INTERVENTIONS	RATIONALE
	Encourage patient to maintain diversional or recreational activities, exercise, and social events.	Social isolation and avoiding pleasant activities intensify isolation and reduce ability to cope with vertigo.
	Help patient identify personal strengths and develop coping strategies based on personal strengths, previous positive experiences in dealing with stress, and situational supports.	To enhance patient's strengths that help maintain hope.
	Refer patient to support groups or counseling as indicated.	May help patient feel less alone and isolated.
Diversional activity deficit related to environmental lack of such activity	Assess level and type of diversional activity to plan appropriate activities.	Boredom may be exhibited as well as depression; helps determine tolerances as well as preferences.
	Discuss usual pattern of diversional activities with patient.	To provide information about perceived and actual stressors that influence activity level.
	Suggest opportunities to continue meaningful diversional activities.	To support patient's sense of self-worth and productivity.
Fear related to sensory impairment or phobia	Encourage patient to talk about feelings, personal perception of danger, and perception of own coping skills and limitations.	Expressing feelings can lessen intensity and duration of fear.
	Dispel distorted perceptions and misinformation about vertigo, and provide accurate information.	Realistic appraisal results in problem solving to decrease danger.
	Teach therapeutic treatments of vertigo and what to expect.	Knowledge of what to expect on a sensory level decreases fear of the unknown.
	Refer patient to support groups.	Fear decreases when patient identifies with someone who has successfully dealt with a similar problem.
	Encourage use of such comfort measures as music, religious practices, and family and friends.	To distract self from focusing on fears.
High risk for fluid volume deficit related to increased fluid output, altered intake, and medications	Assess or have patient assess intake and output (including emesis, liquid stools, urine, and diaphoresis).	Accurate records provide basis for fluid replacement.
	Assess indicators of dehydration, including blood pressure (orthostasis), pulse, skin turgor, and mucous membranes.	Prompt recognition of dehydration allows early intervention.

→ > >

NURSING DIAGNOSIS	NURSING INTERVENTIONS	RATIONALE
	Encourage oral fluids as tolerated; discourage beverages containing caffeine.	Oral replacement is begun as soon as possible to replace losses. Caffeine may increase diarrhea.
	Administer or teach administration of antiemetics and antidiarrheal medication as ordered and needed.	Antiemetics reduce nausea and vomiting, reducing fluid losses and improving oral intake. Antidiarrheal medication reduces intestinal motility and fluid losses.
High risk for injury related to altered mobility because of gait disturbance and vertigo	Assess for vertigo (history, onset, description of attacks, duration, any associated symptoms) (see Appendix page 276 for Dizziness Questionnaire).	History provides basis for other interventions and catharsis for patient.
	Assess extent of disability in relation to activities of daily living.	Extent of disability indicates risk of falling.
	Teach or reinforce vestibular/balance therapy as prescribed.	Exercises hasten labyrinthine compensation, which decreases vertigo and gait disturbances.
	Administer or teach administration of antivertiginous medications and/or vestibular sedation medication; instruct patient in side effects.	To alleviate acute symptoms of vertigo.
Powerlessness related to illness regimen and being helpless in certain situations due to vertigo	Assess patient's needs, values, and attitudes and readiness to initiate activities.	Involving patient in planning activities and care enhances potential for mastery.
	Provide opportunities for patient to express feelings (catharsis) about self and illness.	Expressing feelings increases understanding of individual coping styles and defense mechanisms.
	Help patient identify previous coping behaviors that were successful.	Awareness increases understanding of stressors that trigger feeling of powerlessness.
	Help patient identify previous coping behaviors that were sucessful.	Awareness of past successes enhances self-confidence.
Altered auditory sensory perception related to altered state of the ear	Assess hearing acuity and audiogram results.	Hearing may be decreased due to sensorineural hearing loss.
	Speak distinctly without shouting.	Shouting distorts words.
	Assess for tinnitus.	Tinnitus can accompany sensorineural losses.
	Assess history of hearing loss (see Appendix page 275 for Hearing Questionnaire).	History provides basis of other interventions and catharsis for patient.

NURSING DIAGNOSIS	NURSING INTERVENTIONS	RATIONALE
High risk for trauma related to balancing difficulties	Assess for vertigo by history and by examination for nystagmus, positive Romberg, and inability to perform tandem Romberg.	Peripheral vestibular disorders cause these signs and symptoms.
	Assist with ambulation when indicated.	Abnormal gait can predispose patient to unsteadiness and falls.
	Assess for visual acuity and proprioceptive deficits.	Balance depends upon visual, vestibular, and proprioceptor systems.
	Encourage increased activity level with or without use of assistive devices.	Increased activity helps retrain balance system.
	Help identify hazards in home environment.	Adaptation of home environment can reduce risk of falls during rehabilitative process.

5 EVALUATE

PATIENT OUTCOME	DATA INDICATING THAT OUTCOME IS REACHED
Patient exerts maximum control of environment and independence within limits imposed by vertigo.	Patient uses strengths and potentials to engage in the most independent and constructive life-style.
Patient's fear and anxiety about vertiginous attacks have been reduced or eliminated.	Patient has acquired knowledge and skills to deal with vertigo, feels less tension, apprehension, and uncertainty, and demonstrates lack of irritability and crying.
Patient has a positive body image.	Patient verbalizes compensation for the change in ability to estimate spatial relationship of body to environment.
Patient copes effectively with vertigo.	Patient verbalizes less threatening appraisal of situation and is able to identify specific strategies for coping.
Patient engages in diversional activities.	Patient seeks out realistic opportunities for involvement in diversional activities, verbalizes decreased feelings of boredom, and appears alert and animated.
Patient has a normal fluid-electrolyte balance.	Patient is alert and oriented; vital signs are within normal limits; skin turgor is normal; vomiting and/or diarrhea has stopped; mucous membranes are moist; laboratory values for electrolytes are normal; usual oral intake has been resumed.

PATIENT OUTCOME	DATA INDICATING THAT OUTCOME IS REACHED
Patient has no injuries associated with balance problems.	Patient has no injuries and is aware of risk factors associated with vertigo, abnormal gait, and falling.
Patient has an increased sense of control over life and activities despite vertigo.	Patient verbalizes positive feelings about own ability to achieve a sense of power and control.
Patient's hearing has stabilized.	Patient demonstrates knowledge of the cause of the hearing loss and options for rehabilitation.
Patient has adapted home environment or uses rehabilitative devices to reduce risk of falling.	Patient does not fall but is aware of the risks of falling.

PATIENT TEACHING

1. Teach the patient and family about the diagnosis and treatment of chronic vertigo.
2. Stress the importance of maintaining or resuming activities.
3. Stress the importance of regular exercise schedule, including aerobic exercise.
4. Emphasize the importance of diversional or social activities.
5. Teach the patient the names, dosage, frequency, and side effects of prescribed medications.
6. Emphasize the importance of not allowing vertigo to disable or handicap the patient when the vertigo is absent.

Therapeutic Interventions for Ear Disorders

The nursing care given to patients having surgical interventions for ear problems varies predominantly according to the surgical approach and not the specific surgical procedure. The subsequent text is divided into procedures requiring a transcanal approach, procedures requiring a transmastoid approach, and procedures requiring a transcranial approach. A nursing care plan has been developed for each of the surgical approaches. Finally, other medical and minor surgical interventions have been included.

Myringotomy and Transtympanic Tube Placement for Serous Otitis Media

Serous otitis media is not the same as a middle ear infection, although the presence of fluid can lead to such an infection. The cause of serous otitis media is blockage of the eustachian tube from repeated infection, allergy, enlarged adenoids, and other causes. Pressure between the nose and middle ear cannot be equalized, and the ear becomes inflamed. Fluid is formed, and the longer this blockage exists, the more thick and glue-like the fluid becomes. When the middle ear space becomes filled with fluid, sound is not transmitted as well to the inner ear, and a conductive hearing loss occurs.

Myringotomies with or without the placement of transtympanic tubes are performed to regain normal middle ear and eustachian tube function. This goal is

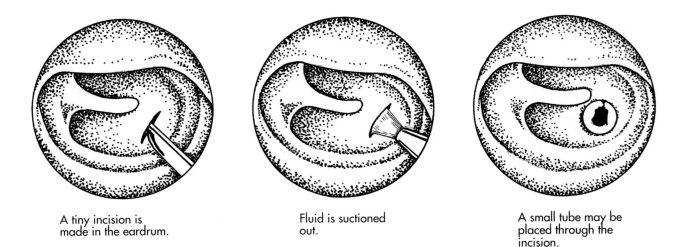

A tiny incision is
made in the eardrum.

Fluid is suctioned
out.

A small tube may be
placed through the
incision.

FIGURE 6-1
Myringotomy and transtympanic tube placement to prevent the
recurrence of fluid in the middle ear.

achieved under local anesthesia by making an incision
in the pars tensa of the tympanic membrane, removing
the fluid by suction, and inserting a tube (Figure 6-1).
There are a wide variety of ventilating tubes; the choice
depends on the surgeon's preference.

The ventilating tube temporarily takes the place of
the eustachian tube in equalizing pressure and remains
in the eardrum for 6 to 9 months. During this time,
the eustachian tube blockage usually subsides. Normally, the tubes come out as the eardrum grows, and
they fall out of the ear canal on their own. After the
tubes come out, the eardrum heals in 99% of patients.
In 1% of patients, a small hole remains which often
serves as a tube. This hole can be repaired at a later
time with a tympanoplasty (surgical reconstruction of
the eardrum).

INDICATIONS

Chronic serous otitis media
Recurrent serous otitis media
Eustachian tube dysfunction with middle ear atelectasis

CONTRAINDICATIONS: None

COMPLICATIONS

Hearing loss
Injury to or dislocation of ossicular chain
Otorrhea
Atrophy of tympanic membrane
Tympanosclerosis of the tympanic membrane
Perforation
Cholesteatoma

DIAGNOSTIC STUDIES AND FINDINGS

Diagnostic test	Findings
Otologic examination	Retracted tympanic membrane with or without bubbles under the drum
Audiometry	Conductive hearing loss
Tympanometry	Flat tympanogram

MEDICAL MANAGEMENT

GENERAL MANAGEMENT

Diet as tolerated. Cotton in ear changed as necessary for first 24 hours.

DRUG THERAPY

Versed: 5 mg IM 1 hr before surgery (2.5 mg for patient ≥70 yr).

Darvocet-N 100:   one tablet q 4-6 h for pain.

Sudafed: 60 mg tid prn for nasal stuffiness.

Cortisporin otic drops: 3 drops tid for 3 days.

PREPROCEDURAL NURSING CARE

1. Explain the technique and purpose of the procedure.
2. Discuss postoperative instructions such as water restrictions.
3. Check operative permission form.
4. Discuss the risks and complications of surgery if appropriate.
5. Administer preoperative medications.

1 ASSESS

ASSESSMENT	OBSERVATIONS
External ear canal	Drainage from myringotomy incision and/or tube such as clear fluid, blood, or pus

2 DIAGNOSE

NURSING DIAGNOSIS	SUBJECTIVE FINDINGS	OBJECTIVE FINDINGS
Acute pain related to myringotomy and tube placement	Complains of sharp pain, dull ache, and discomfort	Crying, grimace, moaning, holding ear
Impaired tissue integrity related to myringotomy	Complains of drainage	Bleeding or drainage of clear fluid or pus from external ear canal

3 PLAN

Patient goals

1. The patient will experience no pain.
2. The patient's incision(s) will heal and normal skin integrity will return without complications.

→ > >

4 IMPLEMENT

NURSING DIAGNOSIS	NURSING INTERVENTION	RATIONALE
Acute pain related to myringotomy and tube placement	Assess and document the intensity and frequency of pain or discomfort.	A small amount of pain is expected. Intense pain should be reported to the surgeon.
	Administer analgesics as ordered.	To provide relief from pain.
Impaired tissue integrity related to myringotomy	Assess for drainage from the external ear canal.	Minimal drainage is expected. Copious drainage should be reported to the surgeon.
	Change cotton ball as necessary.	To assess for amount of drainage.
	Administer antibiotics (oral or topical) as ordered.	Therapeutic or prophylactic therapy can be used.
	Teach water restriction procedure.	Water in the ear can cause infection.

5 EVALUATE

PATIENT OUTCOME	DATE INDICATING THAT OUTCOME IS REACHED
The patient has no pain.	The patient does not complain of pain, there is no holding of the ear, grimacing, moaning, or crying.
The patient demonstrates good skin integrity.	The patient has no drainage from the external ear canal.

PATIENT TEACHING ■

After tube placement

Tubes prevent most ear infections. But if an ear infection develops the ear will drain through the tube without pain. If drainage occurs, notify the surgeon. These tubes cause very little damage to the eardrum or to the hearing. Ear tubes usually come out of the ear by themselves. This will happen in several months to a year, unless permanent tubes have been inserted.

Occasionally, a scar can be seen on the eardrum from the tube placement or from infection, but hearing is not impaired.

Postoperative instructions

1. Advise the patient to use his prescription for ear drops. She should use 3 drops 3 times a day for 3 days in the ear(s) with the tube(s).
2. Inform the patient that there are no physical restrictions except she must not get water in her ears; tell her that she does not have to protect her ear(s) in any other way.
3. **Make sure the patient understands that she must not get any water in her ears.** Provide her with earplugs that are disposable and should be replaced when needed (if they get dirty, etc.). They are available through most drugstores. They can be used for swimming; however, a swim cap is recommended to ensure placement. Advise the patient that a dry piece of cotton in the ear covered by a second piece of cotton that has been saturated with petroleum jelly can be used instead of earplugs to protect the ear from water.
4. Inform the patient that she may have a little bloody drainage the first day. If she has drainage of any kind after this, she should call the physician's office immediately.

Transcanal Surgeries

CANALPLASTY

The otologist is seldom wrong in surmising that a patient with exostoses has been an ardent cold-water swimmer. Exostoses are nodular outgrowths from the bony ear canal; usually several are present in both ears. Exostoses appear as hard, smooth, rounded, whitish nodules of bone that can completely occlude the external ear canal. When exostoses block the ear canal (atresia) so that epidermal debris is retained and conductive hearing loss results, a canalplasty should be performed.

The term *canalplasty* means to create a new ear canal. A general anesthetic is administered, and a transcanal approach is used. The skin and the periosteum covering the exostoses are lifted away, and the growths are drilled with a small, round cutting burr until the normal contour of the external ear canal has been restored. The skin and periosteum are replaced, but if they cannot cover the denuded area, a skin graft can be used.

INDICATIONS

Canal atresia	Postmastoid surgery
Congenital canal atresia	Trauma (acquired canal atresia)
Exostoses	Keloid formation

CONTRAINDICATIONS: None

COMPLICATIONS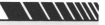

Perforation of tympanic membrane
Facial nerve paralysis

DIAGNOSTIC STUDIES AND FINDINGS

Diagnostic test	Finding
Otologic and microscopic examination of external ear	Hard, smooth, round white nodules protruding from ear canal
Audiometry	Normal or conductive hearing loss
X-ray	Nodular bony growths confined to ear canal

NURSING CARE

See pages 108 to 111.

STAPES REPLACEMENT SURGERY

Otosclerosis is a genetic disorder in which normal bone is replaced by abnormal bone, causing fixation of the stapes and conductive hearing loss, cochlear invasion and sensorineural hearing loss, or both, that is called a mixed loss. Otosclerosis can be bilateral (75% of cases) or unilateral (25% of cases). It is twice as common in women as in men and often progresses during pregnancy. Approximately 5% of all people with hearing problems have otosclerosis. The disorder is associated with van der Hoeve's symptoms (blue sclerae, osteogenesis imperfecta [fragile bones], and stapedial fixation).

Stapes replacement surgery is the treatment of choice for otosclerosis. It involves either the traditional stapedectomy or a stapedotomy. Stapes surgery can be performed with local or general anesthesia but usually is performed with local anesthesia supplemented by intravenous sedation. With this method the patient can communicate with the surgeon during the surgery to report hearing results and dizziness or other symptoms.

The procedure usually is performed transcanal through a speculum, aided by a microscope. A poste-

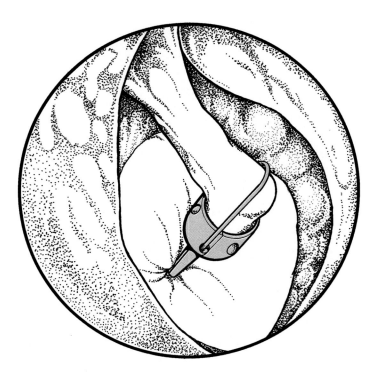

FIGURE 6-2
Stapedectomy with Robinson stainless steel prosthesis in place.

rior tympanomeatal flap is created in the external ear canal, and the tympanic membrane is elevated. Adequate exposure is obtained by curetting the posterior-superior scutum. Care is taken not to injure the chorda tympani nerve, which supplies taste to part of the tongue. A tiny control hole is placed in the footplate of the stapes, and the joint between the incus and stapes is separated. The stapedial tendon is cut, and the superstructure of the stapes is fractured and removed (Figure 6-2). The stapes footplate is removed with picks (a drill is used for thick otosclerosis) and, in a stapedectomy, a graft is placed over the oval window.

The graft can be tissue taken from the tragal perichondrium, temporalis fascia, or a small section of vein from the back of the hand. The graft is harvested before the stapes surgery begins. After placement of the graft, a prosthesis is positioned between the incus and the

covered oval window. Prostheses are made of various materials, and every surgeon has a preference.

In a stapedotomy, after the stapes superstructure has been removed, a laser is used to enlarge the control hole. A Teflon piston prosthesis with a diameter of 0.4 or 0.6 mm is placed in the control hole and crimped over the incus.

In both procedures the tympanic membrane and canal skin are reapproximated and the ear is packed with gelfoam and cotton. Both procedures reestablish a normal sound pathway by replacing the stapes with a prosthesis. The stapes surgery has a high success rate, and the patient notices improved hearing immediately in the operating room. However, hearing diminishes after surgery for some time because of bleeding, edema, and the ear packing.

INDICATIONS

Otosclerosis
Tympanoscleroses of stapes

CONTRAINDICATIONS

Poor speech discrimination thresholds
Small conductive loss
Only hearing ear
Serious medical problems
Perforation of tympanic membrane
Infection

COMPLICATIONS

Hearing loss
Dizziness
Taste disturbance
Mouth dryness
Tinnitus
Facial paralysis
Perforation
Infection
Dislocation of incus
Perilymph gusher
Perilymph fistula

DIAGNOSTIC STUDIES AND FINDINGS

Diagnostic test	Findings
Otologic examination	Normal tympanic membrane
Audiometry	Conductive or mixed hearing loss
Tympanometry	Normal
Stapedial reflex	Usually absent

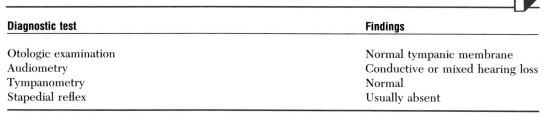

MEDICAL MANAGEMENT

GENERAL MANAGEMENT

Bed rest, maintaining prescribed position if ordered (e.g., operated ear positioned up for several hours). Blood pressure monitoring (put in Trendelenburg's position if pressure falls). Diet as tolerated. Out of bed as tolerated.

DRUG THERAPY

Versed: 5 mg IM 1 hr before surgery (2.5 mg for patient $\geq$70 yr).

Toradol: 30-45 mg IM q 6 h prn for pain.

Darvocet-N 100: q 4 h prn for pain.

Sudafed: 30-60 mg tid prn for nasal stuffiness.

Vistaril: q 6 h IM for restlessness.

Dramamine: 50 mg IM or PO q 4 h prn for vertigo.

Torecan: 10 mg IM tid prn for nausea.

Amoxicillin: 250 mg qid.

PREPROCEDURAL NURSING GUIDELINES

1. Initiate preoperative instruction for the patient and family
   Explain the surgical procedure and the purpose for shaving either above or behind the patient's ear or arm.
   Explain or review the postoperative course.
   Discuss postoperative instructions such as activity restrictions, head movement, and symptoms.
   Encourage the patient to express any anxiety, fears, concerns, and questions.
2. Check the operative permission form.
3. Discuss the risks and complications of surgery if appropriate.
4. Withhold food and water for an appropriate length of time before surgery.
5. Advise the patient to wash hair before surgery.
6. Remove all jewelry, glasses, contact lenses, and hearing aid in operative ear from the patient.
7. Administer preoperative medications.

NURSING CARE

See pages 108 to 111.

TYMPANOTOMY FOR CLOSURE OF A PERILYMPH FISTULA

Leakage of perilymph from the oval window or round window can cause episodic vertigo. Perilymph fistulas can be congenital or acquired. Acquired lesions that are spontaneous or traumatic have vestibular or auditory symptoms or both. Vertigo begins abruptly after a Valsalva maneuver or other times when pressure changes rapidly, such as in diving, airplane descent, or weight lifting. An associated hearing loss that can fluctuate with the vertigo may be present. However, hearing can also be within the normal range with a fistula.

Trauma to the head, previous stapedectomy surgery, or inadvertent entry into the bony labyrinth during mastoid surgery can also cause a perilymphatic fistula. Besides rupturing the oval and round windows, pressure changes can also rupture the intralabyrinthine membrane of the cochlear ductway.

Surgical exploration for a perilymph fistula is performed transcanal using local anesthesia. A tympano-meatal flap is raised, and the oval and round window regions are carefully inspected under high-power magnification. The patient sometimes is placed in Trendelenburg's position and asked to gently perform a Valsalva maneuver. The increase in pressure causes the perilymph to escape. The mucosa in the oval and round window niches are escarified with a pick, and perichondrium, adipose tissue, vein, or fascia graft is placed in these regions. This tissue obliteration often is done even if no fistula is found, because inapparent fistulas have been reported.

If a perilymphatic fistula is diagnosed and treated early, the hearing loss can improve. And even if hearing does not improve, often other aural and vestibular complaints do.

INDICATIONS

History of precipitating event with vertigo and/or sensorineural hearing loss
Poststapedectomy
Postmastoidectomy

CONTRAINDICATIONS

Serious medical problems
Infection

COMPLICATIONS

Meningitis
Infection
Facial nerve paralysis
Tinnitus
Sensorineural hearing loss
Perforation
Dislocation of ossicles
Taste disturbance
Mouth dryness
Permanent balance problem

DIAGNOSTIC STUDIES AND FINDINGS

Diagnostic test	Findings
Otologic examination	Normal tympanic membrane
Audiography	Conductive mixed, sensorineural, or fluctuating hearing loss
Tympanography	Normal
Electronystagmography with fistula test	Unilateral caloric weakness with positive fistula test
Computed tomography (CT) or magnetic resonance imaging (MRI)	Normal

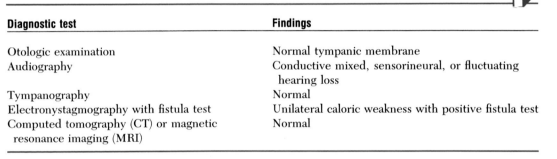

MEDICAL MANAGEMENT

GENERAL MANAGEMENT

Bed rest, maintaining prescribed position if ordered (e.g., operated ear positioned up for several hours). Blood pressure monitoring (put in Trendelenburg's position if pressure falls). Diet as tolerated. Out of bed as tolerated. Assistance with ambulation if necessary.

DRUG THERAPY

Versed: 5 mg IM 1 hr before surgery (2.5 mg for patient ≥70 yr).

Toradol: 30-45 mg IM q 6 h prn for pain.

Darvocet-N 100: 1 tablet q 4 h prn for pain.

MEDICAL MANAGEMENT—cont'd

Sudafed: 30-60 mg tid prn for nasal stuffiness.

Vistaril: q 6 h IM for restlessness.

Dramamine: 50 mg IM or PO q 4 h prn for vertigo.

Torecan: 10 mg IM tid prn for nausea.

Amoxicillin: 250 mg qid.

PREPROCEDURAL NURSING GUIDELINES

1. Initiate preoperative instruction for the patient and family.
   Explain the surgical procedure and the purpose for shaving above and behind the patient's ear.
   Explain or review the postoperative course.
   Discuss postoperative instructions such as activity restrictions, head movement, and symptoms.
   Encourage the patient to express any anxiety, fears, concerns, and questions.

2. Check the operative permission form.
3. Discuss the risks and complications of surgery if appropriate.
4. Withhold food and water for an appropriate length of time before surgery.
5. Wash the patient's hair before surgery.
6. Remove all jewelry, glasses, contact lenses, and hearing aid in the operative ear from the patient.
7. Administer preoperative medications.

NURSING CARE

See pages 108 to 111.

TYMPANOPLASTY

Tympanoplasty is a general term used to describe several surgical procedures for repairing the tympanic membrane. A tympanoplasty is done to treat perforations, retraction pockets, and plaques in the tympanic membrane. Polyps, granulomas, and infection also can be removed from the middle ear through tympanoplasty.

Historically there are five types of tympanoplasties (Figure 6-3). Type I is performed to repair a perforation of the tympanic membrane; type II is done to repair the tympanic membrane and to place a graft on the long process of the incus in cases with dislocation or necrosis of the malleus; type III is done to repair the tympanic membrane and to place graft directly on the head of the stapes in cases with necrosis of both the malleus and the incus; type IV is done to repair the tympanic membrane and to place a graft on the mobile stapes footplate in cases with necrosis of the malleus, incus, and stapes superstructure; type V, which has been replaced by stapes surgery, was performed with stapes footplate fixation by fenestrating the lateral semicircular canal to provide access of sound vibration transmission from the middle ear cavity to the inner ear. Except for type I, all these procedures produced varying degrees of residual conductive hearing loss.

The purposes of a tympanoplasty are (1) to close a perforation of the tympanic membrane; (2) to prevent

> A surgical microscope is used to perform a tympanoplasty. The anesthetic (usually local) is given, and an incision is made above or behind the ear. A piece of muscle covering (fascia) is removed and used to graft the eardrum. The ear is packed to protect the new eardrum. Complete healing of the perforation takes several months.

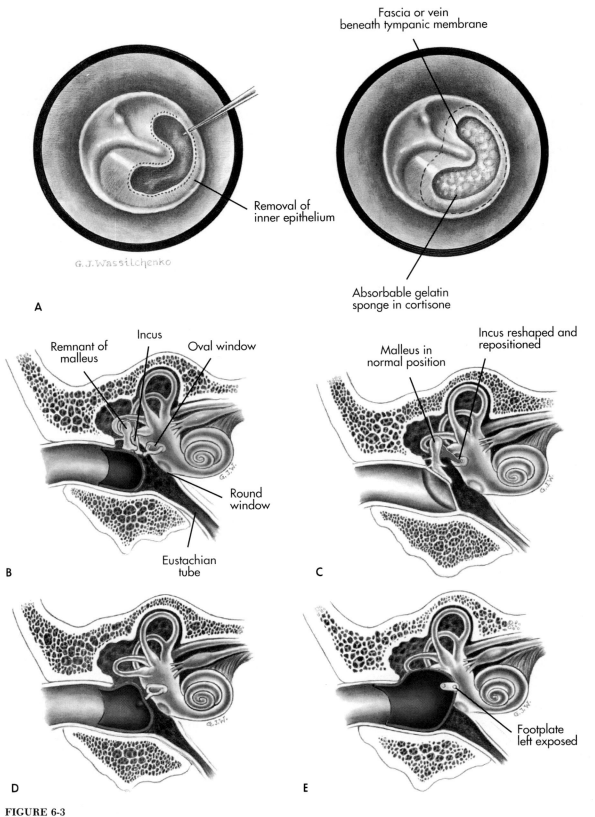

G.J.Wassilchenko

Fascia or vein
beneath tympanic membrane

Removal of
inner epithelium

Absorbable gelatin
sponge in cortisone

A

Remnant of
malleus

Incus

Oval window

Malleus in
normal position

Incus reshaped and
repositioned

Round
window

Eustachian
tube

Footplate
left exposed

B

C

D

E

FIGURE 6-3
Various types of tympanoplasty. **A,** Type I (myringoplasty). **B,**
Type II. **C,** Variation of Type II. **D,** Type III. **E,** Type IV. **F,**
Type V. (From Thompson et al.[71])

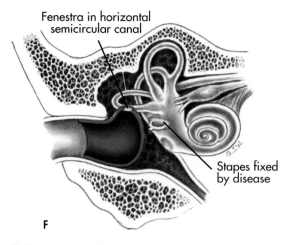

Fenestra in horizontal
semicircular canal

Stapes fixed
by disease

F

FIGURE 6-3, cont'd.

IONTOPHORESIS	

Iontophoresis is a method of numbing the ear canal and the tympanic membrane to lessen the pain of local anesthesia injections.

A solution of 2% lidocaine with epinephrine 1:2000 is placed in the ear canal. An active electrode is then inserted and held in place by a band around the head. An electrical current flows through the electrode, driving the solution through the normally intact skin of the external ear canal and tympanic membrane. The procedure is painless, effective, and takes about 10 minutes.

recurrent infections; (3) to provide adequate aeration of the middle ear; and (4) to improve hearing. Pathologic conditions of the middle ear change the normal transformer mechanism by changing the stiffness of the tympanic membrane, by causing necrosis or fixation of the ossicles, or from a blockage due to polyps or cholesteatoma. Ossicular damage is repaired by means of an ossiculoplasty, which often is performed in conjunction with a tympanoplasty (see page 103).

Ideally, a tympanoplasty is not performed on patients with drainage from the middle ear. Antibiotics are given in the form of ear drops after ear irrigation, and/or orally to eliminate the infection before surgery. Fascia from the temporalis muscle most commonly is used as the graft for the tympanic membrane. However, the grafting techniques for repairing the tympanic membrane and ossiculoplasty vary greatly. Tympanoplasty usually is performed with a local anesthetic.

INDICATIONS

Chronic otitis media
Perforation of tympanic membrane

CONTRAINDICATIONS

Malignant neoplasm
Tuberculosis
Necrotizing external otitis
Several previous tympanoplasty failures
Only hearing ear
Nonfunctioning eustachian tube
Uncooperative patient

COMPLICATIONS

Sensorineural hearing loss	Vertigo
Tinnitus	Facial nerve injuries
Mouth dryness	Infections
Graft failure	Taste disturbance

NURSING CARE

See pages 108 to 111.

DIAGNOSTIC STUDIES AND FINDINGS

Diagnostic test	Findings
Otoscopic and microscopic examination	Perforation of the tympanic membrane with or without cholesteatoma
Audiometry	Normal, conductive, or mixed hearing loss according to size and location of perforation.
Tympanometry	Flat tympanogram

MEDICAL MANAGEMENT

GENERAL MANAGEMENT

Bed rest, maintaining prescribed position if ordered (e.g., operated ear positioned up for several hours). Head or foot of bed elevated for comfort if needed. Modified normal diet the day of surgery.

DRUG THERAPY

PREOPERATIVE

Sudafed: 30-60 mg tid prn for nasal stuffiness.

Versed: 5 mg IM 1 hr before surgery (2.5 mg for patient ≥70 yr).

POSTOPERATIVE

Darvocet-N 100: 1 tablet q 4 h prn for pain.

Toradol: 30-45 mg IM q 4-6 h prn for pain.

Dramamine: 50 mg IM q 4 h prn for nausea and dizziness.

PREPROCEDURAL NURSING GUIDELINES

1. Initiate preoperative instruction for the patient and family
   Explain the surgical procedure and the purpose for shaving above and behind the patient's ear.
   Explain or review the postoperative course.
   Discuss postoperative instructions such as activity restrictions, head movement, and symptoms.
   Encourage the patient to express any anxiety, fears, concerns, and questions.

2. Check the operative permission form if appropriate.
3. Discuss the risks and complications of surgery if appropriate.
4. Withhold food and water for an appropriate length of time before surgery.
5. Advise the patient to wash hair before surgery.
6. Remove all jewelry, glasses, contact lenses, and hearing aid in the operative ear from the patient.
7. Administer preoperative medications.

NURSING CARE

See pages 108 to 111.

OSSICULOPLASTY

Ossiculoplasty is the surgical reconstruction for missing or necrotic ossicles. However, many surgeons use the term *tympanoplasty* (to make or repair an eardrum) to include ossiculoplasty. Reconstruction of the ossicles is not yet an exact science. Various methods and prostheses are used to replace or reposition these tiny ear bones. Prostheses reconnect the ossicles, enabling them to carry sound vibrations to the inner ear.

Prostheses are made of many different materials (e.g., stainless steel, Teflon, polyethylene, hydroxyapatite, and plastipore). However, few synthetic prostheses can guarantee long-term results, because they dislodge or extrude through the tympanic membrane. To try to solve this problem, a tissue such as bone is combined with a prosthesis (producing a semibiologic prosthesis) to reconnect the ossicles and prevent extrusion

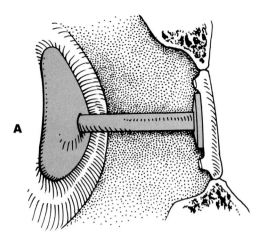

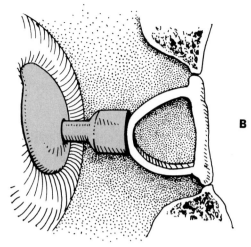

FIGURE 6-4
Middle ear prostheses. **A,** Schuring ossicle columnella prosthesis for total ossicular replacement surgery. **B,** Schuring ossicle cup prosthesis for incus replacement surgery. (From Phipps, Long, Woods, Cassmeyer.[48c])

(Figure 6-4). In rare cases a transplanted ossicle obtained from a bone bank is used. However, the threat of hepatitis and acquired immunodeficiency syndrome (AIDS) has caused a decrease in this practice.

When the ossicular chain is disrupted, neither the area size of the tympanic membrane in relation to the size of the stapes footplate nor the lever ratio of the ossicles contributes to the middle ear transformer mechanism. The tympanic membrane can be perforated or intact with disarticulation of the ossicular chain. If a perforation exists along with disarticulation, a tympanoplasty and an ossiculoplasty (called a tympanossiculoplasty) are performed concurrently.

The purpose of an ossiculoplasty is to restore hearing, and the procedure's success depends on how much damage has been done to the ossicles. The greater the damage, the more reconstruction is necessary, which lowers the success rate. Ossiculoplasty usually is performed with local anesthesia.

INDICATIONS

Partly missing incus (malleus handle and stapes superstructure present)
Defective or missing incus and malleus handle (stapes superstructure present)
Defective or missing incus and stapes superstructure (with or without malleus handle)
Other ossicular problems (e.g., fixed malleus, incus, and stapes)

CONTRAINDICATIONS

Malignant neoplasm
Tuberculosis
Necrotizing external otitis
Several previous ossiculoplasty failures
Only hearing ear
Uncooperative patient

COMPLICATIONS

Infection	Facial paralysis
Cholesteatoma	Taste disturbance
Sensorineural hearing loss	Mouth dryness
Tinnitus	Extrusion
Vertigo	Disarticulation

DIAGNOSTIC STUDIES AND FINDINGS

Diagnostic test	Findings
Otoscopic and microscopic examination	Normal or perforated tympanic membrane with or without cholesteatoma
Audiometry	Conductive or mixed hearing loss according to size and position of perforation and degree of ossicular damage

MEDICAL MANAGEMENT

GENERAL MANAGEMENT

Bed rest with maintenance of prescribed position if ordered (example, operated ear up for first 4 hours) to resist displacement by postural changes.

Head or foot of bed elevated for comfort.

Modified diet the day of surgery.

DRUG THERAPY

Preoperative

Sudafed: 30-60 mg tid prn stuffiness

Versed: 5 mg IM 1 hr pre-op (2.5 mg if over 70 yr)

Postoperative

Darvocet N 100: 1 tablet q 4 h prn pain

Toradol: 30-45 mg IM q 4-6 h prn pain

Dramamine: 50 mg IM q 4 h prn nausea/dizziness

NURSING CARE

See pages 108 to 111.

PREPROCEDURAL NURSING GUIDELINES

1. Initiate preoperative instruction for the patient and family.
   Explain the surgical procedure and the purpose for shaving above and behind the patient's ear.
   Explain or review the postoperative course.
   Discuss postoperative instructions such as activity restrictions, head movement, and symptoms.
   Encourage the patient to express any anxiety, fears, concerns, and questions.
2. Check the operative permission form.
3. Discuss the risks and complications of surgery if appropriate.
4. Withhold food and water for an appropriate length of time before surgery.
5. Wash the patient's hair before surgery.
6. Remove all jewelry, glasses, contact lenses, false teeth, and hearing aid in the operative ear from the patient.
7. Administer preoperative medications.

TRANSCANAL SURGERY CARE PLAN

1 ASSESS

ASSESSMENT	OBSERVATIONS
Vestibular signs/ symptoms	Reports spinning, imbalance, inability to stand or walk unassisted, unsteady or abnormal gait, veering in any direction while walking, altered mobility due to imbalance, history of recent ear surgery, change in ability to estimate spatial relationship of body to environment
Cranial nerve signs/ symptoms	Facial palsies, taste disturbance, mouth dryness, deafness, vertigo

ASSESSMENT	OBSERVATIONS
Auditory signs/ symptoms	Decreased hearing and/or tinnitus in ear that has been operated on, auditory distortion, change in sensory acuity, inattention to communication on affected side
Cardiovascular signs/symptoms	Elevated BP, pulse, and/or respirations
Mental/behavioral factors	Tension, irritability, restlessness, trembling, crying, insomnia
Aural signs/ symptoms	Recent ear surgery with incisions and surgical deficits, elevated temperature, drainage from ear canal or graft site with edema, and/or erythema

2 DIAGNOSE

NURSING DIAGNOSIS	SUBJECTIVE FINDINGS	OBJECTIVE FINDINGS
High risk for infection related to transcanal incisions for ear surgery and incisions at graft site	Reports recent ear surgery with graft sites, complains of fever and ear drainage	Incisions, surgical defects; prophylactic antibiotic therapy; elevated temperature; drainage on pillow; erythema, edema, and drainage from ear or graft site
Acute pain related to physical factor of transcanal ear surgery	Complains of ear pain or discomfort and pain at graft site. Complains of nausea.	Restlessness; increased BP, pulse, and respirations; splinting of pain site; moaning, grimacing, crying; requests pain medication
Altered auditory sensory perception related to ear disorder/ear surgery/ ear packing	Complains of decreased hearing, sensation of fullness or blockage	Inappropriate response to oral communication; inattention to stimulus on affected side; hearing decreased on audiogram; asks that words or phrases be repeated
Impaired skin integrity related to incisions and graft site	Complains of ear or graft site pain, discomfort, tenderness, tingling, and/or burning sensation	Increased risk of infection due to surgical incisions causing a break in the skin
High risk for trauma related to balance difficulties	Complains of vertigo, hearing loss, and feeling faint	Unsteadiness, abnormal gait, poor vision, inability to walk without assistance

3 PLAN

Patient goals

1. The patient will have no signs or symptoms of infection.
2. The patient will have no pain.
3. The patient's hearing will stabilize or increase as a result of ear surgery.
4. The patient's incisions will heal, and normal skin integrity will return without complications.
5. The patient will have no vertigo.

4 IMPLEMENT

NURSING DIAGNOSIS	NURSING INTERVENTIONS	RATIONALE
High risk for infection related to transcanal incisions for ear surgery and incisions of graft site	Assess and document any ear drainage and/or foul odor.	Excessive drainage or odor can indicate an infection.
	Monitor vital signs, especially temperature.	Elevataion of vital signs can indicate infection.
	Administer antibiotics as ordered and document response.	Antibiotics can be prescribed as prophylactic or therapeutic treatment; response determines course of treatment.
	Administer antipyretic as necessary, and document response.	To reduce a temperature and decrease inflammation.
	Instruct patient about water restriction for ear and graft site.	Water in the ear can cause infection.
Acute pain related to physical factor of transcanal ear surgery	Assess and document intensity and frequency of otalgia.	Some incisional pain is expected; a sudden change or severe pain may indicate complications.
	Observe for ear drainage, bleeding, and inflammation or swelling at graft site.	To document possible causes of ear pain.
	Administer analgesics or narcotics as ordered, and document response.	To relieve ear pain.
Altered auditory sensory perception related to ear disorder/ear surgery/ear packing	Assess and document hearing acuity.	Hearing may be decreased due to surgery, ear canal packing, and/or edema.
	Speak distinctly and without shouting. Reassure patient that ear packing can block hearing.	Shouting can distort speech. Patients who have had reconstructive ear surgery can have decreased hearing because of ear packing.
	Assess for hearing aid function.	Hearing aid can be worn in unoperated ear.
Impaired skin integrity related to incisions and graft site	Assess ear canal for pain, discomfort, drainage, and paresthesia.	May indicate developing problem.
	Assess graft site for erythema, edema, and tenderness.	A stitch abscess or infection can occur postoperatively.
High risk for trauma related to balance difficulties	Assess for vertigo by interview, and examine for nystagmus and abnormal gait.	Inadvertent trauma to inner ear during surgery can cause vertigo.
	Provide assistance with ambulation when indicated.	Unsteadiness and abnormal gait predisposes patient to falls.
	Assess for visual and proprioceptor deficits.	Balance depends on vestibular, visual, and proprioceptor sensory input.
	Administer antivertiginous medication as ordered, and document results.	To relieve symptoms of vertigo.

5 EVALUATE

PATIENT OUTCOME	DATA INDICATING THAT OUTCOME IS REACHED
Patient has no signs or symptoms of infection.	Temperature is normal; there is no drainage from ear canal; there is no erythema, edema, or drainage from graft site.
Patient has no pain.	Patient does not complain of pain and does not splint incisional sites; patient shows no grimacing, moaning, or crying.
Patient's hearing has stabilized or increased.	Patient understands goal for hearing and status of that goal as it relates to specific surgical procedure.
Patient demonstrates good skin integrity.	Incisions for surgery and graft site have healed without complications of tissue breakdown or infection.
Patient demonstrates no injury or trauma secondary to vertigo.	Patient does not complain of vertigo and shows no unsteadiness or abnormal gait.

PATIENT TEACHING

1. Instruct the patient to sneeze or cough with the mouth open for 1 week after surgery to prevent dislodgement of grafts and/or prostheses.
2. Instruct the patient to blow the nose gently one side at a time for 1 week after surgery to prevent dislodgement of grafts and/or prostheses.
3. Instruct the patient to perform no physical activity for 1 week, even though she may feel well, and then to resume all normal activities.
4. Tell the patient she may return to work after 1 week. If her work is strenuous or if she lifts more than 20 pounds, she should return to work in 2 to 3 weeks.
5. Inform the patient that she may hear a variety of noises such as cracking or popping; reassure her that this is normal.
6. Tell the patient that the ear packing decreases hearing in the affected ear, and it can seem as if she is talking in a barrel.
7. Reassure the patient that minor ear discomfort is expected, and urge her to take the prescribed pain medication. Stress that excessive ear pain should be reported to the ear surgeon.
8. Occasionally a small amount of bleeding from the ear occurs; reassure the patient that this is normal. Warn her to report excessive ear drainage to the ear surgeon.
9. Remind the patient to change the cotton ball in her ear as ordered.
10. Tell the patient that she must not get water in her ear for several weeks; she may not shampoo her hair for 1 week. She should protect the ear with two pieces of cotton, the outer one saturated with petroleum jelly.
11. Tell the patient that the graft site should be protected for 1 week; usually there are no sutures to be removed.
12. Urge the patient to take antibiotics as prescribed.
13. Remind the patient to wear noise defenders or cotton with petroleum jelly if she works around loud noises.
14. Tell the patient to check with the ear surgeon about instructions for flying.

Postoperative instructions for transcanal surgery vary greatly among ear surgeons. These guidelines are only suggested areas for patient teaching.

Transmastoid Surgeries

MASTOID SURGERY

Infection of the mastoid cells of the temporal bone (called mastoiditis) usually is a complication of chronic otitis media, and the infection can be acute or chronic in onset. The development of antibiotics has reduced the incidence of mastoiditis. Use of the operating microscope and the development of microsurgical techniques have improved mastoid and middle ear surgery. Most cases of mastoiditis today are found in patients who did not receive adequate ear care in childhood and had untreated ear infections. Poverty also plays a role in the treatment of chronic otitis media.

Cholesteatoma is a complication of chronic otitis media in the middle ear as well as the mastoid. Squamous epithelium of the external ear canal and outer layer of the tympanic membrane grows into the middle ear cleft through a perforation. This skin can form a sac that fills with debris such as degenerated skin and sebaceous material. This sac destroys structures in the middle ear and mastoid by pressure necrosis.

Mastoid surgery is performed to eradicate infection and eliminate cholesteatoma and to create access to neural structures in neurotologic procedures. The basic objectives of any mastoid surgery are to remove the causes of disease and restore hearing. There are several different types of mastoid surgery, all of which require general anesthesia and a transmastoid approach through a postauricular incision. All procedures require drilling of the mastoid and removal of the causes of disease.

Simple mastoidectomy. A simple mastoidectomy is performed to enlarge and clean the mastoid cavity.

Radical mastoidectomy. A radical mastoidectomy is performed to clean and completely exteriorize the mastoid cavity, which sacrifices the middle ear for hearing.

Modified radical mastoidectomy. A modified radical mastoidectomy is performed to clean and partly exteriorize the mastoid cavity, which preserves the middle ear and hearing.

Tympanomastoidectomy. A tympanomastoidectomy is performed to clean but preserve the mastoid cavity, which restores the middle ear and hearing. A tympanomastoidectomy combines mastoid surgery with tympanoplasty and ossiculoplasty.

INDICATIONS

Chronic otitis media
Chronic mastoiditis
Cholesteatoma
Transmastoid labyrinthectomy
Cochlear implantation

CONTRAINDICATIONS

Age
Malignant neoplasm
Infectious systemic diseases
Necrotizing external otitis
Only hearing ear
Serious medical problems
Tuberculosis

COMPLICATIONS

Infection
Hearing loss/dead ear
Dislocation of stapes
Facial nerve paralysis
Vertigo
Taste disturbance
Dry mouth
Meningitis
Hemorrhage
Cerebrospinal fluid leak
Abscess of central nervous system
Septicemia
Perforation of tympanic membrane

DIAGNOSTIC STUDIES AND FINDINGS

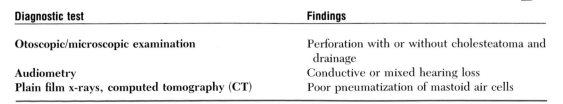

Diagnostic test	Findings
Otoscopic/microscopic examination	Perforation with or without cholesteatoma and drainage
Audiometry	Conductive or mixed hearing loss
Plain film x-rays, computed tomography (CT)	Poor pneumatization of mastoid air cells

MEDICAL MANAGEMENT

GENERAL MANAGEMENT

Bed rest, maintaining prescribed position if ordered (e.g., operated ear positioned up for first several hours). Head of bed elevated for comfort if needed. Out of bed with help. Diet as tolerated. Mastoid dressing removed on postoperative day 1.

DRUG THERAPY

Preoperative medications and sedative per anesthesia.

Amoxicillin: 250 mg 1 tablet qid.

Darvocet-N 100: q 4 h prn for pain.

Sudafed: 30-60 mg tid prn for nasal stuffiness.

Cepacol throat lozenges: prn for sore throat.

Toradol: 30-45 mg IM prn for pain.

Dramamine: 50 mg IM or PO q 4 h prn for nausea or vomiting.

Nembutal: 100 mg HS prn (*Dalmane*, 15 mg for patient >70 yr).

PREPROCEDURAL NURSING GUIDELINES

1. Initiate preoperative instruction for the patient and family.
   Explain the surgical procedure and the purpose for shaving above and behind the ear.
   Explain or review the postoperative course.
   Discuss postoperative instructions such as activity and water restrictions, head movements, and symptoms.

NURSING CARE

See pages 117 to 121.

Encourage the patient to express any anxiety, fears, concerns, or questions.
2. Check the operative permission form.
3. Discuss the risks and complications of surgery.
4. Withhold food and water for an appropriate length of time before surgery.
5. Wash the patient's hair before surgery.
6. Remove all jewelry, glasses, contact lenses, false teeth, and hearing aids from the patient.
7. Administer preoperative medications.

COCHLEAR IMPLANTATION

The purpose of cochlear implants is to provide auditory sensation to patients with severe to profound binaural sensorineural hearing loss who cannot benefit from conventional hearing aids. The hearing loss may be either acquired or congenital. Every candidate must fulfill these requirements: (1) be able to give informed consent; (2) have no useful hearing in either ear; (3) be emotionally stable; (4) be reasonably intelligent; (5) be in good health; (6) be noninstitutionalized; and (7) have an intact auditory nerve and central auditory pathway.

With a cochlear implant, a microphone picks up environmental and speech sounds. The sounds are sent to a sound processing unit, which filters the broad range of acoustic stimuli. The auditory stimuli (mechanical sound waves) are converted into an electrical code, which is transmitted to an external transmitter unit.

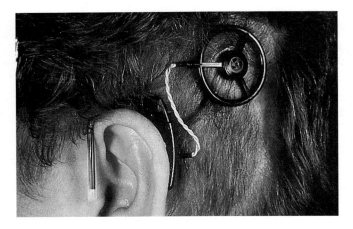

FIGURE 6-5
Cochlear implant in place.

The unit is worn over an internal receiver, which is held in place by a set of magnets in each unit. The magnets attract across the skin. The internal receiver converts the electrical code into electrical stimuli, which are transmitted to the cochlea by an electrode. In multichannel cochlear implants, 22 electrodes are inserted at varying distances along the cochlear partition. Each electrode is individually stimulated to discharge a particular portion of the cochlear nerve fibers.

Preparations for the surgical procedure are the same as those for mastoid surgery. A C-shaped incision is made transmastoid postauricularly. A complete mastoidectomy is performed, with the canal wall left intact. The facial recess is identified and removed to visualize the round window niche. A bed is created for the internal receiver, and a groove for the electrode is constructed from the implant bed to the inner ear. The active electrode is placed directly into the basal turn of the cochlea, either through the round window or through a separate fenestra created in the cochlea. To prevent leakage of perilymphatic fluid, a piece of temporalis fascia can be placed over the opening. The implant is then secured, and the incision is closed. The external equipment is applied after healing, and the extensive cochlear rehabilitation program begins (Figure 6-5). The signals will become more recognizable with time.

INDICATIONS

Totally deaf patients who cannot benefit from a hearing
  aid

CONTRAINDICATIONS

Age (only 5 "research sites" in the United States are authorized to perform cochlear implants on children)
Serious medical problems
Intact auditory nerve

COMPLICATIONS

Perforation of the cochlea	Paralysis of facial
Infection/otorrhea	nerve
Meningitis	Lump behind ear
Cerebrospinal fluid leak	Failure of device,
Vertigo	requiring removal
Perilymphatic fluid leak	Taste disturbances
Hemorrhage	Tinnitus

DIAGNOSTIC STUDIES AND FINDINGS

Diagnostic test	Findings
Otologic examination	Normal tympanic membrane
Auditory and speech evaluation	Total sensorineural hearing loss bilaterally
Promontory stimulation	Auditory response
Psychological evaluation	Shows emotional stability
Computed tomography	Within normal limits

MEDICAL MANAGEMENT

GENERAL MANAGEMENT

Bed rest, maintaining prescribed position if ordered (e.g., operated ear positioned up for first several hours). Head of bed may be elevated. May get out of bed with help. Diet as tolerated. Mastoid dressing removed on postoperative day 1.

MEDICAL MANAGEMENT—cont'd

DRUG THERAPY

Preoperative medications and sedative per anesthesia.

Amoxicillin: 250 mg 1 tablet qid

Darvocet-N 100: q 4 h prn for pain.

Sudafed: 30-60 mg tid prn for nasal stuffiness.

Cepacol throat lozenges: prn for sore throat.

Toradol: 30-45 mg IM prn for pain.

Dramamine: 50 mg IM or PO q 4 h prn for nausea or vomiting.

Nembutal: 100 mg HS prn (*Dalmane*, 15 mg for patient >70 yr).

PREPROCEDURAL NURSING GUIDELINES

1. Initiate preoperative instruction for the patient and family
   Explain the surgical procedure and the purpose for shaving above and behind the ear.
   Explain or review the surgical procedure and postoperative course.
   Discuss postoperative instructions such as activity and water restrictions, head movements, and symptoms.

NURSING CARE

See pages 117 to 121.

Encourage the patient to express any anxiety, fears, concerns, or questions.
2. Check the operative permission form.
3. Discuss the risks and complications of surgery if appropriate.
4. Withhold food and water for an appropriate length of time before surgery.
5. Wash the patient's hair before surgery.
6. Remove all jewelry, glasses, contact lenses, false teeth, and hearing aids from the patient.
7. Administer preoperative medications.

LABYRINTHECTOMY

All labyrinthectomy procedures are destructive and designed to rid the patient of vertigo by completely destroying the vestibular and auditory functions of the labyrinth.

TRANSCANAL LABYRINTHECTOMY

Using local anesthesia, a tympanomeatal flap is raised and the oval and round windows are exposed. The stapes is removed, and a hook is introduced into the vestibule. As much membranous labyrinth as possible is removed, and ototoxic drugs can be instilled into the vestibule. Some surgeons advocate drilling off the promontory to connect the oval and round windows and ensure complete removal of the contents of the vestibule. The tympanomeatal flap is then replaced. Vertigo often recurs because the transcanal approach allows only incomplete removal of the membranous labyrinth.

TRANSLABYRINTHINE LABYRINTHECTOMY

Using general anesthesia, a transmastoid, translabyrinthine approach is made (this approach allows more extensive removal of the membranous labyrinth). A simple mastoidectomy is performed, and each of the three semicircular canals is drilled away. The utricle and saccule are removed with a hook. In this way all neuroepithelium is removed. The postauricular incision is then closed.

INDICATIONS

Ménière's disease
Paroxysmal positional vertigo
Postoperative and traumatic vertigo
Perilymphatic fistula
Vestibular neuronitis
Vestibular labyrinthitis

CONTRAINDICATIONS

Only hearing ear
Serious medical problems
Infection

COMPLICATIONS

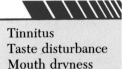

Meningitis
Infection
Cerebrospinal fluid leak
Facial nerve paralysis

Tinnitus
Taste disturbance
Mouth dryness

DIAGNOSTIC STUDIES AND FINDINGS

Diagnostic test	Findings
Otologic examination	Normal tympanic membrane
Audiometry	Varying degrees of sensorineural hearing loss
Tympanometry	Within normal limits
Electronystagmography	Unilateral caloric weakness
Rotary chair	Asymmetry

MEDICAL MANAGEMENT

GENERAL MANAGEMENT

Bed rest, maintaining prescribed position if ordered (e.g., operated ear up for several hours). Blood pressure monitoring (put in Trendelenburg's position if pressure falls). Diet as tolerated. Out of bed as tolerated. Assistance with ambulation if necessary.

DRUG THERAPY

Versed: 5 mg IM 1 hr before surgery (2.5 mg for patient ≥70 yr).

Toradol: 30-45 mg IM q 6 h prn for pain.

Darvocet-N 100: q 4 h prn for pain.

Sudafed: 30-60 mg tid prn for nasal stuffiness.

Vistaril: q 6 h IM for restlessness.

Dramamine: 50 mg IM or PO q 4 h prn for vertigo.

Torecan: 10 mg IM tid prn for nausea.

Amoxicillin: 250 mg qid.

PREPROCEDURAL NURSING GUIDELINES

1. Initiate preoperative instruction for the patient and family.

   Explain the surgical procedure and the purpose for shaving above and behind the patient's ear.

   Explain or review the postoperative course.

   Discuss postoperative instructions such as activity restrictions, head movement, and symptoms.

   Encourage the patient to express any anxiety, fears, concerns, and questions.

2. Check the operative permission form.
3. Discuss the risks and complications of surgery if appropriate.
4. Withhold food and water for an appropriate length of time before surgery.
5. Wash the patient's hair before surgery.
6. Remove all jewelry, glasses, contact lenses, and hearing aid in the operative ear from the patient.
7. Administer preoperative medications.

TRANSMASTOID SURGERY CARE PLAN

1 ASSESS

ASSESSMENT	OBSERVATIONS
Cardiovascular signs/symptoms	Increased BP, pulse, and/or respirations
Cranial nerve signs/symptoms	Partial to total loss of feeling or sensation and/or partial to total facial paralysis on same side of face as ear surgery; taste disturbance; mouth dryness; vertigo; partial to total loss of hearing; tinnitus
Auditory signs/symptoms	Decreased hearing and/or tinnitus in operated ear, auditory distortion, change in sensory acuity
Vestibular signs/symptoms	Complaints of spinning, imbalance, inability to stand or walk without assistance, unsteady or abnormal gait, veering in any direction while walking, change in ability to estimate spatial relationship of body to environment; history of recent ear surgery
Mental/behavioral factors	Increased tension, anxiety, fear, and stress, insomnia; irritable, limited attention span, withdrawn; restless, crying, trembling, describes lack of control
Aural signs/symptoms	Recent ear surgery with incisions and surgical deficits, elevated temperature, drainage from ear canal or graft site with edema and/or erythema

2 DIAGNOSE

NURSING DIAGNOSIS	SUBJECTIVE FINDINGS	OBJECTIVE FINDINGS
Impaired skin integrity related to ear surgery, incisions, and graft sites	Complains of ear or graft site pain, discomfort, and tenderness Complains of paresthesia	Increased risk of infection and lack of skin integrity due to surgical incisions
Acute pain related to physical factor of transmastoid ear surgery	Complains of pain, discomfort, and tenderness of ear canal and/or postauricular incisions; complains of nausea	Restlessness, elevated BP, pulse, respirations; splinting pain site; moaning, crying, grimacing; requests pain medication

→ ＞ ＞

NURSING DIAGNOSIS	SUBJECTIVE FINDINGS	OBJECTIVE FINDINGS
High risk for infection related to transmastoid approach for ear surgery and placement of grafts, prostheses, and/or electrodes, surgical trauma to surrounding tissues and structures	Reports recent ear surgery; complains of fever and ear drainage	Edema, erythema, and/or drainage of post-auricular incision; ear drainage with or without foul odor, elevated vital signs, especially temperature, prophylactic antibiotic therapy, drainage on pillow
Altered auditory sensory perception related to ear disorder/ear surgery/ear packing	Complains of decreased hearing or deafness, sensation of fullness or blockage	Inappropriate response to oral communication; asks that words and phrases be repeated; inattention to stimulus on affected side; hearing decreased on audiogram
High risk for trauma related to balance difficulties	Complains of vertigo, feeling faint, and hearing loss	Unsteadiness, abnormal gait, poor vision, inability to walk without assistance
Altered sensory perception related to damage to facial nerve (cranial nerve VII) and chorda tympani	Complains of facial numbness, loss of feeling or sensation in and weakness of face; taste disturbance Expresses fear and anxiety related to altered sensory perception	Irritability; reports change in sensory acuity; partial to total facial paralysis on same side of face as ear surgery Mouth dryness
Anxiety related to surgical procedure, loss of hearing and balance, taste disturbance, and/or loss of facial movement	Complains of tension, stress, fear, and lack of control over situation	Increased BP, pulse, respirations; misunderstands instruction; limited attention span, withdrawn demeanor; restlessness; crying

3 PLAN

Patient goals

1. The patient's incisions will heal and normal skin integrity will return without complications.
2. The patient will have no pain.
3. The patient will show no signs or symptoms of infection.
4. The patient's hearing will stabilize or increase as a result of ear surgery.
5. The patient will have no vertigo.
6. The patient will not have or will adjust to altered sensory perception.
7. The patient's anxiety will be reduced.

4 IMPLEMENT

NURSING DIAGNOSIS	NURSING INTERVENTIONS	RATIONALE
Impaired skin integrity related to ear surgery, incisions, and graft sites	Assess ear canal for pain, discomfort, drainage, and paresthesia.	May indicate a developing problem.
	Assess postauricular incision for suture line separation, suture abscess, erythema, edema, drainage, and tenderness.	A broken suture or suture abscess can occur postoperatively.
Acute pain related to physical factor of transmastoid ear surgery	Assess location, intensity, and frequency of otalgia.	Some incisional pain is expected after surgery; a sudden change or severe pain may indicate complications.
	Observe for signs of infection or other complications.	To document possible causes of ear pain.
	Administer analgesics or narcotics as ordered, and document response.	To relieve ear pain.
High risk for infection related to transmastoid approach for ear surgery and placement of grafts, prostheses, and/or electrodes, surgical trauma to surrounding tissues and structures	Assess and document any ear drainage with or without a foul odor.	Excessive drainage and/or odor may indicate an infection.
	Assess and document any erythema, edema, tenderness, or drainage at postauricular incision.	May indicate an infection.
	Monitor and document vital signs, especially temperature.	Elevated vital signs may indicate infection.
	Administer antibiotics as ordered.	Antibiotics are prescribed prophylactically or therapeutically.
	Administer antipyretics as ordered.	Antipyretics reduce a temperature and decrease inflammation.
	Evaluate and document the response to antibiotics and antipyretics.	Response to medication helps determine course of treatment.
	Instruct patient about water restriction for ear and incision site.	Water can cause an infection.
Altered auditory sensory perception related to ear disorder/ear surgery/ear packing	Assess hearing acuity and for presence of tinnitus.	Hearing may be decreased due to surgery or blockage of ear canal by packing and edema.
	Speak distinctly and without shouting. Assess hearing aid function.	Shouting can distort speech. Hearing aid can be worn in unaffected ear.
	Reassure patient that ear packing can block hearing.	With reconstructive ear surgery, hearing is temporarily reduced due to ear packing.
High risk for trauma related to balance difficulties	Assess for vertigo by interview, and examine for nystagmus and abnormal gait.	Inadvertent or anticipated trauma to inner ear causes vertigo after surgery.

→ › ›

NURSING DIAGNOSIS	NURSING INTERVENTIONS	RATIONALE
	Assess for visual and proprioceptive deficits.	Balance depends on vestibular, visual, and proprioceptive sensory input.
	Provide assistance with ambulation when indicated.	Abnormal gait or unsteadiness predisposes patient to falls.
	Administer antivertiginous medication as ordered, and evaluate results.	To relieve symptoms of vertigo.
Altered sensory perception related to damage to facial nerve (cranial nerve VII) and chorda tympani	Assess patient for facial paralysis.	Temporary or permanent facial paralysis is caused by trauma to or resection of cranial nerve VII.
	Assess for taste disturbance and mouth dryness.	Temporary or permanent taste disturbance and mouth dryness are caused by trauma to or resection of the chorda tympani nerve.
	Instruct patient to place food in and chew on unaffected side of mouth; teach patient to manually remove food from affected side, and provide mouth care.	Inability to feel food or debris on affected side of mouth; to remove accumulated food and cleanse the oral cavity.
Anxiety related to surgical procedure, loss of hearing and balance, taste disturbance, and/or loss of facial movement	Assess level of anxiety (ability to concentrate, attention span, ability to comprehend, ability to communicate).	To guide therapeutic interventions and determine readiness for participation in self-care.
	Provide information about expected outcomes of decreased hearing, balance, taste, and facial movement.	Increased knowledge and elimination of incorrect information can decrease anxiety.
	Encourage patient to discuss anxieties and explore concerns about altered sensory perceptions.	To help patient gain awareness and understanding of relationship between anxiety and the behavior.
	Help patient identify coping skills used in the past.	Past coping skills can help relieve anxiety.
	Teach stress management techniques.	Reducing stress often lessens anxiety.
	Refer patient for psychologic consultation for anxiety and depression if necessary.	Anxiety and depression can pose a health problem.

5 EVALUATE

PATIENT OUTCOME	DATA INDICATING THAT OUTCOME IS REACHED
Patient demonstrates good skin integrity.	Incisions for ear surgery have healed without complications of tissue breakdown or infection.

PATIENT OUTCOME	DATA INDICATING THAT OUTCOME IS REACHED
Patient has no pain.	Patient does not complain of pain and does not splint incisions; patient shows no facial grimacing, moaning, or crying.
Patient has no signs or symptoms of infection.	Vital signs are normal; there is no drainage from the ear canal and no erythema, edema, or drainage at the postauricular incision.
Patient's hearing has stabilized or increased.	Patient understands goal for hearing and status of that goal as it relates to specific surgical procedure.
Patient demonstrates no injury or trauma secondary to vertigo.	Patient does not complain of vertigo and shows no unsteadiness or abnormal gait; patient has not fallen.
Patient does not have or has adjusted to altered sensory perception.	Patient is knowledgeable about reason for facial paralysis and numbness, and/or taste disturbance and mouth dryness, and performs necessary self-care tasks.
Patient anxiety about altered sensory perceptions has lessened.	Patient verbalizes and exhibits less stress, tension, and irritability.

PATIENT TEACHING

1. Instruct the patient to sneeze or cough with the mouth open for 1 week after surgery to prevent dislodgement of grafts and/or prostheses.
2. Instruct the patient to blow the nose gently one side at a time for one week after surgery to prevent dislodgement of grafts and/or prostheses.
3. Instruct the patient to perform no physical activity for 1 week even though she may feel well, and then to resume all normal activities.
4. Tell the patient she can return to work after 1 week. If her work is strenuous or if she lifts more than 20 pounds, she can return to work in 2 to 3 weeks.
5. Inform the patient that she may hear a variety of noises such as cracking or popping; reassure her that this is normal.
6. Tell the patient that the ear packing decreases the hearing in the operated ear and it can seem as if she is talking in a barrel.
7. Reassure the patient that minor ear discomfort is expected, and urge her to take the prescribed pain medication. Stress that excessive ear pain should be reported to the ear surgeon.
8. Occasionally, a small amount of bleeding from the ear occurs; reassure the patient that this is normal.

Warn her to report excessive ear drainage to the ear surgeon.

9. Remind the patient to change the cotton ball in her ear as ordered.
10. Tell the patient that she must not get water in her ear for several weeks; she may not shampoo her hair for 1 week. She should protect the ear with two pieces of cotton, the outer one saturated with Vaseline.
11. Tell the patient that the graft site should be protected for 1 week; usually there are no sutures to be removed.
12. Tell the patient to take antibiotics as prescribed.
13. Urge the patient to wear noise defenders or cotton with vaseline if she works around loud noises.
14. Advise the patient to check with her ear surgeon regarding instructions for flying.
15. Inform the patient that temporary facial weakness, taste disturbances, and numbness of the pinna (external ear) can occur, but usually return to normal function.

Postoperative instructions for a transmastoid approach for ear surgeries vary greatly among ear surgeons. These patient teaching guidelines are only suggested areas for education.

Transcranial Surgeries

Acoustic Neuroma Surgery

An acoustic neuroma (neurinoma, neurilemoma, schwannoma) is a benign, encapsulated tumor of the acoustic nerve (cranial nerve VIII), which is divided into the vestibular nerve and the cochlear nerve. Neuromas usually arise from the Schwann cells of the vestibular nerve; only occasionally do they originate in the cochlear nerve. Most acoustic tumors arise from the internal auditory canal, enlarging the meatus and extending into the cerebellopontine angle. A tumor that lies entirely within the internal auditory canal is called a small *intracanalicular* tumor. Acoustic neuromas account for 5% to 10% of all intracranial tumors.

Small tumors measure between 2 and 5 cm; large tumors measure 5 cm or more. After the tumor grows out of the internal auditory canal, it exerts pressure on surrounding structures such as nerves, arteries, and veins, causing many symptoms. Protrusion of this slow-growing, pear-shaped tumor causes cochlear and vestibular symptoms, as well as pressure on the trigeminal and facial nerves (cranial nerves V and VII). Later, the pressure compromises the glossopharyngeal, vagus, accessory, and hypoglossal nerves (cranial nerves IX through XII). Eventually, if the tumor is not removed, hydrocephalus, blindness, and death can occur.

Von Recklinghausen's disease (neurofibromatosis) can also cause acoustic neuromas. These tumors usually are bilateral and expand within the acoustic nerve rather than against it.

Although these tumors can affect both men and women at any age, most occur in middle age, between 40 and 50. The most common symptoms are unilateral tinnitus and hearing loss, or nystagmus with or without dizziness. Some acoustic tumors manifest themselves as sudden sensorineural hearing losses, and others show the classic symptoms of Ménière's disease. The most important feature of acoustic tumors is that they affect only one ear (unilaterality).

Surgical removal of acoustic tumors is the treatment of choice, because these tumors do not respond well to radiation or chemotherapy. The major objective of surgery is to remove the tumor while preserving the facial nerve (when functioning) and the acoustic nerve, and to save the patient's life. Four microsurgical techniques are most often used to remove an acoustic tumor: the middle fossa approach; the translabyrinthine approach; the one-stage, combined translabyrinthine-suboccipital approach; and the suboccipital approach. Most neurosurgeons use the suboccipital approach routinely, whereas most neurotologists select the approach according to the size and location of the tumor and the patient's level of hearing.

Middle fossa approach. The middle fossa approach is used when hearing in the involved ear is normal or near normal, and the tumor is intracanalicular or just protruding from the canal. The patient lies supine with the involved ear up. Using general anesthesia, an incision is made 0.5 to 1 cm anterior to the tragus and carried superiorly for approximately 6 cm.

Translabyrinthine approach. The translabyrinthine approach is used for medium-sized lesions (1.5 to 4 cm) and when the ear has no serviceable hearing. A postauricular incision is made 4 cm behind the postauricular crease, and a simple mastoidectomy is performed.

One-stage, combined translabyrinthine-suboccipital approach. The one-stage, combined translabyrinthine-suboccipital approach is used for large tumors (over 4 cm). A larger postauricular flap is created than with the translabyrinthine approach so as to expose the occipital bone. A complete translabyrinthine dissection is performed, and the occipital bone that overlies the cerebellum is removed. Both approaches are used to remove the tumor.

Suboccipital approach. The suboccipital approach is routinely used by neurosurgeons for tumors of any size. The hearing can be preserved with this approach. A large suboccipital flap is created, and the occipital bone overlying the cerebellum is removed. The major disadvantage of this approach is the lack of a landmark for the facial nerve.

For large acoustic tumors (over 5 cm), special precautions for surgery and anesthesia are needed to prevent neurologic complications. Large tumors can compress the brainstem or cause obstructive hydrocephalus, or both. Failure to recognize these complications can lead to brain herniation. Obviously, large tumors have a higher incidence of morbidity and mortality than do smaller ones.

INDICATIONS

Acoustic neuroma
Neurofibromatosis

CONTRAINDICATIONS

Age
Serious medical problems
Only hearing ear

COMPLICATIONS

Mouth dryness	Facial nerve paralysis
Taste disturbance	Eyelid paralysis
Tinnitus	Hemiparesis
Vertigo	Infection
Hearing loss/dead ear	Transfusion reaction
Extradural and intracranial hemorrhage	Respiratory and circulatory
Cerebral edema	complications
Cerebrospinal fluid leak	Coma
Meningitis	Death

DIAGNOSTIC STUDIES AND FINDINGS

Diagnostic test	Findings
Complete head and neck examination with evaluation of 5th to 12th cranial nerves	Decreased function of the 8th cranial nerve, sometimes the 7th cranial nerve
Cerebellar function examination	Normal to varying degrees of ataxia
Audiometry	Normal to total sensorineural loss
Tympanogram/stapedial test reflex/reflex decay test	Tympanogram is normal; stapedial test reflex is normal or absent; reflex decay test may show that decay is present
Auditory brainstem response	Response is abnormal
Electronystagmography	Unilateral caloric weakness
Imaging: CT with and without enhancement MRI	Mass in internal auditory canal that can extend to cerebellopontine angle

MEDICAL MANAGEMENT

GENERAL MANAGEMENT

Immediate postoperative period

Intensive care monitoring for 24 hours or longer. Hemodynamic and cardiac monitoring to evaluate fluid status and cardiac rhythm.

Intake and output (I&O) charted while patient has intravenous lines.

Frequent monitoring of electrolytes and complete blood counts (CBCs). (A slight state of dehydration is maintained to reduce cerebral edema. The head and abdominal dressings are monitored for excessive drainage from the wounds and reinforced as needed.)

Physical activity, including mostly bed rest and dangle legs over edge of bed or sit in chair on postoperative day 1 if tolerated.

Head of bed maintained at 30-degree angle.

Eye care for irritation or dryness (eye taped when indicated).

Later postoperative care

Diet advanced as tolerated to limit of 2 g of sodium.

Continued.

MEDICAL MANAGEMENT—cont'd

GENERAL MANAGEMENT

Physical activity, such as ambulation, encouraged with assistance.

Head of bed elevated to a maximum of 45 degrees (knees should not be flexed).

Eye care continued as necessary.

DRUG THERAPY

Postoperative

Pain
Demerol: 25 mg IV q 4 h prn immediate postoperative period. *Darvocet-N 100:* 1-2 tablets PO q 4 h prn. *Tylenol:* 650 mg PO q 4 h prn (for pain or fever).

Nausea/vomiting/dizziness

Dramamine: 50 mg IM or PO q 3 h prn. *Milk of Magnesia:* 30 ml PO prn.

Sedation

Dalmane: 15 mg at bedtime prn.

Eye care.

Tearisol: qhs q 1 h prn. *Lacrilube* when indicated.

PREPROCEDURAL NURSING GUIDELINES

1. Initiate preoperative instruction for the patient and family:
   Explain the surgical procedure and the purpose for shaving the patient's head (this is usually done in the operating room).
   Explain or review the postoperative course.
   Discuss suggestions for covering the head after surgery.
   Teach the patient deep breathing exercises.
   Discuss the critical care environment.
   Encourage the patient and family to express their fears and concerns.
   Explain the reason for showering and shampooing with pHisohex soap the night before surgery.
   Fit the patient for thigh-high TED hose.
2. Check the operative permission form.
3. Discuss the risks and complications of surgery if appropriate.
4. Document the patient's baseline neurologic status and all other medical or physical problems.
5. Withhold food and water the night before surgery.
6. Remove all jewelry, glasses, contact lenses, and false teeth from the patient.
7. Insert an IV line.
8. Administer preoperative medications.
9. Apply the TED hose to the patient.

NURSING CARE

See pages 127 to 134.

VESTIBULAR NERVE SECTION

For information on vestibular rehabilitation, see page 137.

Although chronic vertigo, the product of a vestibular disorder, is one of the most common patient complaints, management of vestibular disorders presents a formidable clinical challenge. The ideal surgery would relieve the vertigo safely while preserving hearing. However, any surgery performed on the vestibular system carries a high risk of damage to the auditory system. Any surgery directed toward destroying the vestibular system also carries a high risk of residual or recurring vertigo.

Vestibular nerve surgery is performed for chronic vertigo only after extensive medical trials and treatments have failed and the patient's quality of life has diminished to a level of constant anxiety, uncertainty, and handicapping behavior. The purpose of the surgery is to destroy the vestibular nerve in the affected ear and to preserve hearing when indicated.

Middle fossa vestibular nerve section. The goals of middle fossa vestibular nerve section are to denervate the vestibular nerve and to preserve hearing. The patient lies supine with the involved ear up. Using general anesthesia, the incision is made 0.5 to 1 cm anterior to the tragus and carried superiorly for approximately 6 cm. The vestibular division of the eighth cranial nerve is sectioned, preserving the cochlear division.

Translabyrinthine vestibular nerve section. Using general anesthesia and through a postauricular incision, a transmastoid, translabyrinthine approach is made and the vestibular division of the eighth cranial nerve is sectioned. This surgery is performed when the patient has no serviceable hearing.

Retrosigmoid vestibular nerve section. The retrosigmoid (or suboccipital) approach gives a much more generous exposure of the posterior fossa, allowing more room for manipulation of the surrounding structures.

Using general anesthesia, the vestibular nerve is transsected. Hearing can be preserved.

Retrolabyrinthine vestibular nerve section. Using general anesthesia, a large, U-shaped, postauricular incision is made, and a complete mastoidectomy is performed. The vestibular nerve is sectioned, temporalis fascia is used to reinforce the dural incisions, and abdominal fat is used to obliterate the mastoid cavity. The major disadvantage of a retrolabyrinthine approach is its limited exposure of the posterior fossa.

INDICATIONS

Ménière's disease, uncontrolled vertigo
Other peripheral vestibular disorders, uncontrolled vertigo
Other failed vestibular surgery

CONTRAINDICATIONS

Bilateral Ménière's disease
Serious medical problems
Only hearing ear

COMPLICATIONS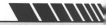

Infection	Facial nerve paralysis
Taste disturbance	Eyelid paralysis
Mouth dryness	Hemiparesis
Vertigo	Transfusion reaction
Respiratory/circulatory complications	Tinnitus
	Coma
Hearing loss/dead ear	Death
Extradural/intradural hemorrhage	Meningitis
Cerebrospinal fluid leak	

DIAGNOSTIC STUDIES AND FINDINGS

Diagnostic test	Findings
Complete head and neck examination with evaluation of 5th to 12th cranial nerves	Decreased function of the 8th cranial nerve
Cerebellar function examination	Within normal limits
Audiometry	Normal to total sensorineural loss
Tympanogram/stapedial reflex test/reflex decay test	Normal tympanogram; normal or absent stapedial test reflex; no decay in the reflex decay test
Auditory brainstem response	Within normal limits
Electronystagmogram	Unilateral caloric weakness
Rotary chair	Assymetry
Imaging CT (with and without enhancement) MRI	Within normal limits

MEDICAL MANAGEMENT

GENERAL MANAGEMENT

Immediate postoperative period

Intensive care monitoring for 24 hours or longer. Hemodynamic and cardiac monitoring to evaluate fluid status and cardiac rhythm.

Intake and output (I&O) charted while patient has intravenous lines.

Frequent monitoring of electrolytes and complete blood counts (CBCs). (A slight state of dehydration is maintained to reduce cerebral edema. The head and abdominal dressings are monitored for excessive drainage from the wounds and reinforced as needed.)

Physical activity, including mostly bed rest and dangle legs over edge of bed or sit in chair on postoperative day 1 if tolerated.

Head of bed maintained at 30-degree angle.

Eye care for irritation or dryness (eye taped when indicated).

Later postoperative care

Diet advanced as tolerated to limit 2 g sodium.

Physical activity, such as ambulation, encouraged with assistance.

Head of bed elevated to a maximum of 45 degrees (knees should not be flexed).

Eye care continued as necessary.

DRUG THERAPY

Postoperative

Pain

Demerol: 25 mg IV q 4 h prn immediate postoperative period. *Darvocet-N 100:* 1 to 2 tablets PO q 4 h prn. *Tylenol:* 650 mg PO q 4 h prn (for pain or fever).

Nausea/vomiting/dizziness

Dramamine: 50 mg IM or PO q 3 h prn. *Milk of Magnesia:* 30 ml PO prn.

Sedation

Dalmane: 15 mg at bedtime prn.

Eye care

Tearisol: qhs 2 drops q 1 h.
Lacrilube when indicated.

PREPROCEDURAL NURSING GUIDELINES

1. Initiate preoperative instruction for the patient and family.
   Explain the surgical procedure and the purpose for shaving the patient's head (this is usually done in the operating room).
   Explain or review the postoperative course.
   Discuss suggestions for covering the head after surgery.
   Teach the patient deep breathing exercises.

PREPROCEDURAL NURSING GUIDELINES (cont'd)

Discuss the critical care environment.

Encourage the patient and family to express their fears and concerns.

Explain the reason for showering and shampooing with pHisohex soap the night before surgery.

Fit the patient for thigh-high TED hose.

2. Check the operative permission form.
3. Discuss the risks and complications of surgery if appropriate.
4. Document the patient's baseline neurologic status and all other medical or physical problems.
5. Withhold food and water the night before surgery.
6. Remove all jewelry, glasses, contact lenses, and false teeth from the patient.
7. Insert an IV line.
8. Administer preoperative medications.
9. Apply the TED hose to the patient.

TRANSCRANIAL SURGERY CARE PLAN

1 ASSESS

ASSESSMENT	OBSERVATIONS
Increased intracranial pressure	Changes in level of consciousness; changes in respiratory patterns; changes in vital signs, including widening pulse pressure, Cushing's response with increased systolic BP, decreased pulse; fluctuations in temperature; impaired pupillary reflex; papilledema; vomiting; seizures; complaints of headaches; hyperactive deep tendon reflexes; cerebellar ataxia
Mentation	Memory loss, personality changes, depression, judgment deficits, mental disorientation
Cranial nerve damage	Pupillary changes, impaired pupillary reflex, visual disturbance, impaired corneal reflex, partial to total loss of hearing or balance, facial paralysis, taste disturbance, mouth dryness, difficulty swallowing, impaired gag reflex
Respiratory signs/ symptoms	Change in respiratory pattern, increased mucous secretions, crackles, rhonchi on auscultation, increased respirations, respiratory depression, abnormal arterial blood gases (ABGs)
Cardiovascular signs/symptoms	Hypertension, hypotension, change in pulse or respiratory rate, cardiac dysrhythmias
Meningeal irritation	Irritability, elevated temperature, nuchal rigidity, increased sensitivity to light, positive Brudzinski's sign, positive Kernig's sign
Fluid-electrolyte status	Excessive bleeding, cerebrospinal fluid drainage, change in gastrointestinal activity, vomiting, diarrhea, altered intake, signs of dehydration (e.g., poor tissue turgor), marked polyuria, change in specific gravity of urine, abnormal serum osmolarity, abnormal serum sodium
Mental/behavioral factors	Increased tension, anxiety, fear, and stress; insomnia; irritable, limited attention span, withdrawn; restless, crying, trembling, describes lack of control

2   DIAGNOSE

NURSING DIAGNOSIS	SUBJECTIVE FINDINGS	OBJECTIVE FINDINGS
High risk for impaired gas exchange related to altered level of consciousness, altered respiratory patterns, effects of anesthetic, increased secretions	Complains of shortness of breath, of anxiety	Increased restlessness, irritability, confusion, changes in respiratory patterns, diminished breath sounds, crackles, rhonchi, arterial blood gases pH <7.35 or >7.45, cyanosis, nasal flaring
Altered cerebral tissue perfusion related to hemorrhage, CSF leak, or hydrocephalus	Complains of increasingly severe headache, palpitations, anxiety	Change in level of consciousness, changes in respiratory patterns and vital signs, pupillary changes, papilledema, restlessness, lethargy, seizures
High risk for infection related to transcranial approach for surgery and trauma to surrounding tissues and structures	Complains of fluid from ear, nose, or dressing over incision; also weakness, chills, and irritability	Elevated temperature; irritability; nuchal rigidity; elevated WBC; tachycardia; leakage of CSF from nose, ear, and/or dressing over incision
Impaired swallowing related to trauma of glossopharyngeal, vagus, and hypoglossal nerves (cranial nerves IX, X, and XII)	Complains of difficulty swallowing, fear of choking	Difficulty swallowing; coughing, choking; collection of food in buccal cavity; evidence of absent gag reflex; facial paralysis
Altered sensory perception related to trauma of trigeminal and facial nerves (cranial nerves V and VII)	Complains of facial numbness and weakness, taste disturbance, difficulty swallowing, difficulty closing eye	Partial to total facial paralysis; inability to close eye or chew on affected side; difficulty swallowing
High risk for fluid volume deficit related to increased fluid output, altered intake, fluid restriction, and diuretics	Complains of fatigue, thirst, dizziness, dry mouth, apprehensiveness	Poor skin turgor, dry mucous membranes, change in urine output, tachycardia, hypotension, hemorrhage, vomiting, CSF drainage, change in mental status, elevated temperature
Acute pain related to physical factors of headache, backache, and/or incisional pain	Complains of headache, eye pain, incisional pain, nausea	Requests pain medication; restless, irritable; elevated BP and heart rate; splinting of pain site; facial grimacing, moaning, crying
High risk for trauma related to trauma to or destruction of vestibular portion of acoustic nerve (cranial nerve VIII)	Complains of vertigo, feeling faint, hearing loss	Unsteadiness, abnormal gait, difficulty focusing, inability to walk without assistance, nystagmus, positive Romberg's sign

NURSING DIAGNOSIS	SUBJECTIVE FINDINGS	OBJECTIVE FINDINGS
Altered auditory sensory perception related to trauma to or destruction of auditory portion of acoustic nerve (cranial nerve VIII)	Complains of decreased hearing or deafness, tinnitus, sensation of fullness or blockage	Inappropriate response to oral communication; inattention to stimulus on affected side; repeatedly asks for clarification of words or phrases
Body image disturbance related to hair loss, surgical incisions, neurologic deficits	Expresses anxiety and negative feelings about hair loss and hearing, balance, and facial problems; refuses to accept changes and appears preoccupied with losses	Change in appearance of face; expresses concern over appearance and about people's reaction to appearance; reluctant to look in mirror; appears depressed, socially isolated
Anxiety related to surgical procedure, loss of hair, decreased hearing, balance, facial function, and/or swallowing on the same side of face as surgery	Expresses tension, stress, fear, and lack of control over situation	Increased BP, pulse, respirations; misunderstands instructions; limited attention span; withdrawn, restless, crying

3 PLAN

Patient goals

1. The patient will have improved ventilation and oxygenation.
2. The patient's cerebral perfusion will be improved.
3. The patient will have no signs or symptoms of infection.
4. The patient will maintain adequate nutrition and hydration.
5. The patient will return to normal facial function or will accept his facial paralysis.
6. The patient will maintain an adequate fluid and electrolyte balance.
7. The patient will have no pain.
8. The patient will not have vertigo.
9. The patient will return to his preoperative hearing level or will accept his hearing loss.
10. The patient will accept the change in his body image.
11. The patient's anxiety about altered sensory perceptions will be reduced.

4 IMPLEMENT

NURSING DIAGNOSIS	NURSING INTERVENTIONS	RATIONALE
High risk for impaired gas exchange related to altered level of consciousness, altered respiratory patterns, effects of anesthetic, and increased secretions	Assess neurologic status q 15 min for first 4 hr, q 1 h for 24 hr, then q 2 h.	To establish a baseline for determining level of consciousness and change in level of consciousness.
	Assess vital signs q 15 min for first 4 hr, q 1 h for 24 hr, then q 2 h.	To detect signs and symptoms of impaired ventilation.
	Auscultate breath sounds.	To determine efficiency of respiratory effort and assess abnormal breath sounds.
	Maintain oxygen at prescribed level.	Supplemental oxygen can be given in immediate postoperative period.

NURSING DIAGNOSIS	NURSING INTERVENTIONS	RATIONALE
	Assess amount, color, consistency, and odor of secretions.	To assess upper airway patency and determine need for suctioning.
	Assess peripheral pulses and capillary refill.	To determine extent of oxygenation to periphery.
	Suction patient as necessary per protocol.	To remove secretions and ensure adequate oxygenation.
Altered cerebral tissue perfusion related to hemorrhage, CSF leak, or hydrocephalus	Assess neurologic status q 15 min for first 4 hr, q 1 h for 24 hr, then q 2 h.	To establish baseline for determining and quantifying changes.
	Assess for signs of increasing cerebral pressure, change in level of consciousness, change in pupillary size, widening pulse pressure, bradycardia, change in respiratory rate.	Cerebral pressure can increase after transcranial surgery due to hemorrhage, CSF leak, or hydrocephalus; brain herniation can occur if increased pressure is not treated promptly.
	Assess vital signs q 15 min for first 4 hr, q 1 h for 24 hr, then q 2 h.	Changes can indicate increased intracranial pressure or potential herniation.
	Maintain head position at appropriate angle; maintain head and neck.	Head of bed should be elevated 30 to 45 degrees to facilitate venous drainage.
	Instruct patient to avoid bending his knees, coughing, and straining at stool when possible.	These activities increase intrathoracic and intraabdominal pressure, which can increase intracranial pressure.
	Assess temperature q 2 h for 24 hr, then q 4 h.	Hyperthermia can change the rate of cerebral metabolism, which can increase intracranial pressure.
	Promote adequate ventilation, and maintain oxygenation.	A decrease in arterial oxygen pressure and an increase in arterial carbon dioxide pressure increases cerebral blood flow and intracranial pressure.
	Assess for seizure activity.	A neurosurgical procedure can precipitate a seizure, resulting in increased intracranial pressure.
	Administer corticosteroids and osmotic diuretics as ordered.	Corticosteroids may reduce cerebral edema; osmotic diuretic draws water from the brain cells to reduce cerebral edema.
High risk for infection related to transcranial approach for surgery and trauma to surrounding tissues and structures	Assess vital signs, including temperature, q 2 h; assess CBC.	Elevated vital signs and WBC can indicate an infection.
	Assess for chills, irritability, complaints of weakness, and change in level of consciousness.	Can be physiologic indicators of an infection.
	Assess head and abdominal dressings; reinforce when necessary.	Excessive drainage can indicate presence of infection.

NURSING DIAGNOSIS	NURSING INTERVENTIONS	RATIONALE
	Observe for CSF drainage from head dressing or nose.	Clear fluid drainage from dressing, wound, ear, or nose is assumed to be CSF; check for sugar with Dextrostix, reinforce dressing, put patient in bed, and notify surgeon.
	Assess for signs and symptoms of meningitis: elevated temperature (38.3° C [101° F]), nausea and vomiting, nuchal rigidity, positive Brudzinski's and Kernig's signs, increased headache, irritability, and photophobia.	Inflammation of the meninges can occur as a result of blood in the subarachnoid space or contamination during surgery.
	Administer antibiotics as ordered, and evaluate response.	Antibiotics can be given as prophylactic or therapeutic treatment after surgery.
	Administer antipyretics as ordered, and evaluate response.	Antipyretics reduce fever.
Impaired swallowing related to trauma of glossopharyngeal, vagus, and hypoglossal nerves (cranial nerves IX, X, and XII)	Assess facial movement, tongue mobility, and ability to swallow.	To determine residual function.
	Assess gag and cough reflex.	To determine patient's ability to protect airway and restore swallowing.
	Consult with dietitian and swallowing therapist when oral feeding begins.	Team members can assist with type of food consistency, placement of food in mouth, and techniques for swallowing.
	Provide a quiet, supervised, nondistracting environment at meals.	To allow patient to focus on eating.
	Tell patient to "think swallow."	Sometimes a conscious thought helps trigger the swallow reflex.
	Place food on unaffected side.	Patient has better movement and sensation for texture and temperature on unaffected side.
	Inspect oral cavity, and provide mouth care after eating.	To remove any accumulated food and cleanse oral cavity.
	Keep patient upright at a 30- to 45-degree angle for 1 hour after eating.	Food could reflux from stomach, causing patient to aspirate.
Altered sensory perception related to trauma of trigeminal and facial nerves (cranial nerves V and VII)	Assess eyes for muscle paralysis, dryness, excessive tearing, ulcerations, and ability to close eyes completely.	To establish extent of function.
	Provide eye care with artificial tears qhs, or tape eye closed and apply lubricant when indicated.	To prevent dryness and irritation of cornea, with subsequent injury.

→ > >

NURSING DIAGNOSIS	NURSING INTERVENTIONS	RATIONALE
	Assess for facial paralysis.	To establish extent of function; temporary or permanent facial paralysis is caused by trauma to or resection of cranial nerve VII.
	Assess for taste disturbance and mouth dryness.	Temporary or permanent disturbances are caused by trauma to or resection of the chorda tympani nerve.
	Instruct patient to place food in and chew on unaffected side of mouth.	Movement and sensation for texture and temperature are better on unaffected side.
	Teach patient to remove food manually from affected side.	Patient will not be able to feel retained food or debris on affected side.
	Inspect oral cavity, and provide mouth care.	To remove any accumulated food and cleanse oral cavity.
High risk for fluid volume deficit related to increased fluid output, altered intake, fluid restriction, and diuretics	Assess intake and output, specific gravity, and color of urine q 2 h.	Accurate records provide basis for treatment and fluid replacement.
	Assess for indicators of dehydration (orthostasis, polydipsia, dry mucous membranes, poor skin turgor, fatigue, dizziness, apprehension).	These are physiologic indicators of fluid volume depletion; prompt recognition of dehydration allows early intervention.
	Administer IV or oral fluid replacement as prescribed; encourage ice chips and fluid as tolerated.	Fluid replacement is done judiciously.
	Administer antiemetics and/or antidiarrheal drugs as ordered whenever necessary.	To reduce nausea, vomiting, and diarrhea, and to improve oral intake.
Acute pain related to physical factors of headache, backache, and/or incisional pain	Assess location, frequency, and intensity of headache or incisional pain.	Some headache and incisional pain are expected; a sudden change or severe pain may indicate elevating intracranial pressure—report this to the surgeon immediately.
	Assess location, frequency, and intensity of back pain; apply wet heat to back.	Back pain is a common complaint after surgery due to prolonged position on operating table; wet heat helps ease severe back pain.
	Administer analgesics or narcotics as ordered, and document response.	To relieve pain.
High risk for trauma related to trauma to or destruction of vestibular portion of acoustic nerve (cranial nerve VIII)	Assess for vertigo, nystagmus, and abnormal gait.	Inadvertent or anticipated trauma to inner ear can cause vertigo postoperatively.
	Assess for visual and proprioceptive deficits.	Balance depends on vestibular, visual, and proprioceptive sensory input.
	Provide assistance with ambulation.	Vertigo, unsteadiness, and abnormal gait predispose patient to falls.

NURSING DIAGNOSIS	NURSING INTERVENTIONS	RATIONALE
	Administer antivertiginous medication as ordered, and evaluate results.	To relieve symptoms of vertigo.
Altered auditory sensory perception related to trauma to or destruction of auditory portion of acoustic nerve (cranial nerve VIII)	Assess for hearing acuity and tinnitus.	Hearing may be decreased due to surgery or blockage of ear canal with packing, edema, and dressing.
	Speak distinctly and without shouting.	Shouting can distort speech.
	Assess for hearing aid and hearing aid function.	Hearing aid can be worn in unaffected ear.
Body image disturbance related to hair loss, surgical incisions, neurologic deficits	Assess patient's awareness and knowledge of reason for change in body image.	To provide baseline for teaching and to identify any misconceptions.
	Encourage patient to discuss implications and concerns of loss or changes.	To help patient identify personal meaning of loss or changes.
	Assess patient's behavioral response (anger, indifference, denial).	These reflect patient's coping style.
	Provide information on a "ready-to-learn" basis regarding hearing loss, balance problem, facial paralysis, and swallowing difficulties.	Increased knowledge and elimination of misconceptions can decrease anxiety.
	Help patient identify successful coping skills used in the past.	Past coping strategies can be used to reduce anxiety.
	Explore potential responses of other people.	To help prepare patient for possible reactions after discharge.
	Refer patient to social worker, psychologist, and/or psychiatrist for severe stress, anxiety, or depression.	To help patient cope with body image alterations.
Anxiety related to surgical procedure, pain, change in body image, and uncertainty about future	Assess level of anxiety (ability to concentrate, attention span, ability to comprehend, ability to communicate).	Provides a baseline for therapeutic interventions and readiness for participation in self-care.
	Provide information about expected outcomes and prognosis.	Increased knowledge can decrease anxiety.
	Encourage patient to discuss anxieties and explore concerns about altered sensory perceptions.	Helps patient gain awareness and understanding of anxieties; catharsis also decreases anxiety.
	Help patient identify coping skills used in the past.	Past coping skills can be used for current problems, which reduces anxiety.
	Refer patient for psychological evaluation of anxiety and depression if needed.	Anxiety and depression can pose health problems.

5 EVALUATE

PATIENT OUTCOME	DATA INDICATING THAT OUTCOME IS REACHED
Patient has adequate ventilation and oxygenation.	Airway is patent; breath sounds are normal; arterial blood gases are within normal limits.
Patient's cerebral perfusion is normal or has improved.	Patient's level of consciousness is stable; there is no evidence of neurologic deficits or seizure activity.
Patient has no signs or symptoms of infection.	Patient is afebrile; WBC is within normal limits; cultures are negative; there is no CSF leakage.
Patient maintains adequate nutrition and hydration.	Patient can swallow; his weight is stable; he shows no evidence of aspiration on swallowing.
Patient has accepted temporary or permanent facial paralysis.	Patient is knowledgeable about prognosis and treatment options for facial paralysis.
Patient has an adequate fluid-electrolyte balance.	Patient is alert and oriented; vital signs are within normal limits; skin turgor and mucous membranes are normal; vomiting and/or diarrhea has stopped; laboratory values are within normal limits; patient has resumed adequate oral intake.
Patient has no pain.	Patient does not complain of pain; he does not splint incisions; he shows no facial grimacing, moaning, or crying.
Patient has no injury or trauma secondary to vertigo.	Patient does not complain of vertigo; he shows no unsteadiness or abnormal gait and does not fall.
Patient's hearing has stabilized or increased.	Patient understands goal for hearing and status of that goal as it relates to specific surgical procedure.
Patient has a positive body image.	Patient expresses acceptance of temporary or permanent change in body image.
Patient's anxiety about altered sensory perceptions has been reduced.	Patient shows decrease in stress, tension, and irritability.

PATIENT TEACHING

1. Reinforce the surgeon's explanation of medical management.
2. Explain the importance of reporting the following signs and symptoms: onset of new motor weakness or sensory loss, increasing headache, stiff neck, elevated temperature, changes in vision, increased sensitivity to light, seizures, drainage from suture line, ear, or nose.
3. Teach skin and suture care: Dressing is removed on the fourth or fifth day after surgery; a cap or hat is recommended after the dressing is removed; after suture removal, the hair can be shampooed, but

scrubbing around the suture line is discouraged.

4. Tell the patient not to blow his nose until his doctor has indicated that the ear is healed. Any accumulated secretions in the nose may be drawn back into the throat and spit out if desired. This is particularly important if the patient develops a cold.

5. Advise the patient not to "pop" his ears by holding his nose and blowing air through the eustachian tube into the ear. If the nose becomes stuffy, the patient should blow his nose very gently one side at a time. If it is necessary to sneeze or cough, the patient should do so with his mouth open.

6. Instruct the patient not to allow water to enter his ear until his doctor has said that the ear is healed. Until that time, cotton may be placed in the ear canal and covered with petroleum jelly before showering or washing the hair. If an incision was made in the skin behind the ear, water should be kept away from this area for 1 week.

7. Warn the patient not to take any unnecessary chance of catching cold, and advise him to avoid undue exposure or fatigue. If he catches a cold, he should treat it as he usually does and report to the doctor if he develops ear symptoms.

8. Reassure the patient that it is normal to notice a certain amount of pulsation, popping, clicking, and other sounds in the ear, and also to have a feeling of fullness. At times it may feel as if there is liquid in the ear.

9. Advise the patient not to plan to drive a car home from the hospital. Air travel is permissible 2 days after surgery and is preferred to automobile or train travel for trips longer than 200 miles. When changing altitude the patient should stay awake and chew gum to stimulate swallowing.

10. Tell the patient to try not to get any water on the incision behind the ear or on the abdomen for 1 week after surgery. There should be no discharge or drainage from the incision after the patient leaves the hospital. The tapes over the incisions may be removed gently when they begin to come off after 7 days. The patient may then clean the incision with peroxide and apply neosporin ointment if necessary. If the patient has any difficulties with the incisions, he should call the doctor.

11. Teach the patient about eye care and eye sling (see Patient Teaching Guide, page 265).

12. Teach the patient the names of medications, dosage, time of administration, and side effects.

13. Emphasize the need for follow-up visits to the doctor.

Incision and Drainage of the External Ear

The external ear is made up of a variety of tissues—skin, cartilage, glands, and the tympanic membrane. All these tissues are subject to disorders that require incision and drainage.

The purpose of incision and drainage (I&D) is to release a pocket of infection or fluid that is causing pain and that may cause the problem to spread. The I&D technique is standard: An incision is made in the affected area deep enough to release the compressed fluid. Because of the anatomy of the external ear, drains are not commonly used. For incision and drainage of the external ear canal or tympanic membrane, an operating microscope normally is used. The primary complication with incision and drainage of the external ear is that the procedure needs to be repeated several times. There are no contraindications or diagnostic studies for this procedure.

Incision and drainage are most often done to treat a small abscess (furuncle) in the ear canal. This bacterial infection may be caused by external otitis or chronic otitis media, or it may be caused by an infected gland. Incision and drainage of the abscess and treatment with antibiotics usually cure a furuncle promptly. Abscesses are rare in other parts of the external ear.

A modified I&D procedure is used to treat bullous myringitis, which is characterized by a painful cystic bleb (bulla) on the tympanic membrane. The bleb is caused either by a virus or by *Mycoplasma* bacteria. Microscope-aided incision and drainage plus antibiotic coverage help the patient to cope during resolution of this self-limiting disorder.

Perichondritis can develop into a very stubborn infection, requiring intravenous antibiotics for control. During the course of perichondritis, abscesses can form and are treated by multiple I&D procedures. Even without abscess formation, I&D procedures are used to drain the infected cartilage.

Trauma of the external ear, especially the pinna,

can cause a hematoma. This disorder is associated primarily with boxing. By performing I&D, the hematoma is drained and infection leading to a perichondritis is averted. Also, I&D lessens the formation of a "cauliflower ear" that results from excessive scar tissue formation (see Figure 4-2).

Rare disorders that necessitate an I&D include blocked sebaceous or cerumen glands; congenital malformation with cystic formation; and infection following chronic ear surgery.

INDICATIONS

Abscesses (furuncles)
Bullous myringitis
Perichondritis
Trauma
Blocked sebaceous glands
Blocked cerumen glands
Postoperative infection

CONTRAINDICATIONS: None

COMPLICATIONS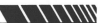

Repeated irrigation and drainages

Ear Irrigation

The ear commonly is irrigated to cleanse the external auditory canal or to remove impacted wax, debris, or foreign bodies. However, because moisture causes vegetable matter to swell, the ear should **never** be irrigated to remove foreign vegetable matter such as beans or corn. Irrigation also is not done if the patient has a history of a perforated eardrum. The irrigating solution (usually water) is warmed to body temperature and placed in the irrigating syringe. The patient's clothes are protected with a plastic drape, and a kidney-shaped basin is placed below the ear to catch the irrigating solution. The patient sits with the ear to be irrigated toward the nurse, with the head tilted toward the opposite ear. The patient should hold the basin beneath the ear and against her face to catch the return solution. In adults the external ear is pulled upward and backward, and the tip of the syringe is directed along the upper wall of the ear canal (Figure 6-6). The syringe should not completely obstruct the canal, to allow for backflow of the solution. In documenting the ear irrigation, the nature of the returned solution (amount, texture, color of cerumen, and type of debris) should be included. Instruct the patient to tell you if she experiences pain, dizziness, or nausea during the procedure.

INDICATIONS

Impacted wax in external ear canal
Foreign body in external ear canal
Debris in external ear canal

CONTRAINDICATIONS

Perforation of tympanic membrane
Vegetable foreign matter in external ear
Infection

COMPLICATIONS

Infection
Trauma
Perforation of tympanic membrane

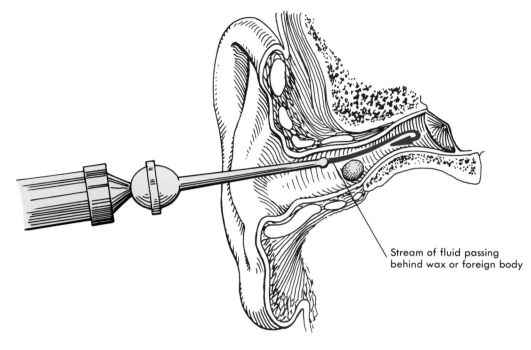

FIGURE 6-6
Ear irrigation. Note that fluid is directed toward upper canal wall so that stream will pass behind wax or object. (From Phipps, Long, Woods, Cassmeyer.[48c])

Vestibular Rehabilitation

Vestibular rehabilitation has emerged as another type of treatment in the management of vestibular disorders. The sophistication of objective vestibular and balance tests has greatly increased the use of vestibular rehabilitation. Research has shown that inactivity retards the rate and degree of compensation achieved after a vestibular disorder. In normal patients prolonged bed rest causes decreased performance on subsequent balance tests, perhaps because vestibular decompensation is associated with inactivity. Thus the therapeutic strategy for vestibular rehabilitation is to actively use the vestibular system.

Vestibular rehabilitation requires a multidisciplinary team approach. In addition to medical and nursing care, stress management, biofeedback, and/or vocational rehabilitation can serve as adjunctive therapy. However, a physical therapist with the appropriate background should be consulted for vestibular rehabilitation.

Several principles should govern the program:

1. Vestibular exercises should exceed the patient's level of capability and should be increased progressively as improvement occurs.
2. An environment should be created that mimics the body movements and environmental conditions that produce the symptoms.
3. The patient should perform self-generated head and eye exercises daily.
4. Sensory reorganization strategies should be used that prevent the patient from becoming dependent on only one of the sensory elements of balance (e.g., standing with feet together, eyes closed; walking on foam with head in air).
5. General aerobic exercise should be encouraged and should exceed the level of exercise the patient now performs.

The initial interview conducted by the physical therapist should include the following:

History

- Description of symptoms
- Onset
- Frequency
- Precipitating factors
- Life-style changes

Assessment of biomechanical factors

- Muscle tone
- Flexibility
- Strength
- Sensation
- Coordination
- Static postural alignment

Assessment of motor coordination

- Ankle, knee, and hip movement
- Ability to step, walk, and jump
- Balance strategies in which one or more sensory element is eliminated
- Evaluation for use of an ambulatory aid (cane, walker)

Vestibular rehabilitation is aimed at helping the patient to (1) achieve functional compensation and (2) adopt strategies for balance control. Exercise programs are developed individually according to each patient's medical condition, diagnosis, strengths, deficits, age, life-style, and needs. Patients are evaluated through demonstration techniques and educational materials and taught the appropriate therapy. The patient is then given a home therapy program for 6 to 8 weeks with monitoring at frequent intervals.

INDICATIONS

Benign paroxysmal positional vertigo
Viral neuronitis
Viral labyrinthitis
Presbyvertigo
Ménière's disease
After surgery for vertigo

CONTRAINDICATIONS

Uncontrolled Ménière's disease
Severe cerebellar-vestibular dysfunction
Acute posttraumatic vertigo

COMPLICATIONS

None

CHAPTER 7

Disorders of the Nose and Sinuses

As air enters the nasal passages, it is prepared for alveolar exchange. For example, the nose can adjust the humidity level of inspired air to as high as 85%; this high humidity enhances gaseous exchange at the alveolar level and prevents drying of the lower airway. Humidity is returned to the nose during exhalation to prevent dryness and thickening of nasal secretions. In areas of low humidity the nose cannot humidify the extremely dry air, and dryness of the nasal mucosa, thick tenacious secretions, and postnasal drip result. Besides providing humidification, the nose also filters particulate matter and warms inspired air through the rich capillary and venous supply of the turbinates, which are composed of highly vascular, erectile tissue. The functions of humidification, warming, and filtration of foreign bodies can be altered by any mechanism that affects the normal upper airway and nasal resistance.

Factors that can affect nasal airway resistance include hypoxia and hypercapnia, nasal obstruction, increased nasal drainage or rhinitis, extrinsic stimuli (e.g., smoke or noxious fumes), and asymmetric pressure to one side of the body, as can be seen in an ipsilateral increase in nasal resistance upon arising in the morning. Most people have a nasal cycle. Edema on one side of the nose increases airway resistance while a concomitant contraction on the other side of the nose decreases airway resistance; thus total airway resistance is maintained at a constant under normal circumstances. The normal airway cycles every 3 to 4 hours.

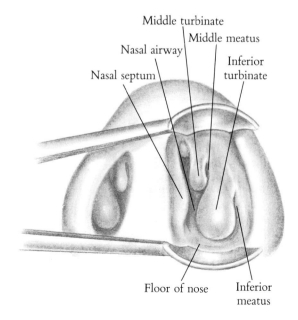

FIGURE 7-1
Nasal polyps. (From Seidel.[58])

Nasal Polyps

Nasal polyps (nasal polyposis) are swellings of the mucous membranes of the sinus mucosa into the cavities of the nose and paranasal sinuses (Figure 7-1).

The incidence of nasal polyps in the general population is unknown, but it is a common condition. Nasal polyps affect men 2:1 over women, and the disorder is found in all age groups. Nasal polyps frequently are associated with allergies, cystic fibrosis, asthma, disorders of ciliary motility, chronic rhinitis, and chronic sinusitis.

PATHOPHYSIOLOGY

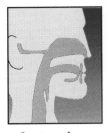

Although the exact cause of nasal polyposis is unknown, many theories have been investigated. An inflammatory response, causing hypertrophic mucosa and edema and thinning of the mucous membrane, may be related to nasal polyps. Patients with chronic viral or bacterial infections have a higher incidence of nasal polyps.

Nasal polyps may be unilateral or bilateral, and several usually occur. The polyps appear as clusters of smooth, gray masses attached by a narrow stalk. Nasal polyps usually arise from the ethmoid air cells and emanate from the middle meatus, where the sinus ostium opens. They are made up of pseudostratified columnar epithelium similar to that of the respiratory mucosa.

Approximately 8% of patients with nasal polyps also have symptoms of asthma and intolerance to aspirin, indomethacin, and the nonsteroidal antiinflammatory medications. The exact cause of this triad of nasal polyps, asthma, and aspirin sensitivity is unknown, but the patient may have an acute exacerbation of asthma in response to infection, anesthesia, surgery, or the administration of aspirin.

DIAGNOSTIC STUDIES AND FINDINGS

Diagnostic test	Findings
Sinus x-rays	Diffuse mucosal disease; may have air-fluid level if sinus is obstructed
Computed tomography (CT) (to evaluate bone and sinuses, especially if endoscopic sinus surgery is possible)	Mucosal swelling, nasal polyps, diffuse mucosal disease, air-fluid level with obstructed sinus
Immunologic assessment (required if allergy is considered causative factor)	Sensitivity to specific allergen

MEDICAL MANAGEMENT

SURGERY

Nasal polypectomy: Removal of polyps.

Functional endoscopic sinus surgery: Removal of polyps with a nasal endoscope.

Caldwell-Luc operation: An incision is made in the gingival buccal sulcus to allow entry into the maxillary sinus so that the polyps can be removed.

DRUG THERAPY

Antihistamines (Seldane, Benadryl): To treat allergic symptoms.

Corticosteroids

Systemic: Used with caution because of side effects; used only with severely obstructed airway.

Local injection into polyp: Temporarily decreases size of polyp.

Local steroid sprays (Beconase, Vancenase, Nasacort): Used for long-term reduction in size of polyps and to prevent recurrence, reduce inflammatory response.

Antibiotics (amoxicillin, erythromycin): Used if infection is present.

1 ASSESS

ASSESSMENT	OBSERVATIONS
Nasal obstruction	Difficulty breathing through nose; mouth breathing; describes foreign body sensation in nose; decreased or absent sense of smell; grayish growths of tissue visible on nasal examination
Rhinorrhea	Watery mucous discharge (yellow or green discoloration indicates infection); sneezing; excessive tearing

2 DIAGNOSE

NURSING DIAGNOSIS	SUBJECTIVE FINDINGS	OBJECTIVE FINDINGS
Ineffective breathing pattern related to nasal obstruction	Complains of difficulty breathing through nose, snoring during sleep, and difficulty blowing nose	Breathes through mouth and has increased nasal discharge; polypoid tissue visible on nasal examination
Altered sensory perception (olfactory, gustatory) related to nasal obstruction	Reports decreased or no sense of smell and/or altered or no sense of taste	Cannot identify common odors (coffee, clove, peppermint); does not maintain weight; caloric intake has decreased
High risk for infection related to nasal obstruction/ obstructed sinus ostia	Complains of yellow-green nasal drainage and "sinus" headache or pain over sinuses	Mucopurulent drainage on nasal examination; elevated temperature; swelling of eyes and area over maxillary sinus

3 PLAN

Patient goals

1. The patient will be able to breathe through his nose with minimal difficulty.
2. The patient will be able to distinguish common odors.
3. The patient will maintain his body weight.
4. The patient will use alternative safety measures to compensate for loss of sense of smell.
5. The patient will have no signs of infection.

4 IMPLEMENT

NURSING DIAGNOSIS	NURSING INTERVENTIONS	RATIONALE
Ineffective breathing pattern related to nasal obstruction	Increase humidification (humidifier, nasal saline spray, increasing fluid intake).	Increasing humidity thins secretions; moistening the air breathed provides comfort to mouth breather.
	Elevate head of bed.	To help reduce nasal edema.

→ > >

NURSING DIAGNOSIS	NURSING INTERVENTIONS	RATIONALE
	Instruct patient to avoid upper respiratory infections.	Upper respiratory infection increases nasal edema, aggravating nasal obstruction; if patient has "triad" condition, upper respiratory infections will exacerbate asthma.
	Administer steroid nasal spray as ordered; nozzle of spray should be aimed toward cheek (sinuses) rather than toward septum. (Steroid nasal sprays must be used for several days before any change in symptomatology is noticed.)	Nasal steroids act directly on nasal mucosa to reduce swelling. Nasal steroid sprays are best used to treat small nasal polyps or to prevent recurrence. For effective absorption, the medication must be absorbed through direct contact with the nasal mucosa (absorption is minimized in patients who do not have a patent nasal airway).
Altered sensory perception (olfactory) related to nasal obstruction	Instruct patient to make appropriate adaptations in living environment (e.g., install smoke detectors; check appearance of stored food for spoiling; routinely check gas lines for leakage; install gas detectors).	People often rely on the sense of smell to detect danger (fire, spoiled food, gas leaks); an individual with an altered sense of smell must rely on other techniques.
Altered sensory perception (gustatory) related to altered sense of smell	Initiate dietary consult; suggest foods with increased visual stimulation; experiment with various spices and additives to food.	With an altered sense of smell, the sense of taste may be affected. Other stimuli should be used to increase appetite, and experimenting with various spices may reveal tastes the patient can detect.
High risk for infection related to nasal obstruction/ obstructed sinus ostia	Instruct patient to avoid upper respiratory infections (e.g., avoid crowds and people known to have an upper respiratory infection).	Upper respiratory infections can increase nasal edema, causing additional blockage of sinus ostia and sinusitis.
	Instruct patient in proper administration of antibiotics, especially side effects, dosage, and administration.	Antibiotics may be used to treat infection; patient must take entire course of drugs to eliminate infection.
	Instruct patient in proper use of antihistamines and decongestants.	Antihistamines can help reduce edema caused by allergy. Decongestants may reduce swelling caused by an upper respiratory infection. Warn the patient about the drowsiness associated with most antihistamines, and tell him to avoid operating machinery, driving, and drinking alcoholic beverages. Decongestants may dry out membranes, requiring increased humidification. Over-the-counter decongestant nasal sprays should be avoided, because a rebound effect results from prolonged use, causing rhinitis medicamentosa.

5   EVALUATE

PATIENT OUTCOME	DATA INDICATING THAT OUTCOME IS REACHED
Patient demonstrates an effective breathing pattern.	Patient can breathe through his nose and can rid his nose of excess mucus by blowing.
Patient has a normal sense of smell.	Patient can distinguish common odors.
Patient maintains his weight.	Patient shows minimal or no weight loss; laboratory blood values are within normal limits.
Patient takes alternate safety measures to compensate for loss of sense of smell.	Patient describes alternate safety measures used (e.g., smoke alarms, gas detectors).
Patient shows no signs of infection.	Patient's temperature is normal; he has no purulent nasal drainage or pain; WBC with differential is within normal limits.

PATIENT TEACHING

1. Teach the patient how to decrease nasal edema to improve nasal breathing (e.g., elevate head of bed).
2. Encourage the patient to increase humidification by using a humidifier and nasal saline sprays and by increasing his fluid intake.
3. Emphasize the importance of avoiding upper respiratory infections (e.g., crowds, other people with upper respiratory infections) and of notifying the physician at the first signs of infection so that appropriate therapy can be instituted.
4. Instruct the patient in the side effects (e.g., drowsiness), proper dosage, and administration of all medications he is to take.
5. Encourage the patient to seek prompt medical attention if signs of polyp recurrence develop.

Rhinitis

Rhinitis is an inflammation of the nasal mucous membranes.

PATHOPHYSIOLOGY

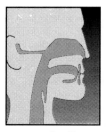

Rhinitis can be classified as allergic, acute, vasomotor, or medicamentosa. **Allergic rhinitis** may be seasonal or perennial. Seasonal allergic rhinitis usually occurs as an acute response to a specific antigen. The patient has symptoms until the specific antigen is no longer present. Seasonal allergies usually are caused by pollen from grass, trees, or flowers. Perennial allergic rhinitis is a more chronic condition usually caused by antigens constantly present in the environment (e.g., dust, animal dander, mold, and foods). Patients with allergic rhinitis also may have a triad of symptoms consisting of asthma, nasal polyps, and aspirin sensitivity.

Acute rhinitis is also known as coryza, or the common cold. Acute rhinitis is most frequently caused by a rhinovirus, adenovirus, or influenza virus, or secondarily by bacterial organisms. Acute viral rhinitis is contagious by droplet infection, most commonly for the first 2 or 3 days of infection.

Vasomotor rhinitis is also known as chronic idiopathic or nonallergic rhinitis. Vasomotor rhinitis is believed to be an abnormality of parasympathetic nervous activity, the cause of which is unknown. Other causes of rhinitis may be tumors, granulomatous disease, septal deviation, nasal polyps, foreign bodies, tuberculosis, or sarcoidosis.

Rhinitis medicamentosa is a form of rhinitis caused by abuse or overuse of topical agents such as Afrin and NeoSynephrine nasal sprays, or intranasal cocaine. Although initially these preparations cause vasoconstriction and decongestion, they have a rebound effect when used habitually. In rhinitis medicamentosa, overuse of the nasal spray causes severe mucosal edema

once the immediate effect of the decongestant has occurred. Patients use nasal sprays frequently during the day to prevent the edema, and a vicious cycle ensues.

For the nose to function properly, the agents causing the rhinitis should be avoided and the symptoms of the rhinitis should be alleviated.

COMPLICATIONS

Serous otitis media
Nasal polyps
Sinus infection
Exacerbation of asthma

DIAGNOSTIC STUDIES AND FINDINGS

Diagnostic test	Findings
Allergy testing	Causative allergen is identified by positive test
Culture of nasal drainage	Organism present
Nasal smear	Eosinophils identified
Rhinoscopy	Edema, drainage
Sinus x-rays/computed tomography (CT) scans	Sinusitis

MEDICAL MANAGEMENT

DRUG THERAPY

Antihistamines: To treat allergic symptoms

Decongestants (oral and topical): To decrease nasal edema

Anticholinergics: Control rhinorrhea

Cromolyn sodium (systemic and topical): Inhibit mast cell degranulation (patients with allergic symptoms)

Corticosteroids (systemic and topical): To decrease nasal edema; reduce mucosal inflammation

Allergic desensitization: To treat allergy

SURGERY

Removal of turbinate: Removal of nasal turbinate

Nasal septoplasty: Straightening of nasal septum

Polypectomy: Removal of polyps

1 ASSESS

ASSESSMENT	OBSERVATIONS

Nasal obstruction
Rhinorrhea/
  postnasal drip
Sneezing; watery,
  itchy eyes and
  nose
Headache, general
  malaise, muscular
  aches, chills
Altered sense of
  smell
	Allergic rhinitis: pale, bluish, edematous nasal mucosa; "allergic salute"—palm of hand rubs nose upward, patient may have nasal crease from repeated action; "allergic shiner"—dark circles under eyes; tearing, periorbital and eyelid edema; difficulty breathing through nose; thin, watery nasal discharge; altered sense of smell
	Vasomotor rhinitis: altered sense of smell; boggy, swollen mucous membrane; thin, watery nasal discharge; difficulty breathing through nose
	Infectious, viral, or bacterial rhinitis (acute rhinitis/coryza/upper respiratory tract infection): mucopurulent, thick nasal secretions; difficulty breathing through nose; red, swollen, boggy nasal mucosa; altered sense of smell
	NARES syndrome (Nonallergic rhinitis with eosinophilia): same symptoms as allergic rhinitis with negative results on allergy testing

2 DIAGNOSE

NURSING DIAGNOSIS	SUBJECTIVE FINDINGS	OBJECTIVE FINDINGS
Ineffective airway clearance related to nasal obstruction	Complains of difficulty breathing through nose and nasal drainage	Breathes through mouth; increased nasal discharge; edematous nasal membranes; pale, swollen turbinates; clear, watery nasal discharge (allergic); red, swollen turbinates; mucopurulent nasal discharge (acute)
Altered sensory perception (olfactory) related to edema of nasal mucosa	Complains of decreased or altered sense of smell	Cannot identify common odors

3 PLAN

Patient goals

1. The patient will be able to breathe through her nose with little difficulty.
2. The patient will be able to distinguish common smells.
3. The patient will use alternative safety measures to compensate for lack of sense of smell.

4 IMPLEMENT

NURSING DIAGNOSIS	NURSING INTERVENTIONS	RATIONALE
Ineffective airway clearance related to nasal obstruction	Elevate head of bed.	May decrease nasal edema and facilitate mucous drainage.
	Increase humidification (humidifier, nasal saline spray, increased fluid intake).	Humidifying air makes nasal secretions less viscous, allowing them to be removed by blowing; forcing fluids is important if fever is present.

→ > >

NURSING DIAGNOSIS	NURSING INTERVENTIONS	RATIONALE
	Instruct patient how to use decongestants, antihistamines, and nasal sprays properly.	Medications to treat rhinitis may cause drowsiness, insomnia, and rebound effects if not properly used and monitored.
	Instruct patient in environmental control measures to decrease exposure to allergens.	Controlling allergens in the environment may decrease symptoms.
	Identify drugs that may have caused rhinitis.	Certain medications (antihypertensives, nasal spray abuse, oral contraceptives) may affect the vascular channels of the nose, causing vasodilation and engorgement of the mucous membrane.
	Identify other medical conditions that may play a role in nasal stuffiness.	Pregnancy, menstruation, and birth control pills increase the estrogen level, causing vascular engorgement of mucous membranes (uterus, nose). Hypothyroidism results in a hypoactive sympathetic nervous system with a predominance of parasympathetic activity, causing vasodilation and nasal obstruction.
Altered sensory perception (olfactory) related to edema of nasal mucosa	Instruct patient to make appropriate changes in living environment (e.g., use smoke detectors); to observe appearance of stored food for spoilage; and to routinely check gas lines for leaks.	Sense of smell helps detect some dangerous occurrences (e.g., fires, spoiled food, gas leaks).

5 EVALUATE

PATIENT OUTCOME	DATA INDICATING THAT OUTCOME IS REACHED
Patient demonstrates effective breathing pattern.	Patient can breathe through the nose; she maintains adequate oxygenation, as demonstrated by pink nail beds and mucous membranes.
Patient demonstrates normal sense of smell.	Patient can distinguish common odors.
Patient uses alternate safety measures to compensate for decrease in sense of smell.	Patient describes alternate safety measures used (e.g., smoke alarms, gas detectors).

PATIENT TEACHING

1. Teach the patient how to take medications properly (e.g., route, dosage, frequency, action, and side effects). Instruct her to avoid activities that require alertness, such as driving or operating machinery, while taking medications known to cause drowsiness.
2. Help the patient identify the cause of her rhinitis, and help her develop strategies for avoiding those causes (e.g., *pollens*—avoid outdoor activities such as lawn work; keep doors and windows closed during high pollen seasons; install electrostatic air filters to filter pollen; plan vacation during peak pollen season; *molds*—control dampness in homes to minimize mold growth; avoid heavy vegetation around house, which increases humidity in the house; *dust*—control household dust; avoid carpeting; avoid down or feather comforters and pillows; vacuum mattress frequently; *animal dander*—avoid furred or feathered animals).
3. Help the patient identify medications that may have caused the rhinitis (e.g., antihypertensive drugs, birth control pills, decongestant nasal sprays).
4. Advise the patient to avoid crowds and people known to have an upper respiratory tract infection.

Deviated Nasal Septum/Nasal Fractures

Deviated nasal septum is a deflection of the normally straight nasal septum, a condition that may result in obstruction to nasal breathing. Septal deviation usually is caused by trauma, such as injury during birth, a nasal fracture, or some other direct injury to the nose.

PATHOPHYSIOLOGY

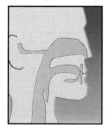

The nasal septum is composed of cartilage and bone joined by a fibrous attachment. It separates the nose into two cavities, provides support, and acts as a shock absorber for the floor of the frontal fossa. Causes of nasal septal deviation include congenital disproportion, in which the cartilaginous septum is too large for the area, or trauma to the nasal septum. Repeated trauma may result in a fibrous growth of tissue that fills in the fractures; this produces an overgrowth, causing bowing of the septum and obstruction. Abnormalities in the bones of the face also may cause displacement of the septum.

CLINICAL MANIFESTATIONS

The main clinical symptom of a deviated nasal septum or nasal fracture is obstruction to nasal breathing. Because nasal breathing is a subjective process, only the patient can gauge the degree of obstruction and the amount of difficulty it causes. Another consideration in

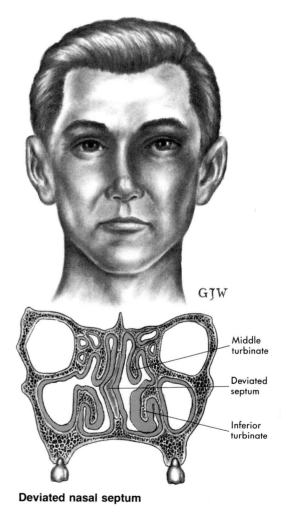

GJW

Middle turbinate

Deviated septum

Inferior turbinate

Deviated nasal septum

nasal obstruction is the nasal valving mechanism. The nasal valve is a space located anterior to the upper lateral cartilage and the nasal septum. This valve changes the shape of air currents entering the nose, thus controlling the amount of resistance and the velocity of the air currents. A deviated septum may block or enlarge the nasal valve, resulting in a loss of inspiratory control of air. The nose also is continuously exposed to irritants, but the normal design of the nose and nasal septum allows for equal distribution of air with accompanying irritants; septal deviation can affect this function as well.

The nasal functions of maintaining temperature and humidification and filtering of foreign substances are essential for pulmonary function, and the nasal septum is designed to perform these roles. A deviated septum changes the velocity of air, altering normal nasal activity and resulting in dryness of the mucosa, crusting, nasal bleeding, and changes in the lining membranes of the nose.

A severely deviated septum, with or without concurrent nasal edema, may block the normal sinus ostia. Because mucus is produced by the sinuses, obstructing the flow of mucus through the openings into the nose results in stagnation of the secretions, with possible sinus infection.

COMPLICATIONS

Obstruction of nasal breathing
Epistaxis
Cosmetic nasal deformity
Sinusitis

DIAGNOSTIC STUDIES AND FINDINGS

Diagnostic tests	Findings
Plain x-rays	Nasal fracture, deviation of nasal septum
Skull x-rays	To rule out skull fracture

MEDICAL MANAGEMENT

DRUG THERAPY

Decongestants: To decrease nasal edema

Nasal steroid sprays: To decrease nasal edema

SURGERY

Reduction of nasal fractures: Replaces normal placement of fracture

Nasal septoplasty: Straightening of nasal septum

Rhinoplasty: Cosmetic surgery of nose

1 ASSESS

ASSESSMENT	OBSERVATIONS
Nasal obstruction	Difficulty breathing through nose; mouth breathing; deflection of nasal septum, resulting in narrow nasal passage; edema of nasal mucosa
Dryness of nasal mucosa	Cracked or fissured mucosa, excoriation and crusting of nasal mucosa

ASSESSMENT	OBSERVATIONS
Nasal bleeding	Excoriation of nasal mucosa, areas of bleeding nasal mucosa
Edema of nose, eyes, face	Swelling and ecchymosis of midface from recent trauma

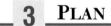 **2 DIAGNOSE**

NURSING DIAGNOSIS	SUBJECTIVE FINDINGS	OBJECTIVE FINDINGS
Ineffective breathing pattern related to nasal obstruction	Complains of difficulty breathing through nose, snoring during sleep, and headaches	Breathes through mouth; twisted nasal septum, causing deflection of septum into nasal cavity; hypertrophy of nasal mucosa; if injury is recent, patient may exhibit ecchymosis of skin over nose and eyes and edema of nose, face, and eyes
High risk for fluid volume deficit related to nasal bleeding	Complains of nasal bleeding	Blood or blood-tinged mucus in nasal cavity; area of excoriation or bleeding on nasal septum

3 PLAN

Patient goals

1. The patient will be able to breathe through his nose.
2. The patient will maintain adequate air exchange, as evidenced by respiratory rate of 16 to 20 respirations per minute.
3. The patient will have minimal or no nasal bleeding.
4. The nasal fracture will be reduced within 1 to 2 hours of injury, before edema develops.

4 IMPLEMENT

NURSING DIAGNOSIS	NURSING INTERVENTIONS	RATIONALE
Ineffective breathing pattern related to nasal obstruction	Elevate head of bed.	May reduce nasal edema.
	Administer decongestants and nasal sprays as ordered.	Decongestants, decongestant nasal sprays, and steroid nasal sprays reduce edema of nasal mucosa to improve nasal breathing.
High risk for fluid volume deficit related to nasal bleeding	Apply ice compresses to nose after acute injury.	To promote vasoconstriction of bleeding vessels.
	Pinch nostrils at tip for minimum of 10 min.	Direct pressure on bleeding vessels stops bleeding from superficial vessels.

NURSING DIAGNOSIS	NURSING INTERVENTIONS	RATIONALE
	Encourage use of bedside humidifier; instill normal saline solution spray prn; insert small amount of ointment into nasal cavity to lubricate nasal mucosa.	Increasing humidification reduces nasal dryness and mucous crusting to prevent nasal bleeding and obstruction of breathing passages from dry mucus.

5 EVALUATE

PATIENT OUTCOME	DATA INDICATING OUTCOME REACHED
Patient demonstrates effective breathing pattern.	Patient can breathe through his nose; if nasal breathing is still ineffective, patient understands need for surgical repair of nasal septum or cosmetic correction.
Patient has minimal or no nasal bleeding.	Patient has normal fluid volume, Hb, and Hct.

PATIENT TEACHING ■■■■■■■■■■■■■■■■■■■■■■■■■■■■■■■■■■■■

1. Instruct the patient in ways to minimize nasal edema (e.g., elevate head of bed).
2. Explain techniques of nasal humidification (e.g., bedside humidifier; normal saline sprays and irrigations; apply ointment in nose to lubricate membranes).
3. Inform the patient about side effects of medications, such as drowsiness.
4. Caution the patient against using decongestant nasal sprays continuously because of rebound effects (rhinitis medicamentosa).

Epistaxis

Epistaxis is bleeding from the nose. It may be caused by trauma, foreign bodies, infection, inflammation, blood or coagulation disorders, or tumors.

Epistaxis occurs in all age groups, and men and women are affected about equally. Children and young adults have a tendency to develop anterior nasal bleeding, whereas older people more commonly have posterior nasal bleeding. Anterior nasal bleeding usually stops spontaneously or can be self-treated, but posterior nasal bleeding may require medical care.

PATHOPHYSIOLOGY

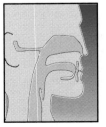

The nose is an extremely vascular structure. Normal deviation of the septum may alter the air currents, causing crust formation and making the vessels of the nose more vulnerable to bleeding. Anterior nasal bleeding occurs most frequently in Little's area on the anterior nasal septum, which is the area where the anterior ethmoid, sphenopalatine, and superior labial arteries anasto-

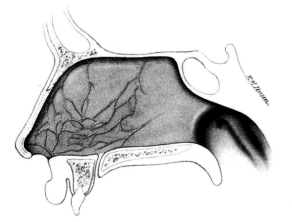

FIGURE 7-2
Kiesselbach's plexus. (From DeWeese.[16])

mose. Within Little's area is Kiesselbach's plexus (Figure 7-2), which is the venous plexus on the anterior septum that is vulnerable to trauma. Other areas commonly affected during anterior nasal bleeding are the cartilaginous septum, the inferior turbinates, the anterior portion of the middle meatus, and the area of the anterior ethmoid artery. Posterior epistaxis usually occurs high on the nasal septum. A common area of bleeding is Woodruff's plexus, an area under the posterior portion of the inferior turbinate. In addition, the sphenopalatine recess and the posterior portion of the middle meatus may be sites of posterior nasal bleeding.

Blood is supplied to the nose by the internal and external carotid arteries. The internal carotid artery branches into the ophthalmic artery and then into the anterior and posterior ethmoid arteries, which go into the posterior ethmoid sinus, joining the sphenopalatine artery, which supplies the anterior ethmoid cells, frontal sinus dura, anterior septum, and lateral nasal walls. The external carotid artery branches into the maxillary artery and the facial artery. The maxillary artery supplies the nose by way of the sphenopalatine and the pharyngeal arteries. The sphenopalatine artery supplies

the turbinates, the ethmoid and maxillary sinuses, and the posterior septum. The facial artery branches into the superior facial artery, covering the anterior septum, and the alar branch of the facial artery supplies the nasal alae.

Trauma is the leading cause of epistaxis. Trauma can be caused by many factors, such as a direct blow to the nose, causing a nasal fracture, or insertion of a foreign body, including use or abuse of nasal cocaine and nasal picking. It can also be a result of nasal surgery. Infection produces an inflamed, hyperemic, friable nasal mucosa that bleeds easily.

Hereditary hemorrhagic telangiectasia, or Rendu-Osler-Weber syndrome, is an autosomal dominant disorder passed by either parent to either sex child. In these individuals the walls of the blood vessels lack contractility, resulting in frequent bleeding. The most common sites of hereditary hemorrhagic telangiectasias are the nose, gastrointestinal tract, and lungs.

Blood disorders that aggravate or prolong bleeding play a role in epistaxis. Disorders such as hemophilia or lymphoproliferative disorders, alcoholism, and immunodeficiencies all decrease clotting factors and platelet counts. Patients who have had chemotherapy or who take aspirin or nonsteroidal antiinflammatory drugs may also notice an increase in epistaxis because of prolonged bleeding. It is estimated that 5% of epistaxis is due to coagulopathy.

Although not causative factors, atherosclerotic vascular disease and hypertension are thought to be contributing factors to posterior epistaxis, because they alter blood vessel contraction.

COMPLICATIONS

Otitis media
Sinusitis
Toxic shock syndrome
Hypoventilation
Hypoxia
Cardiac arrest

Table 7-1

INSERTING POSTERIOR NASAL PACKING

1. Put on gloves, goggles, gown, and mask.
2. Assemble the supplies needed: red rubber catheter, nasopharyngeal pack coated with antibiotic ointment, curved Kelly hemostat, and anterior nasal packing coated with antibiotic ointment.
3. Arrange adequate lighting. Then, insert the catheter through the nose and into the nasopharynx.
4. Pull the catheter through the oral cavity with the Kelly hemostat.
5. Tie the strings of the posterior pack to the catheter.
6. Withdraw the catheter through the nose to position the pack in the nasopharynx.
7. Insert anterior nasal packing in both nares.
8. Untie the strings of the posterior plug from the catheter, and tie them over the tonsil sponge to secure the packing.

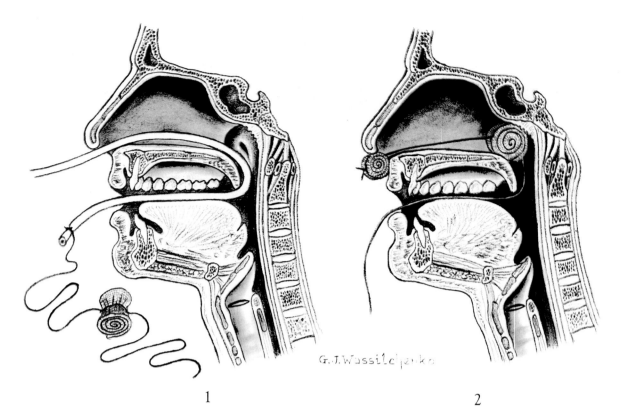

FIGURE 7-3
Postnasal packing for epistaxis. (From Thompson.[71])

DIAGNOSTIC STUDIES AND FINDINGS

Diagnostic test	Findings
Rhinoscopy	Blood in nasal cavity and oropharynx
Nasopharyngoscopy	Blood in nasal cavity and oropharynx

MEDICAL MANAGEMENT

SURGERY

Ligation of ethmoid, maxillary, or carotid artery: Clip or ligature to arterial supply of area of bleeding.

Endoscopic cautery: Chemical or electrical cauterization of bleeding vessel visualized by nasal endoscope.

Laser photocoagulation for Rendu-Osler-Weber syndrome: Use of laser to cauterize bleeding area.

Skin graft to nasal septum and lateral nasal walls for Rendu-Osler-Weber syndrome: Application of skin graft to telangiectasias.

Angiogram with embolization: Embolization of bleeding vessels in patients unable to undergo surgery.

1 ASSESS

ASSESSMENT	OBSERVATIONS
Cardiovascular	Bright red blood from nares, hypertension or hypotension, increased pulse rate
Respiratory	Blood in nasal cavity and oropharynx; mouth breathing; swollen nasal mucosa, with blood obstructing nasal cavity

2 DIAGNOSE

NURSING DIAGNOSIS	SUBJECTIVE FINDINGS	OBJECTIVE FINDINGS
High risk for fluid volume deficit related to nasal bleeding	Complains of bright red blood from nose, frequent swallowing, taste of blood, fatigue, and feeling of fullness in nose	Bright red blood from nares; blood in oropharynx; Hb and Hct below normal
High risk for aspiration related to nasal bleeding	Complains of frequent swallowing, fear of choking, and frequent coughing and clearing of throat	Blood in oropharynx; swallows and/or gags often; emesis with bright red blood or coffee-ground material
High risk for infection related to nasal packing	Complains of headache, lethargy, fever, nausea with or without vomiting, myalgia (toxic shock syndrome), foul odor, and foul smell	Elevated temperature and WBC; hypotension; tachycardia; foul odor
Ineffective breathing pattern related to nasal bleeding, nasal packing	Complains of inability to breathe through nose	Mouth breathing; blood in nasal cavity
Fear related to exsanguination	Expresses fear of bleeding to death; is concerned that any activity may increase bleeding or bleeding potential; fears treatment procedures	Elevated BP; increased pulse and respiratory rate; diaphoresis

3 PLAN

Patient goals

1. The patient will be able to control nasal bleeding.
2. The patient will not aspirate blood.
3. The patient will have no infection.
4. Nasal breathing will be restored, and the patient will maintain a normal breathing pattern.
5. The patient's fears will be resolved.

4 IMPLEMENT

NURSING DIAGNOSIS	NURSING INTERVENTIONS	RATIONALE
High risk for fluid volume deficit related to nasal bleeding	Practice universal precautions (goggles, gloves, mask, gown).	Patient will be expectorating blood, causing particle spray; protective equipment is mandatory to avoid exposure to blood.

→ > >

NURSING DIAGNOSIS	NURSING INTERVENTIONS	RATIONALE
	Identify source of bleeding; provide good illumination (headlight or head mirror) and suction equipment.	Source of bleeding must be identified before initiating treatment; using a headlight or head mirror leaves both hands free for the examination; to remove excess blood and visualize the area of bleeding, use suction or have patient blow her nose.
	Keep patient in sitting position.	To prevent aspiration of blood.
	Administer medications as ordered (e.g., morphine, Valium).	To provide vasoconstriction, allay anxiety, and relieve discomfort.
	Observe patient for signs of respiratory depression, tachycardia, and hypertension by monitoring BP, pulse, and respiratory rate.	Possible side effects of drugs include respiratory depression and hypertension.
	Prepare topical agents (e.g., 4% cocaine hydrochloride; epinephrine 1:1,000; oxymetazoline) to be sprayed into nose or applied to cotton pledgets for insertion into nose.	Topical vasoconstrictors and anesthetics are used to stop bleeding before instituting treatment.
	Prepare patient for treatment to stop bleeding: cellular preparation (Surgicel, Merocel); topical thrombin; cautery of bleeding vessel—silver nitrate, electrocautery, laser (for patients with Rendu-Osler-Weber syndrome); microfibrillar collagen, a compressed polymer made into a tampon and inserted into the nose, which expands with moisture.	Cellular preparations and topical thrombin promote clotting and provide a barrier to the bleeding site; bleeding vessel is cauterized by applying topical hemostasis; microfibrillar collagen tampon applies pressure to bleeding sites as it expands (it is used in immunocompromised and thrombocytopenic patients, because it dissolves and does not require removal).
	Insert anterior nasal packing (½- to 1-inch plain ribbon gauze impregnated with antibiotic ointment); gauze is inserted tightly into anterior nasal cavity and remains in place for 48 to 72 hours.	For nasal tamponade if previous measures fail; antibiotic ointment prevents local infection caused by stasis and lack of normal drainage.
	Apply nasal sling (2 × 2 gauze pad folded into thirds with tape placed tightly on either side of nose).	To prevent anterior slipping of packing and to apply pressure from outside; placing tape on nose prevents facial movement from loosening sling.
	Inspect oral cavity for palatal bulging (may indicate overpacking).	Overpacking can put excessive pressure on delicate membranes, resulting in pressure necrosis.
	Insert posterior packing (14 or 16 F Foley catheter, rolled lambswool or gauze). (See Table 7-1 for guidelines in proper posterior packing insertion.) (Figure 7-3)	Used for posterior nasal bleeding to enhance anterior packing.
	Examine nasal columella for excoriation and laceration.	Anterior securing of posterior packing over nasal columella may cause necrosis.

NURSING DIAGNOSIS	NURSING INTERVENTIONS	RATIONALE
	Monitor fluid, electrolyte, and hematologic values.	In patients with nasal bleeding, Hb and Hct drop and fluid and electrolyte imbalance may develop; blood values help in estimating the amount of blood loss.
	Assess BP, pulse, and level of consciousness.	To determine circulating blood volume and to detect hypotension or hypertension.
	Administer IV hydration and blood products as ordered.	To restore blood and fluid and electrolyte values.
	Elevate head of bed.	To prevent aspiration of blood; to decrease nasal edema
	Apply ice compresses to nose and face.	To minimize edema and cause vasoconstriction of nasal blood vessels.
	Encourage patient to minimize activity.	To prevent reactivation of nasal bleeding.
High risk for aspiration related to nasal bleeding	Elevate head of bed; keep patient in sitting position.	To allow blood to drain through anterior nares and to promote expectoration of posterior bleeding.
	Help patient with suctioning as needed during emesis.	Many patients swallow blood initially, resulting in blood-tinged or coffee-ground emesis; blood in the stomach is an irritant that causes vomiting.
High risk for infection related to nasal packing	Take axillary, rectal, or otic temperatures q4h.	Elevated temperature may indicate infection; nasal congestion or nasal packing necessitates mouth breathing, preventing accurate oral temperature recordings.
	Apply antibiotic ointment to nasal packing before insertion; administer antibiotics as ordered.	Infection, primarily otitis media and sinusitis, may be caused by retained blood in the nasal cavity, altered integrity of the mucous membranes, an alteration in mucociliary transport, and blocking of the normal sinus ostia, which prevents drainage of mucus and causes obstruction of the eustachian tube orifice, preventing equalization of pressure.
	Observe patient for symptoms of toxic shock syndrome (nausea, vomiting, headache, myalgia, fever, hypotension, tachycardia); obtain physician's order for blood cultures if TSS is suspected.	Nasal packing may promote production of an endotoxin produced by certain strains of *Staphylococcus aureus* that may be present in the nasal cavity: absorption of these endotoxins may result in TSS.
Ineffective breathing pattern related to nasal bleeding, nasal packing	Monitor rate and rhythm of respirations; monitor pulse oximetry and/or arterial blood gases (ABGs) as ordered.	A patient with nasal packing, especially a combination of anterior and posterior packing, is at risk for hypoventilation and hypoxia with resultant cardiac dysrhythmia and cardiac arrest.

→ 〉 〉

NURSING DIAGNOSIS	NURSING INTERVENTIONS	RATIONALE
	Administer supplemental humidified oxygen (usually at a 40% concentration) as ordered by face mask.	The patient will have obligatory mouth breathing, causing dryness of the mucous membranes of the oral cavity and oropharynx.
	Monitor patient receiving supplemental oxygen for possible respiratory depression.	Some patients, especially those with chronic obstructive pulmonary disease (COPD), will have a respiratory depression while receiving oxygen as a result of removal of the respiratory drive by lowering of the partial pressure of carbon dioxide (P_{CO_2}).
	Evaluate lips and oral membranes for signs of dryness, irritation, and ulceration; provide and encourage frequent oral hygiene; provide adequate hydration.	Obligatory mouth breathing bypasses the normal humidification system of the nose, producing dryness of the mucous membranes.
	Advise patient not to use oral hygiene products containing glycerine or alcohol (e.g., most commercial mouthwashes).	Glycerine and alcohol enhance dryness and may irritate the mucosa.
Fear related to exsanguination	Allay patient's anxiety by thoroughly explaining all procedures.	To help minimize fear of the unknown.
	Offer reassurance.	Patients are frightened that they are bleeding to death and require constant reassurance.
	Monitor respiratory status closely if sedatives or antianxiety medications are given.	Respiratory depression is a side effect of many sedatives and antianxiety medications.
	Investigate causes of fear and anxieties.	Pain and hypoxia can cause agitation; it is imperative to know the cause before initiating treatment.

5 EVALUATE

PATIENT OUTCOME	DATA INDICATING OUTCOME REACHED
Nasal bleeding has been controlled.	Fluid volume is maintained, and blood and fluid and electrolyte values are normal.
No aspiration is noted.	Bleeding has been controlled, and patient has no emesis.
There are no signs of infection.	Temperature, BP, and pulse are normal; WBC is normal; mucous membranes have healed and there is no evidence of ulceration or excoriation; nasal mucous drainage is clear and has no signs of blood, purulence, or odor.
Nasal breathing has been restored, and patient maintains a normal breathing pattern.	Bleeding has been controlled and packing has been removed; blood oxygen levels are normal, as demonstrated by pulse oximetry and/or ABGs.
Patient's fears have been resolved.	Patient can discuss fear and redirect energy.

PATIENT TEACHING ■

1. Teach the patient ways to enhance nasal humidity (e.g., use a bedside humidifier; use nasal saline sprays; apply a small amount of ointment to the anterior nasal cavity).
2. Encourage the patient to stop using nasal decongestant sprays.
3. Instruct the patient to avoid vigorous nose blowing and to sneeze with her mouth open.
4. Encourage the patient to avoid nasal trauma, especially nose picking.
5. Instruct the patient to avoid strenuous activity, lifting, straining, for 4 to 6 weeks after nasal bleeding.
6. Encourage the patient to control concomitant medical conditions (e.g., hypertension).
7. Instruct the patient to minimize or avoid, if possible, use of aspirin, aspirin-containing products, and nonsteroidal antiinflammatory drugs.
8. If nasal bleeding occurs, the patient and family should be instructed to:
   a. Pinch the nostrils tightly closed for 10 minutes.
   b. Apply ice compresses.
   c. Have the patient sit upright with her head tilted forward.
   d. Instill nasal decongestant spray (NeoSynephrine) to prompt vasoconstriction, per physician's order.

Sinusitis

Sinusitis is an infection of one or more of the paranasal sinuses.

PATHOPHYSIOLOGY

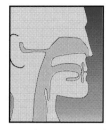 The paranasal sinuses are sterile, air-filled cavities located within the bones of the skull. They consist of the maxillary sinuses (in the cheeks), the ethmoid sinuses (between the eyes), the frontal sinuses (above the eyebrows), and the sphenoid sinus (behind the eyes and ethmoid sinuses). The paranasal sinuses normally are kept sterile by mucociliary transport. Anything that alters this transport, including anatomic variations of the nasal cavity, can lead to sinusitis. Anatomic variations such as nasal edema from allergy, nasal polyps, or a deviated nasal septum may obstruct sinus drainage. Inflammation, generally an upper respiratory infection, results in increased secretions and edema of the nasal mucosa. Secretions are retained in the sinuses as a result of altered ciliary activity and obstruction of the normally open sinus ostia. When secretions are retained in the sinus cavity, normal oxygen from the sinuses can be absorbed and the fluid accumulation can result in negative pressure, causing pain and a breeding ground for organisms. Additional causes of infection of the paranasal sinuses are swimming and diving, which may allow a massive influx of contaminated material to enter the sinuses, and dental manipulation, such as a dental abscess or a root canal procedure on teeth with roots in the maxillary sinus. Indwelling nasal tubes have also been associated with acute sinusitis. Prolonged use of large nasogastric or nasotracheal tubes causes increased irritation and edema of the nasal mucosa, resulting in obstruction of the sinus ostia.

Sinusitis can be bacterial, viral, or fungal in origin and may be classified as acute or chronic.

Bacterial sinusitis most commonly is associated with *Streptococcus pneumoniae, Haemophilus influenzae,* and *Moraxella catarrhalis.* The latter two organisms may produce beta-lactamase, causing a resistance to penicillin antibiotics.

Acute sinusitis usually is the result of an upper respiratory infection, allergic rhinitis, swimming, or dental manipulation, all of which can cause inflammatory changes and retention of secretions, providing a medium for bacterial infection. **Viral sinusitis** is believed to follow an upper respiratory infection in which the virus penetrates the normal mucous membrane, decreasing ciliary transport. Most cases of acute rhinosinusitis are of viral origin. The stasis that results from immobility of cilia and osteal edema may result in a bacterial superinfection. Chronic sinusitis is a persistent infection usually associated with allergy and nasal polyps. Patients with chronic sinusitis generally have had repeated episodes of acute sinusitis, resulting in an irreversible loss of the normal ciliated epithelium lining the sinus cavity.

Fungal sinusitis is uncommon and is found more often in patients who are immunocompromised or in a debilitated state, such as patients with uncontrolled diabetes or patients who are immunosuppressed because of chemotherapy or organ transplantation. The most common types of fungal sinusitis are aspergillosis, mucormycosis, candidiasis, histoplasmosis, and coccidioidomycosis. The organisms that cause these infections are spores that normally are found in the soil. They enter the respiratory tract through inhalation, and in a person with a normal immune system are promptly eliminated. However, in an immunocompromised or debilitated patient, a fungal infection may begin.

Aspergillosis sinusitis produces dark, thick secretions, and the patient has a mucopurulent discharge and nasal edema. Aspergillosis may be associated with allergic rhinitis.

Mucormycosis is almost exclusively seen in immunocompromised, chronically ill patients. It thrives in an acid, glucose-rich environment and therefore is seen with increased incidence in patients with uncontrolled diabetes with ketoacidosis. Mucormycosis results in vascular thrombosis, which causes necrosis of the turbinates. Necrotic turbinates appear dark red or black. These patients complain of a bloody discharge, rather than the mucopurulent drainage seen in other forms of sinusitis. Because mucormycosis may cause erosion of the bone of the sinuses and the orbit, it is a more destructive form of sinusitis and will lead to death if not treated aggressively.

COMPLICATIONS

Orbital/periorbital cellulitis
Orbital/periorbital abscess
Cavernous sinus thrombosis
Bacteremia/septicemia
Osteomyelitis
Brain abscess
Meningitis

Table 7-2

SINUS IRRIGATION

1. Observe universal precautions (gown, gloves, goggles, and mask).
2. Apply local anesthesia to the nasal cavity (e.g., cocaine hydrochloride, 1% lidocaine with epinephrine, 4% topical lidocaine).
3. Place a trocar with inserter into the maxillary sinus through the ostium under the inferior turbinate.
4. Attach a 20 to 50 ml syringe.
5. Aspirate the sinus to obtain exudate for culture; if no exudate is aspirated, 3 to 5 ml of normal saline solution may be inserted and withdrawn for culture.
6. With the patient in a sitting position, head tilted forward and mouth open, inject 50 to 100 ml of room-temperature normal saline solution into the sinus.
7. The solution will exit through the nose and mouth.
8. Remove the trocar.
9. Apply pressure to the nose by pinching the nostrils for 5 to 10 minutes.

DIAGNOSTIC STUDIES AND FINDINGS

Diagnostic test	Findings
Sinus x-rays (plain films); coronal computed tomography (CT) scan (Figure 7-4)	Thickening of mucosal linings, air-fluid level, obstruction of osteomeatal complex, mucocele, paradoxical turbinate, concha bullosa
Sinus endoscopy	Purulent nasal drainage, nasal edema, obstruction of ostia

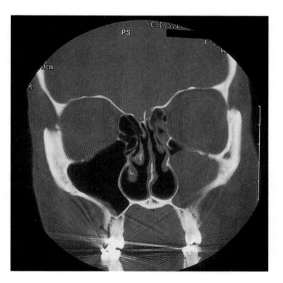

FIGURE 7-4
CT scan showing sinusitis.

MEDICAL MANAGEMENT

SURGERY

Sinus tap and irrigation for acute sinusitis: Insertion of catheter through sinus ostia to irrigate sinus.

Functional endoscopic sinus surgery: Use of sinus endoscopes to enter sinus, remove diseased mucosa, and open sinus ostia.

Caldwell-Luc operation: Incision in gingival buccal sulcus to enter maxillary sinus.

External ethmoidectomy/sphenoethmoidectomy for chronic sinusitis: Incision on lateral nose near inner canthus to enter ethmoid sinus.

Frontal sinusectomy with or without obliteration for chronic sinusitis: Removal of frontal sinus mucosa to remove disease.

1 ASSESS

ASSESSMENT	OBSERVATIONS
Respiratory	Edematous nasal mucosa, mucopurulent drainage in nose and posterior pharynx, opaque sinuses, air-fluid level on x-ray films
Skin	Edema of face and periorbital area, pain
Vital signs	Elevated temperature

2 DIAGNOSE

NURSING DIAGNOSIS	SUBJECTIVE FINDINGS	OBJECTIVE FINDINGS
Ineffective airway clearance related to nasal obstruction	Complains of difficulty or inability to breathe through nose	Swollen nasal mucosa, mouth breathing, opaque sinuses or air-fluid level on x-ray films
High risk for infection related to sinusitis	Complains of purulent nasal drainage, fever, fatigue, and swelling around eyes	Elevated temperature, purulent drainage in nasal cavity, edema of eyelids and periorbital area
Altered sensory perception (olfactory) related to nasal edema	Complains of change in sense of smell	Change in ability to recognize common aromas
Pain (acute) related to sinus infection	Complains of sinus headache and facial pain or discomfort	Facial grimaces, verbalizes pain

3 PLAN

Patient goals
1. Patient will have patent nasal airway.
2. Patient will exhibit no signs of infection.
3. Patient will be able to distinguish common smells.
4. Patient will have no pain.

4 IMPLEMENT

NURSING DIAGNOSIS	NURSING INTERVENTIONS	RATIONALE
Ineffective airway clearance related to nasal obstruction	Increase humidification (use bedside humidifier, increase fluid intake, use nasal saline sprays).	To promote nasal drainage.
	Administer medications as ordered (vasoconstrictors, decongestants, nasal sprays); elevate head of bed.	To reduce nasal edema and promote drainage.

NURSING DIAGNOSIS	NURSING INTERVENTIONS	RATIONALE
High risk for infection related to sinusitis	Assess amount and characteristics of nasal drainage.	To detect infection.
	Monitor temperature.	To detect fever and infection.
	Obtain or assist with obtaining culture of drainage.	To guide choice of medication.
	Perform sinus irrigation (Table 7-2).	To obtain culture of organism; to remove accumulated secretions.
	Observe patient for orbital complications (eyelid/periorbital edema; impaired mobility of eye; anesthesia of skin, cornea, or conjunctivae; protrusion of globe; decreased visual acuity; chemosis [congestion and swelling of conjunctivae]; diplopia; photophobia).	Orbital extension of sinusitis is through open suture lines in the bone, congenital bone openings, via blood vessels, through bone weakened by erosion or necrosis caused by infection, or lymphatics. The sinuses are separated by very thin bone, which can be involved with acute or chronic disease.
	Monitor patient for decrease in pulse rate.	Caused by oculocardiac reflex.
	Monitor patient for signs of intracranial complications (lethargy, anorexia, vomiting, headache, seizure activity, altered level of consciousness, increased intracranial pressure, irritability, somnolence).	Altered sinus physiology resulting from chronic infection, nasal drug abuse, chemical exposure, or trauma may predispose a patient to intracranial complications. All the paranasal sinuses, except the maxillary sinus, share a common wall of thin bone with the cranial cavity. Intracranial extension of sinus disease may occur through erosion of bone, blood/lymphatic extension, or trauma.
	Administer antibiotics and/or antifungal agent as ordered.	To treat infection.
Altered sensory perception (olfactory) related to nasal edema	Instruct the patient to make appropriate adaptations in his living environment (i.e., install smoke detectors, observe appearance of stored food for spoilage, routinely check gas lines for leakage, and install gas detectors).	The patient with an altered sense of smell must rely on alternative techniques to sense dangerous occurrences such as fire, spoiled food, and gas leaks.
Pain (acute) related to sinus infection	Assess amount of pain.	To determine need for analgesics.
	Administer and evaluate effectiveness of analgesics every 4 hours.	To relieve pain and determine effectiveness of analgesics.
	Instruct patient to avoid bending, lifting, stooping.	Increases pressure in sinuses, causing increase in pain.
	Apply warm, moist compresses to sinus area.	To improve drainage and promote comfort.

5   EVALUATE

PATIENT OUTCOME	DATA INDICATING THAT OUTCOME IS REACHED
Patient has no signs or symptoms of sinusitis.	Nasal airway is patent; temperature is normal and nasal drainage is clear; patient has no pain, pressure, headaches. Patient can distinguish common smells.

PATIENT TEACHING

1. Teach the patient and family about the anatomy and physiology of the sinuses; explain how sinusitis develops, possible causative factors, and the proper use and side effects of medications. Also explain any diagnostic procedures that may be performed.
2. Instruct the patient to avoid bending and stooping during the acute phase of sinusitis, because this increases the pain.
3. Instruct the patient to use systemic decongestants 30 to 60 minutes before flying; a decongestant nasal spray should be used 15 to 30 minutes before takeoff and landing to prevent ear discomfort or infection.
4. Encourage the patient to minimize exposure to irritating pollutants (e.g., cigarette smoke).
5. Encourage the patient to avoid contact with people known to have infections.
6. Instruct the patient to increase humidification by using a bedside humidifier or vaporizer and nasal saline sprays and by increasing his fluid intake.
7. Instruct the patient to take medication as prescribed by his physician.
8. Review the signs and symptoms of sinusitis with potential complications, and instruct the patient when to notify his physician.

CHAPTER 8

Surgical and Therapeutic Interventions for Nose and Sinus Disorders

Nasal Surgery

NASAL SEPTOPLASTY/ SEPTORHINOPLASTY

Nasal septal surgery depends on the severity of the patient's symptoms and the patient's desires. Obstruction of the nasal airway, mouth breathing, headaches, nasal bleeding, recurrent rhinosinusitis, and a crooked nose are basically subjective symptoms. The amount of discomfort the symptoms cause is one of the main determinants of whether surgery is performed.

Nasal septal surgery, with or without cosmetic repair (rhinoplasty), involves straightening the nasal septum to restore nasal breathing. An incision is made through the mucosa at the caudal end of the septal cartilage. The mucous membranes are elevated, and the septal cartilage is separated from its bony attachments. Deformities are removed or fixed, and the cartilage is straightened. Current procedures focus on straightening the nasal septum rather than removing it so as to preserve cartilaginous tissue. The septal mucous membranes are carefully reapproximated to prevent any bleeding. If cosmetic changes are desired, a rhinoplasty may be performed after the septoplasty. If cosmetic repair is to be performed, photographs should be taken before surgery and the patient and family should undergo counseling regarding the patient's expectations.

After surgery packing may be inserted, depending on the closure technique the surgeon uses. Packing may be used to prevent a hematoma from forming between the septal flaps and also to help hold the septum in position. Nasal septal splints, which are small pieces of plastic or Silastic, may be inserted into the nose after a septoplasty. These splints help prevent the formation of nasal synechiae, which are scar bands that may form between the surgical site and the lateral nasal wall.

COMPLICATIONS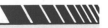

Septal hematoma (leading to cartilage reabsorption
Nasal bleeding
Collapse of the nasal structure
Persistent obstruction caused by incomplete removal of the septum or by intranasal scarring
Intranasal synechiae

Surgery to Control Nasal Bleeding

If epistaxis cannot be controlled through other measures (see Chapter 7), surgery may be required. Early surgical intervention has been advocated by some physicians because it is cost effective (it curtails the need for 5 to 7 days of nasal packing or posterior plugs, or both); it is safer for a patient who is unable to tolerate intranasal packing and posterior packing; and it stops nasal bleeding quickly.

Ligation of the internal maxillary artery is the technique most commonly used. A Caldwell-Luc incision is extended to allow removal of the posterior wall of the maxillary sinus and to gain access to the artery. Sutures or clips are placed on the main trunk of the artery proximal to the descending palatine artery.

Ligation of the external carotid artery may be another means to stop epistaxis. Care must be taken to ligate the external carotid artery and to avoid branches of the vagus nerve. Ligation of the external carotid artery may not control epistaxis, however, because collateral circulation may develop distal to the ligation.

Ligation of the anterior ethmoid artery may be done alone or with ligation of the maxillary artery to control bleeding from the superior part of the nasal cavity. An incision is made at the side of the nose near the inner canthus to gain access to the anterior ethmoid artery. The patient may require nasal packing for 24 to 48 hours after this procedure.

COMPLICATIONS

Paresthesia or anesthesia of the cheek, upper lip, and maxillary teeth	Diplopia Oral-antral fistula Nasal bleeding
Periorbital hematoma	

Sinus Surgery

Functional Endoscopic Sinus Surgery

The main objective of functional endoscopic sinus surgery (FESS) is to reestablish both sinus ventilation and mucociliary clearance. Functional endoscopic sinus surgery emphasizes the removal of tissue from the osteomeatal complex, the area of the anterior ethmoids and middle meatus. FESS can also be used to remove nasal polyps.

Diagnostic evaluation before endoscopic sinus surgery includes nasal endoscopy and coronal computed

Nasal Polypectomy

If medical management of nasal polyps is unsuccessful (see Chapter 7) and the patient continues to complain of obstructed nasal breathing, a nasal polypectomy can be performed. This procedure can be done using local anesthesia with or without sedation. Local anesthesia is the anesthesia of choice because the vasoconstrictive properties of most local anesthetics decrease bleeding during surgery. A snarelike instrument is used to avulse the polyp. The attachment point is cauterized, and packing may or may not be used. Simple polypectomy may be associated with early recurrence, because the polyps originate in the sinuses. If simple polypectomy is insufficient to restore nasal breathing, the polypoid mucous membrane must be removed from the sinuses, because nasal polyps originate in one of the paranasal sinuses (see Chapter 7).

COMPLICATIONS

Nasal bleeding
Recurrence of nasal polyps

NURSING CARE

See pages 167-170.

tomography (CT) scans. Nasal endoscopy can reveal subtle changes in the osteomeatal complex, an area that cannot be seen with anterior rhinoscopy done with a nasal speculum. A coronal CT scan can determine the underlying cause of sinusitis. It is best performed after acute inflammation has subsided and medical treatment has been attempted. Even minor changes in the osteomeatal complex, as seen on CT scanning, can result in sinusitis caused by blockage of the sinus ostia. For example, concha bullosa, an enlargement of an air cell within the middle turbinate, can narrow the middle meatus, preventing mucus from draining. A paradoxical turbinate, which is a lateral convexity of the middle turbinate, also may narrow the middle meatus, resulting in sinusitis. Neither concha bullosa nor paradoxic turbinates can be seen on plain x-ray films of the sinuses, and their role in sinusitis has been recognized only since the use of CT scanning.

Functional endoscopic sinus surgery is done in the operating room using general or local anesthesia and mild sedation. Small nasal endoscopes are used to dissect the diseased mucosa. The physician uses the CT scan as a guide to the nasal and sinus anatomy and to locate diseased tissue. In early sinus disease, the cells are opened through dissection to allow ventilation and drainage; in advanced sinus disease, the cells may be removed.

The surgery is performed on an outpatient basis, and generally, if there is no sign of bleeding or other complication, the patient can be discharged. Intranasal packing may be used for patients with uncontrolled nasal bleeding (especially those with a history of asthma) to prevent postnasal drainage that may result in bronchospasm. Follow-up care of the patient is required. The surgical site should be frequently cleaned of blood, mucus, crusts, hypertrophic mucosa, and bone spicules until the site has healed. If low-grade inflammation or infection is noted during endoscopic examination, antibiotics may be administered. Normal saline sprays may be used beginning 4 or 5 days after surgery to maintain the moisture of the mucosa. Saline irrigations may be necessary for patients with considerable crusting.

With an experienced surgeon, functional endoscopic sinus surgery has few complications. Bleeding is the most common complication and can be avoided through proper vasoconstriction and hemostasis after the procedure. Adequate training in the procedure, good visualization of the area, and proper surgical techniques can prevent orbital hematomas and injury to the optic nerve. Cerebrospinal fluid (CSF) rhinorrhea results from injury to the roof of the ethmoid bone or cribriform plate.

COMPLICATIONS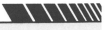

Nasal bleeding
Orbital hematoma
Injury to the optic nerve
Blindness
Cerebrospinal fluid (CSF) rhinorrhea

CALDWELL-LUC OPERATION

A Caldwell-Luc operation is indicated in patients with long-standing maxillary sinusitis that cannot be cured

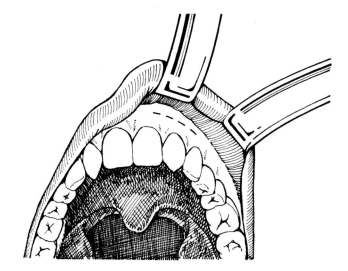

FIGURE 8-1
Caldwell-Luc surgery. The incision is made under the upper lip into the maxillary sinus.

> **For closeups of Caldwell-Luc surgery, see Color Plates 8 and 9, page xi.**

by appropriate antibiotic and other medical therapy. The procedure involves removing diseased mucous membrane and creating a nasal antral window, which is an opening created below the natural sinus ostia. This provides aeration of the sinus and allows infected material to drain. There is some question about the efficacy of a nasal antral window, because sinus drainage has been shown to follow the normal ciliary flow toward the natural sinus ostia rather than through the newly created antral window. However, the increased drainage that occurs during an episode of acute sinusitis may be removed through the larger nasal antral window.

The Caldwell-Luc procedure can be performed using local anesthesia with sedation, but general anesthesia usually is used. An incision is made into the gingival buccal sulcus to allow entry into the anterior wall of the sinus (Figure 8-1). The diseased mucosa is removed, and the nasal antral window is created. Both the maxillary sinus and the nose may be packed. Nasal packing generally is removed after 24 hours and antral packing after 48 to 72 hours.

COMPLICATIONS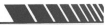

Paresthesia/anesthesia of the cheek, upper lip, maxillary teeth
Oral antral fistula
Nasal bleeding

ETHMOIDECTOMY

Ethmoidectomy is a surgical procedure done to remove diseased mucosa, polyps, or mucoceles from the ethmoid sinus. A mucocele, or mucous cyst, usually is a consequence of repeated infection. Repeated infection causes the sinus ostia from the ethmoid sinus to become blocked by thickened mucosa or scar tissue, and mucus cannot drain. As the mucus builds up, a cyst forms. The mucocele continues to enlarge, causing pressure necrosis to the surrounding bone; this allows the mucocele to be seen as a mass at the medial canthus.

Ethmoidectomy can be performed transnasally, by an external approach, or by a transantral approach. Intranasal ethmoidectomy is performed using a headlight and operating microscope or endoscopes. General or local anesthesia with sedation may be used. The procedure most commonly is performed to remove nasal polyps arising in the ethmoid sinus. The ethmoid cells are removed, creating a single large cavity. After surgery, the cavity is packed for 24 to 48 hours. The patient usually is given intranasal steroids to prevent recurrence of the nasal polyps. Intranasal ethmoidectomy can be technically difficult, and complications to the orbit or entry through the cribriform plate, resulting in CSF rhinorrhea, can occur.

External ethmoidectomy is performed through an incision lateral to the medial canthus of the eye near the dorsum of the nose. Diseased mucosa or mucoceles can be removed through this incision. A pressure dressing generally is applied over the eye to prevent postoperative edema.

Transantral ethmoidectomy is performed through a Caldwell-Luc incision. The ethmoid cells are identified and removed from below. This approach makes it difficult to remove the anterior ethmoid cells, and a combined intranasal and transantral approach may be necessary. After the transantral procedure, anesthesia or paresthesia of the infraorbital nerve (numbness of the lip or upper teeth) may be noted.

COMPLICATIONS

Periorbital hematoma
Diplopia
CSF rhinorrhea
Paresthesia/anesthesia of cheek, upper lip, maxillary teeth

FRONTAL SINUS SURGERY

Acute frontal sinusitis initially is treated medically. Intravenous antibiotics, topical vasoconstrictors, analgesics, and heat are prescribed when frontal sinusitis has been diagnosed. If the disease continues and the patient remains symptomatic, frontal sinus trephination can be done to drain the infection. A small incision is made in the medial aspect of the upper eyelid. The frontal sinus is entered from the bottom, and the sinus is drained. A small catheter may be inserted through the incision to irrigate and drain the sinus. The catheter is irrigated daily and removed once the irrigation fluid drains through the nose. Nasal drainage of the irrigation fluid indicates opening of the sinus ostium.

Osteoplastic frontal sinusectomy is the usual procedure for chronic frontal sinusitis. The frontal sinus is approached through either a butterfly incision above the eyebrows or a more cosmetically acceptable coronal incision in the hairline. A template is made by outlining the sinus on a 6-foot Caldwell view of the sinuses to facilitate opening of the front wall of the sinus. The sinus is entered, and all diseased mucosa is removed. If an adipose obliteration of the sinus is to be performed, all frontal sinus mucosa is removed. Adipose tissue is taken from the abdomen and placed within the sinus to completely obliterate the frontal sinus. A pressure dressing is placed over the area to minimize postoperative swelling.

SPHENOID SINUS SURGERY

Sphenoid sinus surgery can be accomplished using an endoscopic technique, an external or transantral ethmoidectomy approach, or a transseptal approach. The ethmoid sinus generally is removed and the anterior wall of the sphenoid sinus opened. As with other sinus surgery, the diseased tissue is removed, along with the mucous membrane lining the sinus. The sinus ostium is opened wide to facilitate drainage directly into the nasopharynx.

COMPLICATIONS

CSF leak
Periorbital edema
Infection of adipose tissue

1 ASSESS

ASSESSMENT	OBSERVATIONS
Fluid balance	Nausea, vomiting (hematemesis), decreased fluid intake, bleeding from the nose, frequent swallowing
Respiratory	Mouth breathing, shortness of breath
Vision	Edema of eyelids, double vision, blurred vision

2 DIAGNOSE

NURSING DIAGNOSIS	SUBJECTIVE FINDINGS	OBJECTIVE FINDINGS
High risk for fluid volume deficit related to nasal bleeding, inadequate intake	Complains of nasal bleeding, difficulty swallowing, nausea, vomiting, anorexia	Bloody drainage from nose, blood in oropharynx, poor skin turgor
Ineffective breathing pattern related to nasal edema, nasal packing, and/or intranasal splints	Complains of inability to breathe through nose, mouth breathing, shortness of breath, swelling of nose and face	Breathes through mouth, has nasal packing and/or nasal splints; labored breathing, nasal and facial edema
Pain (acute) related to surgery	Complains of pain in ears, nose, face, and throat; has headache and nasal and facial tightness; requests pain medication	Elevated BP, pulse, respirations; facial grimaces; nasal and facial swelling
High risk for infection related to surgical procedure	Complains of increased pain, foul odor, swelling of nose and cheeks, swelling of lips, discoloration of nose and lips	Increased nasal, facial, and lip edema; redness and discoloration of skin of nose, face, and lips; elevated WBC; elevated temperature
Altered sensory perception (visual) related to surgical procedure or complications	Complains of eyelid edema, double vision, and blurred or no vision	Partial or total loss of vision; edema, redness of eyelid; diplopia

3 PLAN

Patient goals
1. The patient will have adequate hydration.
2. The patient will have no postoperative nasal bleeding; if bleeding occurs, it will be treated promptly.
3. The patient will maintain adequate ventilation.
4. The patient's postoperative pain will be relieved.
5. The patient will have no postoperative infection.
6. The patient will have no visual disturbances.

4   IMPLEMENT

NURSING DIAGNOSIS	NURSING INTERVENTIONS	RATIONALE
High risk for fluid volume deficit related to nasal bleeding, inadequate intake	Monitor for signs of nasal bleeding (increased blood on drip pad; blood in oropharynx; frequent swallowing); monitor vital signs, and check laboratory values.	Hemostasis is achieved before surgery is completed and packing is inserted. Due to the vasculature of the nose, minimal bleeding is anticipated for 24 to 48 hours. Blood-tinged mucus is expected for an additional 48 to 72 hours. If hemostasis is not maintained, nasal bleeding through packing, anterior or posterior, may be noted by visible blood or swallowing of blood. Decreased BP and increased pulse rate may indicate blood loss. Decreases in Hb and Hct indicate substantial blood loss.
	Continue IV fluids until patient is awake and alert; monitor intake and output; encourage oral fluids.	Patient will be NPO for 8 hours before surgery and until she has recovered from the anesthetic; fluid intake must be maintained until an oral diet is tolerated.
	Evaluate emesis and stool for bleeding; give guaiac test as indicated.	Patient may swallow blood during surgery and if actively bleeding; positive result on guaiac test indicates blood.
	Administer antiemetics as prescribed.	To prevent vomiting, which may increase nasal pressure and stimulate additional bleeding.
	Instruct patient to avoid activities that increase intranasal pressure for 10 to 14 days: nose blowing (instead, sniff and swallow or expectorate); lifting; exercise; sneezing with mouth closed (instead, sneeze with mouth open).	Increased intranasal pressure may stimulate bleeding.
Ineffective breathing pattern related to nasal edema, nasal packing, and/or intranasal splints	Elevate head of bed.	To minimize edema.
	Apply ice compresses to nasal and cheek area.	To promote vasoconstriction.
	Increase nasal humidification by using bedside humidifier or humidified air via face mask.	Nasal breathing is bypassed because of edema and packing, causing the patient to breathe through her mouth; supplemental humidification is necessary.
	Monitor respiratory rate and rhythm; monitor pulse oximetry as ordered (should be maintained at >90%).	Nasal packing forces obligatory mouth breathing; patient is at risk for hypoventilation and hypoxia, with resultant cardiac dysrhythmia and cardiac arrest.
Pain (acute) related to surgery	Administer analgesics as ordered, and evaluate effectiveness.	To minimize or eliminate postoperative pain and discomfort; if analgesic is not effective, a complication may have developed.

NURSING DIAGNOSIS	NURSING INTERVENTIONS	RATIONALE
	Instruct patient not to use aspirin or non-steroidal antiinflammatory drugs.	Aspirin and nonsteroidal antiinflammatory drugs reduce blood clotting and may promote bleeding.
	Administer analgesics 30 minutes before removal of packing.	After a Caldwell-Luc procedure, antral packing is inserted; it is removed 24 to 48 hours later through the nasal-antral window, and removal is uncomfortable.
High risk for infection related to surgical procedure	Observe for increased drainage, foul odor, increased edema, and pain; monitor blood parameters, especially WBC.	To detect signs and symptoms of infection.
	Monitor temperature by rectal, axillary, or otic routes.	Mouth breathing necessitates alternative routes for measuring temperature.
	Observe for increased or abnormal swelling, pain, and discoloration of the nose, cheeks, and upper lip.	Septal hematoma is a complication of nasal surgery. Bleeding occurs within the intranasal tissues and dissects into tissues at the base of the nose (upper lip). No frank bleeding is noted, because blood is trapped in tissues. Hematoma of the nasal septum deprives the cartilage of its blood supply, resulting in destruction and absorption of cartilage.
	Report signs of septal hematoma to physician.	Immediate incision and drainage of septal hematoma will prevent cartilage destruction.
	Provide frequent mouth care; evaluate lips and oral cavity for signs of dryness and irritation.	Mouth breathing bypasses normal humidification, resulting in dryness of the oral mucosa.
	Instruct patient not to use oral hygiene products containing glycerine or alcohol.	Alcohol and glycerine promote dryness and may irritate the oral mucosa.
	Evaluate oral cavity incision (transantral ligation; Caldwell-Luc procedure.)	Intraoral incision has greater potential for infection because of the constant presence of saliva.
	Provide mouth rinses of ½ hydrogen peroxide and ½ water or saline q 4 h; rinse with water or saline.	Good oral hygiene decreases bacteria.
	Encourage patient to continue to brush teeth but to avoid incisional area; caution patient about lack of sensation in upper teeth on side of incision.	Incision into gingival buccal sulcus above lateral incisors gives access to maxillary sinus; stretching of the nerve results in paresthesia or anesthesia of the upper teeth, cheek, or gingiva.
	Observe oral cavity for oral-antral fistula.	Separation of sutures or opening of the incision may result in a connection between the maxillary sinus and the mouth.

NURSING DIAGNOSIS	NURSING INTERVENTIONS	RATIONALE
Altered sensory perception (visual) related to surgical procedure or complications	Apply ice compresses to eye; maintain pressure patch over incision and eye; elevate head of bed.	To minimize eyelid edema.
	Report altered vision immediately to physician.	May indicate orbital hematoma and/or injury to optic nerve, which require emergency surgical intervention.

5 EVALUATE

PATIENT OUTCOME	DATA INDICATING THAT OUTCOME IS REACHED
Fluid volume is maintained.	Patient has no nasal bleeding; blood parameters are normal. Vital signs are within normal limits. Skin turgor is normal.
Patient has no nasal bleeding.	Patient has no nasal bleeding; Hb and Hct are normal.
Nasal breathing is restored, and patient maintains adequate ventilation.	Packing has been removed and edema has subsided; pulse oximetry is >90%; patient has no signs of respiratory distress.
Patient has no pain.	Patient reports no discomfort or relieves discomfort with analgesics.
Patient has no signs of infection.	Temperature, BP, and pulse are normal; WBC is normal; nasal drainage is clear and has no odor or evidence of infection.
Patient has no visual disturbances.	Eyelid edema has subsided, and visual acuity has returned to presurgical status.

PATIENT TEACHING

1. Describe the normal postoperative course: nasal edema will persist for 10 to 14 days; minimal blood-tinged mucous drainage will be present for 10 to 14 days; discomfort can be expected for 7 to 10 days, but actual pain should be reported to the physician.
2. Instruct the patient to change the drip pad as needed to avoid wiping her nose.
3. Encourage the patient not to blow her nose for 10 days. She should sniff the secretions to the back of the nose and swallow or expectorate.
4. Instruct the patient to sneeze with her mouth open to avoid increasing intranasal pressure and bleeding.
5. Encourage the patient to increase humidification by using a bedside humidifier, steam inhalation, and nasal saline spray.
6. Instruct the patient to avoid lifting, straining, and exercise for at least 14 days or as instructed by her physician.
7. Encourage the patient to avoid smoking and other noxious fumes that may irritate the nose.

CHAPTER 9

Disorders of the Oral Cavity, Oropharynx, and Larynx

Pharyngitis

Pharyngitis is an acute inflammation of the pharyngeal walls. It may include the tonsils, palate, and uvula.

PATHOPHYSIOLOGY

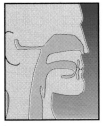

Although the exact incidence of pharyngitis is unknown, inflammatory disorders of the oropharynx are among the most common reasons for visits to health care facilities by both children and adults.

Bacteria, viruses, and fungi can cause acute pharyngitis. A thorough history and physical examination may indicate the cause even before a culture is done. Beta-hemolytic streptococci account for 15% to 20% of acute pharyngeal episodes. *Neisseria gonorrhoeae* and *Corynebacterium diphtheriae* are other bacterial organisms that may infect the pharynx. Viral pharyngitis accounts for approximately 70% of acute pharyngitis cases.

Although all forms of pharyngitis cause throat discomfort, the appearance of the throat may vary, depending on the causative organism. Streptococcal pharyngitis may produce a uniform infection of the pharyngeal walls. Purulent exudate and edema of the lymphoid tissue may be present, especially around the palate, tonsils, and uvula. A patient with a streptococcal infection may complain of throat discomfort, malaise, and a slightly elevated temperature. Diphtherial pharyngitis is caused by the release of a toxin produced by *C. diphtheriae*. This toxin causes local inflammation, formation of exudate, and cellular necrosis. The main characteristic of diphtherial pharyngitis is a gray or white membrane that covers the pharyngeal and tonsillar regions. Attempts to remove this membrane may cause bleeding, which is not seen in other types of pharyngitis. Patients with gonococcal pharyngitis may complain of minimal discomfort. Since this type of in-

> A close-up of tonsils covered with exudate in mononucleosis appears in Color Plate 14, page xii.

chronic debilitation. Candidiasis is recognized not only by pain and dysphagia but also by adherent white plaques in the oral cavity or on the pharyngeal walls.

All forms of pharyngitis are communicable by droplet or direct contact. Mononucleosis is transmitted by oral contact and sometimes is referred to as the "kissing disease." Instituting prompt, appropriate treatment requires culture and sensitivity testing of the pharyngeal mucosa. If the nursing history indicates exposure to diphtheria or gonorrhea, the laboratory should be alerted to evaluate the specimen for these two organisms. Mononucleosis is not diagnosed by throat culture; however, the peripheral blood is examined by means of heterophil agglutination antibody (Monospot) test and WBC count to determine whether large, atypical lymphocytes and an elevated total peripheral white blood count are present.

Because of the lymphatic supply to the retropharyngeal and parapharyngeal spaces, pharyngitis may result in an inflammation of these areas (Figure 9-1). The retropharyngeal space extends from the base of the skull to the mediastinum. The parapharyngeal space is located lateral to the pharynx and extends from the base of the skull to the hyoid bone. Pharyngitis that does not respond to antimicrobial therapy may cause either a retropharyngeal abscess or a parapharyngeal abscess. A patient with a retropharyngeal abscess complains of dyspnea and dysphagia and may have a palpable mass in the posterior pharyngeal wall. A patient with a parapharyngeal abscess may complain of pain in both the throat and the neck, may have edema at the angle of the mandible, and may have difficulty opening the mouth (trismus) as a result of inflammation and edema of the pterygoid muscles. Once the symptoms become evident, computed tomography (CT) scans may help identify the exact location of the abscess. Administration of intravenous antibiotics followed by surgical incision and drainage is the treatment of choice for both parapharyngeal and retropharyngeal abscesses.

> **Candidiasis is shown in Color Plate 15, page xii.**

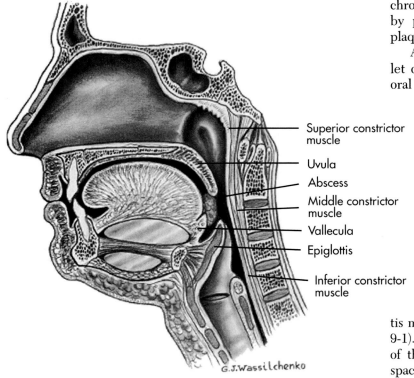

Superior constrictor muscle

Uvula

Abscess

Middle constrictor muscle

Vallecula

Epiglottis

Inferior constrictor muscle

G.J.Wassilchenko

FIGURE 9-1
Retropharyngeal abscess. (From Thompson.[71])

fection is becoming more common, a thorough history covering exposure to gonorrhea may alert the health care professional to request specific cultures for the organism, as well as additional tests for other sexually transmitted diseases.

Patients with viral pharyngitis may complain of a fever and diffuse sore throat, and vesicles may be present on the pharyngeal walls and tonsils. Infectious mononucleosis, caused by the Epstein-Barr virus, may also produce pharyngitis. Patients with mononucleosis may complain of sore throat, cervical lymphadenopathy, and fever, and exudate will be present on the pharyngeal walls and tonsils. The spleen may also become enlarged.

Fungal pharyngitis, especially candidiasis (thrush), can develop with prolonged use of antibiotics in an immunosuppressed patient, especially those who have the human immunodeficiency virus (HIV), who are receiving radiation therapy or chemotherapy, or who show

Tonsillitis

Tonsillitis is an inflammation of the palatine tonsils.

PATHOPHYSIOLOGY

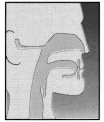

The palatine tonsils are part of a collection of lymphoid tissue in the oropharynx. Waldeyer's ring is a band of lymphoid tissue that includes the palatine tonsils, the lingual tonsils, the pharyngeal bands, the nasopharynx, and the adenoids. Blood is supplied to the palatine tonsils by the ascending and descending palatine arteries. The nerve supply is by way of the lesser palatine nerves, the pterygopalatine ganglion, and the glossopharyngeal nerve. Involvement of the glossopharyngeal nerve by way of the tympanic branch accounts for the referred ear pain commonly seen in patients with acute or chronic tonsillitis. The lymphatic drainage system from the tonsils goes to the upper deep cervical lymph nodes and then to the jugulodigastric lymph nodes.

Approximately 30% of tonsillitis cases are caused by group A beta-hemolytic streptococci or staphylococci. Less commonly, other organisms such as pneumococci, gram-negative organisms, or viruses may be the causative agents.

A patient with tonsillitis has red, swollen tonsils and yellow or white exudate, especially found in the crypts of the tonsils. The patient will complain of a dry throat, malaise, fever, a feeling of fullness in the throat, dysphagia, otalgia, and swollen lymph nodes in the upper part of the neck.

COMPLICATIONS

Retropharyngeal abscess
Parapharyngeal abscess
Glomerulonephritis
Subacute bacterial endocarditis

DIAGNOSTIC STUDIES AND FINDINGS

Diagnostic test	Findings
Throat culture	Causative organism

MEDICAL MANAGEMENT

SURGERY

Tonsillectomy: Removal of the tonsils

DRUG THERAPY

Antibiotics

Equine antitoxin (diphtheria)

Antifungal agents (candidiasis)

1 ASSESS

ASSESSMENT	OBSERVATIONS
Pain	Sore throat, difficulty swallowing
Infection	Elevated temperature; redness of pharyngeal wall; purulent exudate; vesicles on pharyngeal wall; cervical lymphadenopathy; edema of palate, uvula, and tonsils
Respiratory	Edema of palate, uvula, and tonsils; dyspnea; tachypnea
General	Malaise, dehydration

2 DIAGNOSE

NURSING DIAGNOSIS	SUBJECTIVE FINDINGS	OBJECTIVE FINDINGS
Pain related to infection	Complains of sore throat, earache, difficulty swallowing, and pain on swallowing	Grimaces when swallowing, looks pale, requests analgesics
Infection related to invasion by microorganisms or viruses	Complains of discomfort, foul taste in mouth, bad breath, general malaise, fever, and swollen glands	Uniformly infected pharynx with generalized redness of pharyngeal walls; fever; purulent exudate on tonsils and pharyngeal walls; edema of palate, uvula, and tonsils; cervical lymphadenopathy; vesicle formation on pharynx
Ineffective airway clearance related to edema	Complains of a foreign body sensation, feeling of fullness in the throat, and mouth breathing	Mouth breathing; edema of palate, uvula, and pharyngeal walls; fullness palpated in pharyngeal wall
Impaired swallowing related to edema and pain **High risk for fluid volume deficit** related to impaired swallowing.	Reports difficulty swallowing, pain on swallowing, and drooling	Grimaces when swallowing, drools, unable to swallow regular food

3 PLAN

Patient goals
1. The patient will have no pain and will be able to swallow.
2. The patient will have no signs of infection.
3. The patient will exhibit effective airway clearance.
4. The patient will maintain hydration.

4 IMPLEMENT

NURSING DIAGNOSIS	NURSING INTERVENTIONS	RATIONALE
Pain related to infection	Assess degree of patient's pain.	To determine need for analgesics.

NURSING DIAGNOSIS	NURSING INTERVENTIONS	RATIONALE
	Administer analgesics q4h, and assess their effectiveness.	To relieve pain and determine use of analgesics.
	Provide warm saline throat irrigations.	To soothe irritated pharynx and localize infection.
Infection related to invasion by microorganisms, viruses, or fungi	Obtain nursing history.	To detect exposure to gonorrhea, diphtheria, or immunosuppressive agents before culture.
	Assist with or perform throat culture as ordered.	To determine causative organism so that appropriate treatment can be prescribed.
	Administer medications as ordered.	Antibiotics and antifungal agents are the treatments to eliminate causative organism.
	Observe patient for adverse reaction to antibiotic (urticaria, dyspnea, shortness of breath, gastrointestinal upset).	Penicillin is the usual antibiotic of choice, but it may cause an allergic reaction.
	Monitor vital signs, especially temperature, q 4 h.	Elevated temperature indicates infection; a return to normal temperature indicates a response to therapy.
	Inform patient about need to finish entire course of antibiotic.	Failure to complete course of antibiotic may result in inadequate treatment, causing recurrent infection or abscess formation.
	Encourage bed rest or frequent rest periods; have patient avoid strenuous activity.	Infection lowers general body immunity; rest is necessary to restore resistance.
Ineffective airway clearance related to edema	Inspect oropharynx for edema.	Edema of palate and uvula may occur with acute pharyngitis, resulting in obstruction of airway; fullness of pharyngeal wall may indicate abscess.
	Increase humidification (use humidifier and encourage oral fluid intake).	Mouth breathing (caused by edema) results in dryness of mucous membranes.
	Apply lubricant to lips, and provide frequent oral hygiene.	To prevent dryness of lips and oral cavity from obligatory mouth breathing.
Impaired swallowing related to edema and pain	Assess patient's hydration status (measure intake and output; evaluate skin turgor and dryness).	Decreased oral intake (resulting from edema and pain) may cause dehydration; early detection of decreased fluid intake allows medical intervention.
High risk for fluid volume deficit related to impaired swallowing	Monitor blood parameters, and assess mucous membranes (oral cavity and lips).	To prevent problems and complications.
	Encourage oral fluid intake, and evaluate swallowing ability; if IV fluid replacement is necessary, monitor flow rate.	If patient has trouble swallowing, IV fluid replacement is necessary.

→ > >

5 EVALUATE

PATIENT OUTCOME	DATA INDICATING THAT OUTCOME IS REACHED
Patient shows no signs of infection thereby exhibiting effective airway clearance, normal swallowing, and adequate hydration.	Pharyngeal mucous membrane appears normal and has no purulent exudate; temperature and WBC are normal; no cervical lymphadenopathy is palpated.

PATIENT TEACHING

1. Explain to the patient the need to complete the entire prescribed course of antibiotics.
2. Teach the patient the symptoms of pharyngitis and tonsillitis, and warn her of the potential for complications; advise her to seek medical attention if symptoms reappear.
3. Instruct the patient to avoid smoking and use of alcohol, which may exacerbate symptoms.

Peritonsillar Abscess (Quinsy)

Peritonsillar abscess (quinsy) develops when purulent exudate forms between the tonsillar bed and the capsule around the tonsillar pillar. The condition usually is the result of inadequate treatment of tonsillitis.

PATHOPHYSIOLOGY

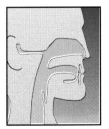

Peritonsillar abscess is the main complication of tonsillitis, especially in patients with chronic tonsillitis. The abscess usually is unilateral. The patient complains of both local and referred pain, and there is edema of the pharyngeal wall and tonsil, resulting in odynophagia, dysphagia, drooling, and inability to swallow. The patient also may have lymphadenopathy, trismus, an elevated temperature, and malaise.

A physical examination will show gross unilateral edema of the palate and anterior tonsillar pillar, with displacement of the tonsil downward and medially. The edema may displace the uvula toward the opposite side.

The treatment of choice for acute episodes of peritonsillar abscess is surgical incision and drainage or needle aspiration of the abscess followed by the administration of intravenous antibiotics. A tonsillectomy may be performed once the acute infection has subsided; however, many physicians advocate a tonsillectomy (quinsy tonsillectomy) during the episode.

Systemic complications include glomerulonephritis and subacute bacterial endocarditis with group A beta-hemolytic streptococci. Immediate treatment of tonsillitis with antibiotics is mandatory to prevent these conditions.

COMPLICATIONS

Aspiration	Glomerulonephritis
Parapharyngeal abscess	Subacute bacterial
Internal phlegmon	endocarditis
Dehydration	

DIAGNOSTIC STUDIES AND FINDINGS

Diagnostic test	Findings
Computed tomography (CT) scan	Abscess

MEDICAL MANAGEMENT

SURGERY

Needle aspiration of abscess

Incision and drainage of abscess

Tonsillectomy: Acute removal of tonsils or elective removal of tonsils after resolution of infection

DRUG THERAPY

Antibiotics

1 ASSESS

ASSESSMENT	OBSERVATIONS
Infection	Elevated temperature and WBC; sialorrhea; oral odor; cervical lymphadenopathy; and edema and redness of the oropharynx
Pain	Dysphagia, severe throat pain with otalgia, trismus, and guarding of neck
Respiratory	Stridor; cough; dyspnea; change in respiratory depth; tachypnea; and edema of pharynx, palate, and uvula

2 DIAGNOSE

NURSING DIAGNOSIS	SUBJECTIVE FINDINGS	OBJECTIVE FINDINGS
Infection related to invasion by microorganisms	Complains of fever, foul taste in mouth, bad breath, and discomfort; has swollen glands and muffled voice and recent history of tonsillitis	Elevated temperature and WBC, oral fetor, edema of pharynx and tonsil with displacement of uvula, cervical lymphadenopathy, characteristic "hot potato" voice
Pain related to abscess	Complains of pain in throat and ear, pain on swallowing, and difficulty opening mouth; has tender lymph nodes	Facial grimaces, guarding of neck, trismus
High risk for ineffective breathing pattern related to edema	Complains of fullness in throat, noisy breathing, rapid breathing, cough, and anxiety	Stridor, dyspnea, tachypnea, edema of oropharynx (especially with bilateral abscesses), anxiety, increased pulse

→ > >

NURSING DIAGNOSIS	SUBJECTIVE FINDINGS	OBJECTIVE FINDINGS
High risk for fluid volume deficit related to pain and edema	Complains of dry mouth, inability to swallow, pain on swallowing	Dry mucous membranes, poor skin turgor, tachycardia, hypotension, increased urine specific gravity, altered blood parameters (electrolyte imbalance, elevated Hb and Hct)

3 PLAN

Patient goals

1. The patient will have no signs of infection.
2. Complications will be minimized or avoided.
3. The patient will have no pain.

4. The patient will have no airway distress.
5. The patient will show no signs of dehydration.

4 IMPLEMENT

NURSING DIAGNOSIS	NURSING INTERVENTIONS	RATIONALE
Infection related to invasion by microorganisms	Assess oral cavity for edema, exudate, and drainage.	To determine extent of disease and response to treatment, and to detect spontaneous rupture of abscess.
	Monitor blood parameters and temperature (rectal or otic).	To determine response to therapy (temperature is not taken orally to avoid accidentally rupturing abscess).
	Administer antibiotics as ordered, and monitor for adverse effects.	IV antibiotics are the treatment of choice; therapy is most effective when blood levels of the antibiotic are constant.
	Encourage oral hygiene q 4 h; advise patient to avoid gargling.	To rid mouth of exudate and avoid inadvertent rupture of abscess.
Pain related to abscess	Monitor pain level and factors that increase pain.	To determine need for analgesics and to avoid circumstances that increase pain.
	Administer analgesics, and evaluate their effectiveness.	To minimize pain.
	Apply ice collar.	To reduce pain and edema.
	Help patient find a comfortable position by supporting head, neck, and shoulders.	Spasm of neck and shoulders increases pain caused by guarding posture.
High risk for ineffective breathing pattern related to edema	Assess respiratory rate and depth and breath sounds.	To detect ineffective breathing.
	Monitor edema of oropharynx.	Increased edema, especially with bilateral peritonsillar abscess, can compromise breathing.

NURSING DIAGNOSIS	NURSING INTERVENTIONS	RATIONALE
	Elevate head of bed.	May decrease edema and prevent aspiration of purulent drainage if spontaneous rupture occurs.
	Have oral suction equipment available at bedside.	To suction oral cavity if spontaneous rupture occurs, preventing aspiration of purulent drainage.
	Have emergency equipment available at bedside (endotracheal intubation set, emergency tracheostomy set).	For emergency management of airway distress.
High risk for fluid volume deficit related to pain and edema	Administer analgesics.	Severe pain on swallowing is one cause of fluid deficit.
	Encourage cool, bland liquids, nonacidic juices; popsicles; fruit; gelatin	To minimize discomfort on swallowing.
	Observe for signs of dehydration (evaluate skin turgor and mucous membranes; monitor intake and output; monitor and record vital signs).	Prevention or early detection of dehydration helps prevent complications.
	Administer IV fluids as ordered.	If swallowing becomes too difficult, IV fluids will be needed to prevent dehydration.

5 EVALUATE

PATIENT OUTCOME	DATA INDICATING THAT OUTCOME IS REACHED
Patient shows no signs of infection.	Edema has subsided; temperature and WBC are normal.
Patient has minimal or no pain.	Pain relieved with analgesics; no swallowing difficulty.
Patient has normal breathing.	Respiratory rate and depth are within normal limits; edema has subsided.
Patient is able to swallow without difficulty.	Eats normal food; patient exhibits normal skin turgor.

PATIENT TEACHING

1. Encourage the patient to complete antibiotic therapy, even after symptoms have subsided.
2. Review the signs and symptoms of peritonsillar abscess. Encourage the patient to seek immediate medical attention if symptoms recur.
3. Prepare the patient for a tonsillectomy once the acute infection has subsided.

Adenoid Hypertrophy

Adenoid hypertrophy is enlargement of the adenoid tissue.

PATHOPHYSIOLOGY

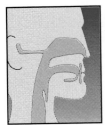

The adenoids, or pharyngeal tonsils, are areas of lymphoid tissue in the nasopharynx. At birth the adenoids are very small; however, they continue to enlarge as a result of chronic infection. Symptoms of adenoid hypertrophy may include mouth breathing and snoring (because of the inability to breathe through the nose); otitis media (resulting from blockage or swelling of the eustachian tube orifice); hyponasal or hypernasal speech, and adenoid facies (from chronic nasal obstruction and mouth breathing), which is characterized by a pinched appearance of the nose, open mouth, an inverted lower lip, and a short, protruding upper lip. Recurrent infection of the adenoids results in adenoid hypertrophy and is treated with antibiotics. If medical management is not effective, adenoidectomy is indicated.

COMPLICATIONS

Otitis media
Obstructive sleep apnea
Right-sided heart failure
Cor pulmonale

DIAGNOSTIC STUDIES AND FINDINGS

Diagnostic test	Findings
Nasopharyngoscopy	Lymphoid hypertrophy in nasopharynx
Lateral neck and naso-pharynx x-rays	Lymphoid hypertrophy in nasopharynx

MEDICAL MANAGEMENT

SURGERY

Adenoidectomy: Removal of adenoids

DRUG THERAPY

Antibiotics: to treat infection

Decongestants: to decrease edema

---

1 ASSESS

ASSESSMENT	OBSERVATIONS
Respiratory	Obstruction to nasal breathing, mouth breathing, sleep apnea, snoring, rhinorrhea
Ear	Recurrent ear infection (otitis media with effusion)

2 DIAGNOSE

NURSING DIAGNOSIS	SUBJECTIVE FINDINGS	OBJECTIVE FINDINGS
Ineffective breathing pattern related to nasal obstruction	Complains of difficulty breathing through nose, mouth breathing, snoring, and sleep problems	Abnormal tissue in nasopharynx, mouth breathing, documented breath-holding episodes during sleep, snoring during sleep, hyponasal speech

NURSING DIAGNOSIS	SUBJECTIVE FINDINGS	OBJECTIVE FINDINGS
Sleep pattern disturbance related to sleep apnea	Complains of snoring, sleep disturbance, daytime sleepiness, and fatigue	Snoring, documented apneic episodes with decreased oxygen saturation
High risk for infection related to nasal and/or eustachian tube obstruction	Complains of nasal stuffiness, nasal discharge, bad breath, frequent ear infections, fever, and hearing loss	Abnormal tissue in nasopharynx, purulent rhinorrhea, halitosis, otitis media with effusion, elevated temperature, hearing loss, flat tympanometric pattern

3 PLAN

Patient goals

1. The patient will have a clear nasal airway.
2. The patient will have restful sleep with normal oxygen saturation.
3. The patient will have no infection.
4. The patient will have no complications from adenoid hypertrophy or infection.

4 IMPLEMENT

NURSING DIAGNOSIS	NURSING INTERVENTIONS	RATIONALE
Ineffective breathing pattern related to nasal obstruction	Elevate head of bed.	To minimize nasal edema.
	Increase humidification.	To thin secretions.
Sleep pattern disturbance related to sleep apnea	Evaluate and document sleep apnea and snoring (question patient about breath-holding during sleep; tape-record sleep sessions; arrange sleep evaluation studies with documentation of oxygen saturation).	To determine presence and severity of sleep disturbance
High risk for infection related to nasal and/or eustachian tube obstruction	Administer antibiotic and/or decongestant as ordered.	Adenoiditis and otitis media with effusion initially are treated with antibiotics and decongestants.

5 EVALUATE

PATIENT OUTCOME	DATA INDICATING THAT OUTCOME IS REACHED
Nasal airway is clear.	Nasal breathing has been restored; patient does not use mouth breathing; edema in nasopharynx has been reduced; there is no purulent discharge in nose or nasopharynx.
Patient has restful sleep with no decrease in oxygen saturation.	Snoring has subsided; patient has no apneic episodes; oxygen saturation is >90%; daytime somnolence has been eliminated.

→ > >

PATIENT OUTCOME	DATA INDICATING THAT OUTCOME IS REACHED
Patient has no evidence of infection.	There is no purulent drainage; patient's hearing has returned to normal; tympanic membrane is not retracted.
Patient has no complications.	There are no signs of infection; nasal breathing is restored; no evidence of sleep apnea; no symptoms of cardiac dysfunction.

PATIENT TEACHING

1. Instruct the patient and family about possible complications of adenoid hypertrophy (e.g., right-sided heart failure, cor pulmonale).
2. Teach the patient the signs of infection and when to seek medical attention.
3. Encourage the patient to complete the entire course of antibiotics; warn him about the potential side effects of antibiotics and decongestants.
4. Reinforce information about surgical interventions (adenoidectomy, myringotomy with tubes).

Dysphonia

> **Close-up views of vocal cord polyps, nodules, and paralysis appear in Color Plates 16, 17, and 18 on page xii.**

Dysphonia refers to any abnormal speech.

PATHOPHYSIOLOGY

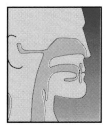

Speech is produced when air flows from the lungs, through the subglottis, and then through the glottis, causing the vocal folds to vibrate. The amount of vibration is related to the tension of the vocal cords. Anything that alters the tension or motion of the vocal cords causes a speech abnormality.

Laryngitis

Laryngitis is an inflammation of the vocal cords. The inflammatory response causes edema of the vocal cords which restricts movement. Causes of laryngitis include vocal abuse, smoking, upper respiratory infection, and reflux esophagitis (gastroesophageal reflux).

Vocal Cord Paresis and Paralysis

Partial paralysis of the vocal cords (paresis) or total paralysis of the cords results when movement is lost in one or both vocal cords. The condition can be caused by injury or inflammation of the vagus nerve, most commonly the recurrent laryngeal nerve or, less often, the superior laryngeal nerve. The left recurrent laryngeal nerve follows a longer course, from its exit at the base of the skull, through the neck, and into the mediastinum before returning to the neck and innervating the larynx. The right recurrent laryngeal nerve passes around the subclavian artery, located below the clavicle, before innervating the larynx. The longer course of the left recurrent laryngeal nerve puts it at greater risk of injury. Paresis or paralysis of the vocal cords affects the amplitude and velocity of airflow through the cords. The vocal cords close slowly and with less force, causing a leak of unaltered air; this produces the breathy quality to the voice that is characteristic of unilateral vocal cord paralysis.

Spasmodic Dysphonia

Spasmodic dysphonia is a hyperfunctional neuromuscular disorder. The patient is unable to maintain uniform vibration of the vocal cords, which gives the voice a spastic quality.

Presbylaryngeus

Dysphonia may also be seen in older people, as a condition known as presbylaryngeus. Presbylaryngeus causes a loss of muscle tone, resulting in weakened closure or bowing of the vocal cords. The voice produced by presbylaryngeus is lower in volume and has an audible escape of air.

Vocal Cord Lesions

Lesions of the vocal cord cause irregular vibrations of the cords. In addition, any abnormality on a vocal cord prevents the cords from touching, resulting in air escape and a hoarse quality to the voice.

Vocal cord polyps are edematous mucous membrane attached to the vocal cord. Pedunculated polyps may hang under the vocal cord and cause intermittent symptoms (hoarseness, breathy voice), whereas broad-based polyps on the cords produce constant symptoms. Vocal cord polyps may be caused by chronic voice abuse, allergies, heavy smoking, or acute infection.

Vocal cord nodules, also known as singer's nodules, are caused by chronic voice abuse. These nodules are benign growths that resemble calluses on the vocal cords. Since they occur on the free margin of the vocal cords, they prevent the cords from touching, thereby producing a hoarse, breathy voice.

COMPLICATIONS

Aspiration pneumonia
Airway distress

DIAGNOSTIC STUDIES AND FINDINGS

Diagnostic test	Findings
Indirect laryngoscopy	Vocal cord abnormality
Videostroboscopy (**to observe vocal cord vibration during phonation**) (Videostroboscopy is the use of fiberoptic laryngoscopy attached to a videotape to record actual vocal cord motion)	Abnormal vibrations
Electromyography (**to determine innervation of vocal cord**)	Poor movement
Computed tomography (**CT**) scan (**to determine cause of vocal cord paresis or paralysis**)	Tumor, aneurysm along course of recurrent laryngeal nerve

MEDICAL MANAGEMENT

SURGERY

Direct laryngoscopy with microlaryngoscopy: To visualize vocal cords.

Excision of nodules or polyps with or without laser: To remove vocal lesion.

Injection of Gelfoam or Teflon into vocal cord: To provide bulk to paralyzed cord.

Thyroplasty: Insertion of stent to reapproximate vocal cord.

DRUG THERAPY

Antacids: To treat gastroesophageal reflux by neutralizing acid

H$_2$ inhibitors: To treat gastroesophageal reflux by reducing acid

Antibiotics: To treat infection

Systemic steroids: To reduce swelling

Botulinum injection: To paralyze spastic movement

1   ASSESS

ASSESSMENT	OBSERVATIONS
Communication	Dysphonia (hoarseness, aphonia, breathy quality to voice, huskiness)
Respiratory	Dyspnea; shortness of breath; thick, tenacious secretions; throat clearing; altered respiratory rate; cough; restlessness; aspiration on swallowing; and rhonchi and/or rales upon auscultation

2   DIAGNOSE

NURSING DIAGNOSIS	SUBJECTIVE FINDINGS	OBJECTIVE FINDINGS
Impaired verbal communication related to vocal cord abnormality	Complains of change in voice pattern	Hoarseness, dysphonia, aphonia; edema, redness of vocal cords; paresis or paralysis of vocal cord; spastic movement of vocal cords; lesion on vocal cord
High risk for ineffective airway clearance related to vocal cord abnormality	Complains of dyspnea, shortness of breath, thick mucous secretions, frequent throat clearing	Edema of larynx, dyspnea, thick secretions, stridor, decrease in breath sounds, altered rate and depth of respirations, nasal flaring, abnormal blood gas (ABG) measurements
High risk for aspiration related to vocal cord paresis or paralysis	Reports coughing when swallowing	Aspiration when swallowing, rales or rhonchi upon auscultation

3   PLAN

Patient goals
1. The patient will regain a normal speaking voice.
2. The patient will understand the causes of her dysphonia and ways to prevent it.
3. The patient will have no signs of infection.
4. The patient will have no airway distress.

4   IMPLEMENT

NURSING DIAGNOSIS	NURSING INTERVENTIONS	RATIONALE
Impaired verbal communication related to vocal cord abnormality	Assess factors that may have contributed to dysphonia (vocal cord abuse, smoking, upper respiratory infection, exposure to noxious fumes, gastroesophageal reflux).	To teach patient how to prevent recurrence of dysphonia.
	Monitor voice use (range, pitch, abuse).	To identify problem areas that may contribute to dysphonia.

NURSING DIAGNOSIS	NURSING INTERVENTIONS	RATIONALE
	Encourage breathing and speech exercises suggested by speech pathologist.	Chronic dysphonia may result in abnormal speech patterns, which should be assessed by a speech pathologist; proper use of speech and breathing patterns and exercises must be practiced.
	Encourage voice rest; provide alternative communication aids during voice rest.	Laryngeal edema caused by inflammation or voice abuse responds to voice rest.
	Tell patient to avoid whispering during voice rest.	Whispering causes movement of cords and does not provide voice rest.
	Provide increased humidification (humidifier, steam inhalation).	To thin tenacious secretions, allow for easier removal of secretions, and promote comfort.
	If gastroesophageal reflux is a cause, promote antireflux activity (elevate head of bed on blocks; instruct patient to avoid eating or drinking for 3 hours before going to bed; instruct her to avoid caffeine, smoking, peppermint, chocolate, alcohol, and other foods and drinks that produce acid; if she is overweight, encourage her to lose weight; have her avoid tight-fitting clothing).	To reduce acid production and prevent reflux of gastric acid, which reduces chronic irritation of larynx.
	Have patient take antacids between meals and at bedtime.	To neutralize acid.
	If these measures fail, H_2 inhibitors may be used.	To minimize production of acid.
	Encourage referral to gastroenterologist.	If noninvasive measures do not prevent symptoms, additional testing and treatment may be required.
	Instruct patient in proper use and adverse effects of medications, if indicated (antibiotics, steroids, mucolytic agents).	If dysphonia is caused by an infection, antibiotics may be prescribed; patient should complete entire course. If edema is substantial and voice use is mandatory, a short course of steroids, tapered over 5 days, may be used. Mucolytic agents may be used to thin tenacious secretions.
High risk for ineffective airway clearance related to vocal cord abnormality	Assess breath sounds, ABGs, pulse oximetry level, and rate and depth of respirations.	To determine whether breathing is adequate.
	Increase humidification.	To thin secretions and promote comfort.
	Elevate head of bed.	To minimize edema.

NURSING DIAGNOSIS	NURSING INTERVENTIONS	RATIONALE
	Encourage bed rest; have patient avoid strenuous activity.	To minimize oxygen use until airway edema subsides.
	Keep emergency equipment available (endotracheal intubation set, emergency tracheostomy tray).	For immediate use if patient develops acute airway distress.
	Provide ice collar, throat irrigations, and cold fluids.	To promote comfort.
	Instruct patient to avoid crowds and people with upper respiratory infections (especially if patient has bilateral vocal cord paralysis).	Midline bilateral vocal cord paralysis provides only a minimal airway; any additional edema may result in acute airway distress.
High risk for aspiration related to vocal cord paresis or paralyses	Urge patient to avoid thin liquids and to eat foods with more substance that can be controlled during the swallowing process.	Thin liquids are aspirated more often than thicker, more solid foods.

5 EVALUATE

PATIENT OUTCOME	DATA INDICATING THAT OUTCOME IS REACHED
Patient has a normal speaking voice.	Voice will return to normal quality.
Patient understands causes of dysphonia and ways to prevent it.	Patient can identify causative factors and discusses plans to change her environment to prevent recurrence.
Patient has no signs of infection.	Temperature and WBC are normal; discomfort has been alleviated.
Patient has no airway distress.	Pulse oximetry is >90%; respiratory rate and depth are adequate; patient has no dyspnea, shortness of breath, or stridor.

PATIENT TEACHING

1. Instruct the patient to avoid smoking, smoke-filled environment, and noxious fumes.
2. Help the patient identify causative factors and develop a plan to avoid those causes; include appropriate referrals (e.g., smoking cessation program).
3. Encourage follow-up medical visits as indicated (physician, speech pathologist or voice clinic, gastroenterologist).
4. Encourage the patient to increase environmental humidity, especially during upper respiratory infections and during dry seasons or in dry environments.
5. Teach the patient how to take drugs properly; instruct her in the side effects to watch for.
6. Encourage the patient to rest her voice and avoid abusing it.
7. Encourage the patient to avoid crowds and people with upper respiratory infections, as well as strenuous activity (especially patients with bilateral vocal cord paralysis), because these can increase airway edema, resulting in airway distress.

Ludwig's Angina

Ludwig's angina is an infection or cellulitis of the submental, sublingual, and submandibular spaces (Figure 9-2).

PATHOPHYSIOLOGY

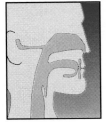

Ludwig's angina is an infection of dental origin. Trauma, dental extraction, and periapical abscess or periodontal disease around the mandibular teeth may cause infection to spread directly from the teeth and bone into the submental, sublingual, and submandibular spaces. The infection is caused by mixed oral flora, including oral anaerobes. Dental infection that goes untreated or dental infection in an immunocompromised patient is more likely to result in Ludwig's angina.

COMPLICATION

Airway distress

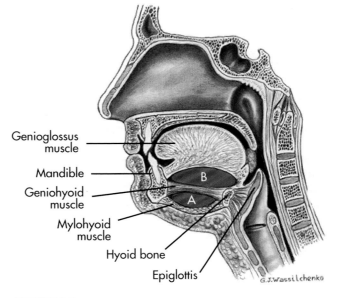

FIGURE 9-2
Ludwig's angina. *A* and *B* indicate spaces in which infection may start. (From Thompson.[71])

DIAGNOSTIC STUDIES AND FINDINGS

Diagnostic test	Findings
Computed tomography (CT) scan	Abscess in submental, sublingual, or submaxillary spaces

MEDICAL MANAGEMENT

SURGERY

Incision and drainage of abscess: to remove purulent abscess and reduce swelling

DRUG THERAPY

Penicillin, Clindamycin, Cephalosporins: antibiotics of choice to treat infection

Analgesics: to control pain

1 ASSESS

ASSESSMENT	OBSERVATIONS
Oral cavity	Pain, tenderness, infection of mandibular teeth; swelling of floor of mouth; elevation of tongue; trismus; muffled voice; dysphagia; inability to swallow saliva; drooling
Respiratory	Dyspnea, stridor; muffled voice; tachypnea; shortness of breath; lowered partial pressure of oxygen (P_{O_2}); restlessness; anxiety
Infection	Elevated temperature and WBC, halitosis

2 DIAGNOSE

NURSING DIAGNOSIS	SUBJECTIVE FINDINGS	OBJECTIVE FINDINGS
High risk for infection related to invasion of soft tissue by pathogens	Complains of fever and malaise; has history of dental infection or trauma; swelling visible under tongue and neck; has bad breath and difficulty opening mouth	Elevated temperature and WBC; edema of floor of mouth, tongue, and neck; inflammation or trauma of mandibular teeth; mouth odor; trismus
Ineffective breathing pattern related to edema	Complains of shortness of breath	Dyspnea, decreased PO_2, restlessness, anxiety, tachypnea, shallow breathing
Pain (acute) related to infection	Complains of dental, neck, and mouth pain	Facial grimaces, tachypnea, tachycardia, elevated BP
Altered nutrition: less than body requirements related to edema and pain	Complains of inability to swallow or pain on swallowing, drooling, weight loss, and fatigue	Edema of floor of mouth and tongue, inability to handle saliva, weight loss, abnormal blood parameters, inability to swallow
Anxiety related to upper airway edema	Complains of nervousness	Increased pulse and respiratory rate, tense or anxious appearance, short attention span

3 PLAN

Patient goals

1. The infection will resolve without complications.
2. The patient's pain will be relieved.
3. The patient will have no respiratory distress.
4. The patient will maintain hydration and nutritional parameters.
5. The patient's anxiety will be relieved.

4 IMPLEMENT

NURSING DIAGNOSIS	NURSING INTERVENTIONS	RATIONALE
High risk for infection related to invasion of soft tissue by pathogens	Assess temperature and monitor laboratory values.	To detect infection and determine response to treatment.
	Administer antibiotics as ordered and observe for side effects.	IV antibiotics are initial treatment for infection.

NURSING DIAGNOSIS	NURSING INTERVENTIONS	RATIONALE
	Perform oral hygiene q 4 h with hydrogen peroxide and water or saline.	To provide comfort and minimize oral organisms.
	Administer antipyretics as ordered.	To reduce fever.
Ineffective breathing pattern related to edema	Observe for signs of airway obstruction (restlessness, shortness of breath, stridor, dyspnea, decreased oxygen level via pulse oximetry, tachypnea, tachycardia).	Early diagnosis of airway problems prevents acute airway distress and death; allow for early surgical intervention (i.e., endotracheal intubation or tracheostomy).
	Suction oral secretions gently.	To remove excess saliva and to prevent drooling and aspiration of secretions.
	Have emergency endotracheal intubation and tracheostomy sets available at bedside.	To permit emergency measures at bedside in case of acute respiratory distress.
	Elevate head of bed.	To help minimize edema and to prevent aspiration of secretions.
	Provide supplemental oxygen with humidification.	To thin secretions, prevent dryness, maintain oxygenation, and enhance comfort.
Pain (acute) related to infection	Assess degree of pain.	To determine need for analgesics.
	Administer analgesic, and evaluate effectiveness.	To relieve pain and improve comfort.
Altered nutrition: less than body requirements related to edema and pain	Monitor oral intake and output.	To assess hydration status.
	Monitor blood parameters (i.e., serum albumin, serum ferritin, leukocyte count, Hb, and Hct).	To assess nutritional status.
	Provide IV fluids as ordered.	To prevent dehydration.
	Assess swallowing ability, especially with foods of various consistencies.	To allow oral feedings if possible.
	Weigh daily, and record weight.	To detect any weight loss, allowing prompt intervention.
	Perform caloric assessment; consult with nutritionist.	To ensure adequate caloric intake.
Anxiety related to upper airway edema	Explain all procedures, progress, and areas of concern.	To ease anxiety and patient's fear of unknown; allow patient to participate in his care by having him alert medical personnel of increase in symptoms.
	Offer consistent reassurance; respond to patient's needs, and check him frequently.	To reduce anxiety.

→ › ›

5   EVALUATE

PATIENT OUTCOME	DATA INDICATING THAT OUTCOME IS REACHED
Infection has resolved.	Temperature and WBC have returned to normal, and edema has subsided.
Patient's anxiety has been reduced.	Dental disease has been treated effectively; patient understands causes and symptoms of Ludwig's angina and the need for medical follow-up.

PATIENT TEACHING

1. Explain the need for prophylactic dental care (i.e., prevention and treatment of dental caries, gingivitis, periodontal disease, and dental abscesses).

2. Encourage the patient to finish entire course of antibiotics.

Epiglottitis

Epiglottitis is an infection of the supraglottic larynx.

PATHOPHYSIOLOGY

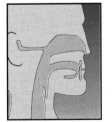

The supraglottis includes the epiglottis, aryepiglottic folds, and false vocal cords. Epiglottitis usually is caused by *Haemophilus influenzae*, type B, and less commonly by pneumococci, streptococci, or a virus. Epiglottitis is seen more often in the winter. Patients may have a positive result on blood culture, indicating systemic disease.

COMPLICATION

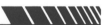

Respiratory arrest

DIAGNOSTIC STUDIES AND FINDINGS

Diagnostic test	Findings
Indirect or direct laryngoscopy	Red epiglottis, edema of supraglottis

MEDICAL MANAGEMENT

SURGERY

Nasotracheal intubation; Tracheostomy: To relieve upper airway distress

DRUG THERAPY

Antibiotics: Ampicillin, chloramphenicol, moxalactam—to treat infection

Steroids: To reduce inflammation and edema

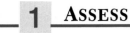
1 ASSESS

ASSESSMENT	OBSERVATIONS
Respiratory	Inspiratory stridor, upright posture, drooling, thi
Infection	Elevated temperature and WBC, positive res throat

2 DIAGNOSE

NURSING DIAGNOSIS	SUBJECTIVE FINDINGS	OBJECTIVE FINDINGS
Ineffective breathing pattern related to infection and edema	Complains of difficulty in breathing and noisy breathing	Dyspnea, inspiratory stridor, sits upright to breathe, history of acute onset, edema of larynx with cherry red appearance
High risk for infection related to invasion of upper airway by microorganisms	Complains of fever, rapid onset of infection and related symptoms, difficulty swallowing, drooling, thick secretions	Elevated temperature and WBC; edema of supraglottis with inflammation, resulting in difficulty swallowing; presence of thick secretions

3 PLAN

Patient goals

1. The patient will not have respiratory distress.
2. The upper airway edema will subside without complications.
3. The infection will resolve.

4 IMPLEMENT

NURSING DIAGNOSIS	NURSING INTERVENTIONS	RATIONALE
Ineffective breathing pattern related to infection and edema	Assess airway (monitor breath sounds; observe respiratory rate, depth, and effort; monitor oxygen concentration via pulse oximetry; monitor arterial blood gases [ABGs]).	To detect early changes in breathing, for early management and prevention of acute airway distress.
	Provide supplemental oxygen.	To improve oxygenation.
	Increase humidification (humidified oxygen or air, bedside humidifier, increased fluid intake).	To thin secretions and improve patient's comfort.

➜ ❯ ❯

	NURSING INTERVENTIONS	RATIONALE
	Place patient in high Fowler's position.	To reduce edema, improve comfort, facilitate breathing, and facilitate swallowing (to prevent aspiration).
	Keep emergency equipment available.	For immediate intervention in event of acute obstruction.
k for infec- lated to inva- f upper airway icroorganisms	Monitor temperature and WBC.	To determine progression of infection.
	Administer antibiotics, antipyretics, and steroids as ordered.	To treat infection and to reduce fever and edema.
	Increase fluid intake (oral fluids, parenteral fluids).	To thin secretions, reduce fever, and maintain hydration.

5 EVALUATE

PATIENT OUTCOME	DATA INDICATING THAT OUTCOME IS REACHED
Infection has resolved.	Temperature and WBC are normal; supraglottic edema has subsided; mucous membrane appears normal; secretions are thin and clear.
No airway distress is experienced.	Patient has a normal breathing pattern.
Upper airway edema subsides.	Supraglottic edema has subsided.

PATIENT TEACHING

1. Instruct the patient to seek medical attention if symptoms recur (i.e., shortness of breath elevated temperature, difficulty swallowing).
2. Instruct the patient to increase humidification by using a bedside humidifier or steam inhalation and by increasing her fluid intake.
3. Instruct the patient to complete the entire course of prescribed antibiotics.

Foreign Body in Upper Aerodigestive Tract

A **foreign body** is the presence of any object that is not common to the upper aerodigestive tract.

PATHOPHYSIOLOGY

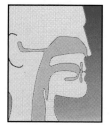 Both children and adults can accidentally ingest a foreign body (only foreign bodies in adults are addressed in this text). Foreign bodies in the upper aerodigestive tract are most frequently seen in the area of the tonsil, pyriform sinus, larynx, and esophagus, or in the main bronchus (the right main stem bronchus is affected more often than the left). Patients generally report eating food that may contain a bone or foreign particle, most commonly fish or chicken, which contain fine bones. Also, a large piece of food may lodge in the esophagus or be aspirated into the airway.

COMPLICATIONS

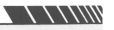

Infection
Airway distress

DIAGNOSTIC STUDIES AND FINDINGS

Diagnostic test	Findings
Computed tomography (CT) scan	Foreign body, edema
Barium swallow	Foreign body, edema
Soft tissue x-rays	Foreign body, edema

MEDICAL MANAGEMENT

Heimlich maneuver (Figure 9-3)

SURGERY

Surgical removal by way of direct laryngoscopy, bronchoscopy, or esophagoscopy

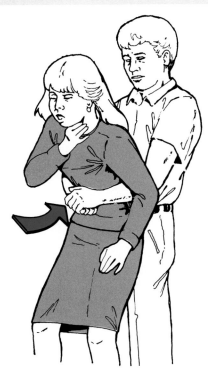
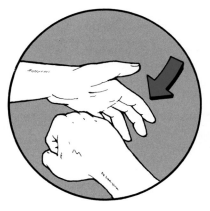
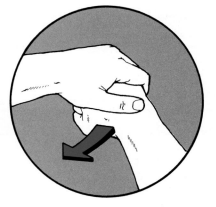

FIGURE 9-3
Heimlich maneuver.

1 ASSESS

ASSESSMENT	OBSERVATIONS
Respiratory function	Ineffective breathing, inability to vocalize, airway distress, hemoptysis
Swallowing	Recently swallowed foreign body (i.e., chicken, fish, unknown object), inability to swallow, drooling of saliva, pain and foreign body sensation in throat, edema

2 DIAGNOSE

NURSING DIAGNOSIS	SUBJECTIVE FINDINGS	OBJECTIVE FINDINGS
Ineffective breathing pattern related to foreign body in airway	Demonstrates international distress signal, unable to speak, difficulty breathing, coughing and spitting blood	Ineffective breathing, unable to vocalize, hemoptysis
Impaired swallowing related to obstruction by food and edema from trauma of foreign body	Complains of pain, difficulty swallowing, drooling, inability to swallow saliva, sore throat	Unable to swallow, drooling, edema of oropharynx and esophagus
Anxiety related to breathing difficulty	Appears nervous and anxious; expresses fear	Restlessness, frightened look on face, increased diaphoresis, tachycardia, tachypnea

3 PLAN

Patient goals

1. The foreign body will be removed without complications.

2. The patient will not develop a postremoval infection.

4 IMPLEMENT

NURSING DIAGNOSIS	NURSING INTERVENTIONS	RATIONALE
Ineffective breathing pattern related to foreign body in airway	Instruct patient to try to speak.	To determine degree of airway obstruction and institute appropriate treatment; if patient can speak, partial obstruction is suspected; if no speech is possible, obstruction is total.
	For partial obstruction: instruct patient to cough deeply. If patient needs assistance, have patient lean over table, loosen constricting clothes, and have him cough deeply.	To remove obstruction and restore airway.

NURSING DIAGNOSIS	NURSING INTERVENTIONS	RATIONALE
	For total obstruction: perform Heimlich maneuver; repeat if necessary.	To remove obstruction and restore airway.
	After removal of the foreign body, assess respiratory rate and depth, breath sounds, and ABGs; pulse oximetry should be >90%.	To determine whether airway has been cleared and oxygenation is adequate.
Impaired swallowing related to obstruction by food and edema from trauma of foreign body	Keep patient NPO.	If removal of foreign body is required, NPO status will be necessary to prevent aspiration during procedure.
	If foreign body is partially obstructive or has been passed, force oral fluids.	To rehydrate patient, thin secretions, and force foreign body to pass.
	Administer topical or systemic analgesics before meals as ordered.	To relieve pain and improve swallowing.
	Consult with dietitian.	To determine food consistencies with adequate caloric intake.
	Place patient in high Fowler's position.	To decrease edema, facilitate swallowing, and minimize aspiration.
Anxiety related to breathing difficulty	Explain all procedures, remain with patient, and offer reassurance.	To allay anxiety.

5 EVALUATE

PATIENT OUTCOME	DATA INDICATING THAT OUTCOME IS REACHED
Foreign body has been removed without complications.	Normal breathing has been restored, patient can speak, and swallowing is normal.
Patient will not develop a post-removal infection.	Temperature and WBC within normal limits; no discomfort in swallowing or breathing.

PATIENT TEACHING

1. Instruct the patient and family in proper use of the Heimlich maneuver (see Figure 9-3).
2. Instruct the patient to seek medical attention if symptoms of shortness of breath, difficulty swallowing, or infection occur.
3. Review dietary considerations (i.e., eat soft, bland foods; drink lots of fluids, and be sure to get an adequate caloric intake until swelling has subsided).

Zenker's Diverticulum

Zenker's diverticulum is a herniation of mucosa and submucosa through a defect in the posterior pharyngeal muscular wall, creating a pouch or sac.

PATHOPHYSIOLOGY

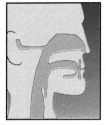

The exact cause of Zenker's diverticulum is unknown; however, many theories exist. One common theory is that a weakened area develops in the pharyngeal wall above the cricopharyngeus muscle. The cricopharyngeus muscle normally is in a state of tonic contraction, but during the swallowing process, it relaxes and pressures decrease. Patients with a weakened area and abnormally high pressure may develop a Zenker's diverticulum, or herniation of the mucosa, with increased pressures. The two most frequent causes of Zenker's diverticulum are irritation of the muscle caused by gastroesophageal reflux and neurologic abnormalities.

Zenker's diverticulum is most commonly seen in the elderly, with most patients ranging from 60 to 90 years of age. Men tend to be affected more often than women.

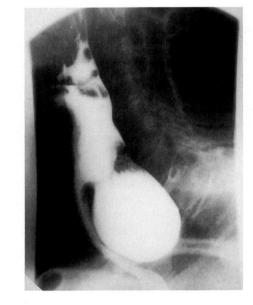

FIGURE 9-4
Barium esophagogram demonstrating Zenker's diverticulum.

COMPLICATIONS

Aspiration
Recurrent pneumonia
Lung abscess

DIAGNOSTIC STUDIES AND FINDINGS

Diagnostic test	Findings
Barium esophagogram (Figure 9-4)	Prominent cricopharyngeus muscle, herniations of mucosa, diverticulum

MEDICAL MANAGEMENT

SURGERY

Cricopharyngeal myotomy: Cutting of cricopharyngeus muscle (sufficient for small diverticula).

Cricopharyngeal myotomy with excision of diverticulum: Removal of pouch (recommended for larger Zenker's diverticula).

Cricopharyngeal myotomy with diverticulopexy: Suspending pouch for drainage (recommended for larger Zenker's diverticula).

1 ASSESS

ASSESSMENT	OBSERVATIONS
Respiratory	Recurrent aspiration, pneumonia, labored breathing
Gastrointestinal	Foreign body sensation, local discomfort, regurgitation of undigested food, dysphagia, hypersalivation

2 DIAGNOSE

NURSING DIAGNOSIS	SUBJECTIVE FINDINGS	OBJECTIVE FINDINGS
High risk for aspiration related to regurgitation of undigested food, saliva	Complains of increased mucus production, coughing, and vomiting of undigested food	Increased mucus, productive cough, rales, rhonchi, regurgitation of undigested food
High risk for infection related to aspiration of food, secretions collected in diverticulum	Complains of fever and weakness	Elevated temperature and WBC, malaise

3 PLAN

Patient goals

1. The patient will understand how to minimize chances of aspiration.
2. The patient will not develop pneumonia.
3. The patient's airway will be clear.

4 IMPLEMENT

NURSING DIAGNOSIS	NURSING INTERVENTIONS	RATIONALE
High risk for aspiration related to regurgitation of undigested food, saliva	Instruct patient to avoid eating for 3-4 hours before going to bed.	To prevent regurgitation of food, with resulting aspiration during sleep.
	Instruct patient to sleep with head of bed elevated.	To minimize aspiration of food collected in diverticulum and to improve breathing.
High risk for infection related to aspiration of food, secretions collected in diverticulum	Encourage deep breathing and coughing.	To aerate lungs and remove secretions from lungs.
	Monitor temperature and blood parameters.	To detect development of pulmonary infection.

→ ❯ ❯

NURSING DIAGNOSIS	NURSING INTERVENTIONS	RATIONALE
	Monitor chest x-ray.	To determine extent and location of pneumonia.
	Administer antibiotics as ordered.	To prevent and treat pneumonia.
	Force fluids.	To reduce temperature and prevent dehydration.
	Administer antipyretics as indicated.	To reduce fever.

5 EVALUATE

PATIENT OUTCOME	DATA INDICATING THAT OUTCOME IS REACHED
Aspiration is minimized.	Patient understands methods to prevent aspiration and shows no signs of pneumonia.
Patient has no symptoms of pneumonia.	Temperature and WBC are normal.
Airway is patent.	Breathing is normal; patient has no dyspnea, rales, or rhonchi.

PATIENT TEACHING

1. Teach the patient deep-breathing and coughing techniques.
2. Teach the patient and family the early signs of pneumonia (fever, shortness of breath, coughing that produces phlegm): instruct patient to notify physician if these symptoms develop.
3. Advise the patient to sleep with the head of the bed elevated.
4. Encourage the patient to avoid eating for 3-4 hours before going to bed.

CHAPTER 10

Therapeutic Interventions for Disorders of the Oral Cavity, Oropharynx, and Larynx

Tonsillectomy

Evaluation of a patient for a possible tonsillectomy involves a thorough history and physical examination. In addition to the history of recurrent infection, general medical conditions should be evaluated. A history of bleeding disorders in the patient or the family should be thoroughly investigated. The patient should be asked whether he or anyone in his family has prolonged bleeding or bruising; sickle cell anemia, hemophilia, or other blood factor deficiencies; or von Willebrand's disease. Neurologic conditions such as cerebral palsy or Down syndrome should also be evaluated, because patients with neurologic disorders have poor coordination of the airway and swallowing, which may result in postoperative complications. Patients with a history of cardiac problems should be thoroughly evaluated before planning any elective surgery, and the need for prophylactic antibiotics should be established.

The patient should not take aspirin or medications containing aspirin for 7 to 10 days before surgery. The patient should take nothing by mouth for a minimum of 8 hours before surgery. A tonsillectomy can be performed using either a local or a general anesthetic, but most patients prefer general anesthesia. In today's economic climate, most tonsillectomies are performed as outpatient or same-day surgery procedures. The patient's previous medical history should be thoroughly evaluated. Individuals identified as high-risk patients should be monitored in the hospital for a longer period after surgery, and this information must be documented for insurance purposes.

The patient is placed in semi-Trendelenburg's position to prevent aspiration during the procedure. Once anesthesia has been achieved, the tonsils can be removed, using sharp and blunt dissection to separate the tonsils from the tonsillar fossae. This procedure may be performed by traditional methods, using a scalpel and scissors, or by using a Bovie cautery or laser. Absolute hemostasis must be achieved before the procedure is completed, and any blood clots should be removed. After the patient has recovered from the anesthetic, he should be given a liquid or soft, bland diet. Fluids should be encouraged to prevent dehydration. Pain can be relieved or controlled with acetaminophen, with or without codeine. Aspirin is still contraindicated during this high-risk time for bleeding.

INDICATIONS

Hypertrophy of the tonsils causing airway obstruction, dysphagia, and speech distortion
Recurrent tonsillitis
Peritonsillar abscess

CONTRAINDICATIONS

None

COMPLICATIONS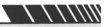

Hemorrhage
Dehydration

NURSING CARE

See pages 201-203.

Adenoidectomy

The choice of adenoidectomy may depend on an examination at the time of the scheduled tonsillectomy, or the adenoidectomy may be scheduled beforehand for patients with known hypertrophy.

General anesthesia is used for an adenoidectomy. The adenoid tissue usually is removed by curettage, although some physicians use a Bovie cautery. The surgery is done as an outpatient or same-day surgery procedure, as was discussed in the patient scheduled for tonsillectomy. High-risk patients must be evaluated separately and concomitant medical conditions must be documented to substantiate the need for an overnight stay.

Postoperative bleeding from the nasopharynx usually is mild and can be controlled with decongestant vasoconstricting nose drops. However, with persistent bleeding the patient may require posterior nasal packing or reexamination in the operating room. Hypernasal speech is related to velopharyngeal insufficiency,

which allows air to escape through the nose. Hypernasality after surgery may be related to pain and usually is limited. However, if the condition persists, speech therapy may be necessary. Naropharyngeal stenosis, which is rare, is related to cicatrix formation (scar contraction).

INDICATIONS

Lymphoid hypertrophy that causes airway obstruction
Chronic infection (e.g., recurrent otitis media or recurrent adenoiditis)

COMPLICATIONS

Bleeding
Hypernasality
Nasopharyngeal stenosis

_1 ASSESS

ASSESSMENT	OBSERVATIONS
Pain	Sore throat, ear pain, grimacing on swallowing, crying, refusal to eat or drink
Fluid intake	Poor skin turgor, dryness of mucous membranes, refusal to eat or drink, elevated temperature, decreased urine output

_2 DIAGNOSE

NURSING DIAGNOSIS	SUBJECTIVE FINDINGS	OBJECTIVE FINDINGS
Pain (acute) related to surgery	Complains of sore throat, ear pain, and difficulty or inability to swallow	Guarding of neck, crying, facial grimaces, drooling, requests pain medication
High risk for fluid volume deficit related to pain; nausea/vomiting	Complains of difficulty or inability to swallow, nausea and vomiting, inability to urinate or minimal urine output, dry mouth	Refuses to eat or drink, drooling, vomiting, inadequate fluid intake by mouth
High risk for aspiration related to bleeding	Complains of frequent swallowing, warm feeling in back of throat, taste of blood	Blood in oral cavity and oropharynx, restlessness, frequent swallowing

_3 PLAN

Patient goals
1. The patient's pain will be eliminated or controlled with analgesics.
2. The patient will maintain his fluid intake.
3. The patient will have no postoperative bleeding or aspiration.

_4 IMPLEMENT

NURSING DIAGNOSIS	NURSING INTERVENTIONS	RATIONALE
Pain (acute) related to surgery	Assess pain (location and amount).	To determine need for analgesics.
	Administer analgesic (acetaminophen with or without codeine), and evaluate effectiveness.	To relieve pain and determine effectiveness of analgesic.
	Encourage cold fluids and chewing gum.	Increased swallowing decreases muscle spasm, thus decreasing pain.
	Apply ice collar.	To minimize edema, reduce bleeding, and provide comfort.

→ > >

NURSING DIAGNOSIS	NURSING INTERVENTIONS	RATIONALE
High risk for fluid volume deficit related to pain; nausea/vomiting	Maintain IV fluids until adequate oral intake is assured.	To prevent dehydration.
	Monitor vital signs and intake and output measurements; assess skin turgor and mucous membranes.	To evaluate hydration status.
	Administer antiemetics as indicated, and evaluate effectiveness.	To prevent vomiting.
	Encourage oral intake (begin with cool liquids; advance to soft, bland diet as tolerated; avoid citrus juices and highly spiced foods).	To prevent dehydration. Citrus fruits and highly spiced foods may aggravate local discomfort.
High risk for aspiration related to bleeding	Assess level of consciousness.	To determine recovery from anesthetic and ability to handle secretions.
	Place patient in side-lying position; arrange oral suction equipment.	To provide for clearance of secretions without aspiration.
	Observe for vomiting; evaluate consistency and color of emesis.	Blood or coffee-ground emesis is from blood swallowed during surgery.
	Administer antiemetic, and evaluate effectiveness.	To prevent vomiting, which increases pressure on surgical site, thus increasing the possibility of bleeding.
	Observe surgical site for bleeding; monitor patient for increased swallowing; monitor vital signs; assess for anxiety and restlessness.	To detect active bleeding.

5 EVALUATE

PATIENT OUTCOME	DATA INDICATING THAT OUTCOME IS REACHED
Patient has no pain, or pain is well controlled with analgesics.	Patient states that pain has been relieved or is well controlled; facial expressions do not reflect pain; patient appears relaxed and comfortable.
Patient maintains fluid intake.	Patient can swallow normally, and fluid intake is not impaired.
Patient has no abnormal bleeding or aspiration.	Inspection reveals no episodes of prolonged bleeding from tonsillar bed.

PATIENT TEACHING

1. Instruct the patient to maintain his fluid intake and to add foods to his diet as tolerated. Bland liquids and soft foods without excess spices are best tolerated for the first few days after surgery. Cold or lukewarm liquids are better tolerated.
2. Inform the patient that throat pain and ear pain are to be expected for 7 to 10 days after surgery. Acetaminophen, with or without codeine, may be taken every 4 to 6 hours for pain. Instruct the patient not to take aspirin or medications containing aspirin.
3. Encourage the patient to rest and avoid strenuous activity for 7 to 10 days.
4. Inform the patient that blood-tinged mucus is normal for 5 to 7 days after surgery. Any increase in bleeding should be reported to the physician. Instruct the patient to avoid coughing or excessive clearing of the throat, which may increase bleeding.
5. Inform the patient that the tonsillar area heals with a yellow or white covering. Increased fluid intake and good oral hygiene measures are necessary to prevent odor from these "scabs," which may last from 7 to 10 days.

Endoscopy

Endoscopy is the direct examination of the aerodigestive tract using a laryngoscope to examine the larynx, a bronchoscope to examine the bronchus and lungs, or an esophagoscope to examine the esophagus.

Both rigid and flexible endoscopy equipment is available. Flexible endoscopy usually is performed with a topical anesthetic. The long, flexible scopes with fiberoptic lighting channels may be passed through the nose or the mouth to examine the upper aerodigestive tract. Flexible scopes are equipped with suction channels for removing mucous secretions, allowing optimum visualization. Rigid endoscopy can be performed with a local anesthetic, with or without sedation, or with a general anesthetic.

Benign or malignant lesions of the upper aerodigestive tract can be biopsied or removed using a forceps or laser. The carbon dioxide and argon lasers are most commonly used in the upper aerodigestive tract. In addition to routine surgical precautions, special care must be taken for both the patient and personnel when a laser is used. To avoid laser ignition of the endotracheal tube, metal endotracheal tubes or specially wrapped tubes should be used. Both the patient and the medical personnel in the room must wear eye protection. The laser must not be used unless the staff has been specifically trained in the use of laser equipment.

If the esophagus is perforated or the vocal cords are injured during endoscopic surgery, the damage is repaired immediately. If there is concern that these complications may occur, the patient should be closely observed for symptoms.

INDICATIONS

To assess the aerodigestive tract
To obtain biopsies
To remove foreign bodies, mucous plugs, and benign lesions

CONTRAINDICATIONS

None.

COMPLICATIONS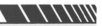

Laryngospasm or bronchospasm during extubation
Perforation of the esophagus (especially with use of a rigid esophagoscope and removal of foreign bodies)
Injury to the vocal cords

1 ASSESS

ASSESSMENT	OBSERVATIONS
Respiration	Increased respirations, shortness of breath, dyspnea, decreased oxygen saturation, restlessness, decreased breath sounds
Infection	Fever, elevated WBC, malaise, bronchorrhea
Nutrition	Decreased oral intake, inability to swallow saliva or liquids, drooling

2 DIAGNOSE

NURSING DIAGNOSIS	SUBJECTIVE FINDINGS	OBJECTIVE FINDINGS
Impaired breathing pattern related to edema	Complains of struggling to breathe, shortness of breath, and noisy breathing; appears anxious	Dyspnea, increased respirations, tachycardia, stridor, decreased breath sounds, oxygen level via pulse oximetry <90%
High risk for infection related to surgical procedure, aspiration	Complains of fever, discomfort in throat, difficulty swallowing or coughing when swallowing	Elevated temperature and WBC, aspiration on swallowing, grimacing when attempting to swallow
Altered nutrition: less than body requirements related to edema, aspiration, perforation of esophagus	Complains of difficulty swallowing and pain on swallowing	Drooling, difficulty swallowing own secretions, poor skin turgor; appears weak
Impaired verbal communication related to edema and surgical procedure	Complains of hoarseness and breathy quality to voice or no audible voice	Hoarseness, breathy or absent voice

3 PLAN

Patient goals

1. The patient will recover from the surgical procedure without impaired breathing or infection.
2. The patient will be able to communicate verbally.

3. The patient will maintain her nutritional status.

4 IMPLEMENT

NURSING DIAGNOSIS	NURSING INTERVENTIONS	RATIONALE
Impaired breathing pattern related to edema	Monitor respiratory rate and depth, pattern of breathing, and stridor; auscultate chest for breath sounds; obtain pulse oximetry measurements as ordered.	To monitor breathing pattern and detect early breathing impairment.

NURSING DIAGNOSIS	NURSING INTERVENTIONS	RATIONALE
	Elevate head of bed once recovery from anesthetic is complete.	To minimize edema.
	Administer humidified oxygen or air as ordered.	To maintain oxygen saturation and prevent obstruction from dry mucus secretions, and to provide comfort.
High risk for infection related to surgical procedure, aspiration	Evaluate patient's temperature, pulse rate, and blood parameters (especially WBC).	To detect infection.
	Monitor breath sounds, and notify physician of rales, rhonchi, or decreased breath sounds.	To detect aspiration pneumonia.
	Instruct patient in proper deep-breathing and coughing techniques.	To rid lungs of accumulated secretions, to promote oxygenation, and to prevent improper coughing technique, which may irritate vocal cords.
	Evaluate any complaints of pain.	Discomfort is expected from intubation and surgical procedure, but significant pain may indicate perforation.
	Observe secretions for color and consistency.	Bronchorrhea, purulent secretions, and odor may indicate infection.
	Administer antibiotics as ordered.	Antibiotics may be used to prevent or treat infection.
Altered nutrition: less than body requirements related to edema, aspiration, perforation of esophagus	Record intake and output.	To determine patient's ability to maintain nutritional status.
	Evaluate patient's ability to swallow (check gag reflex, observe patient's ability to swallow, perform calorie count).	To determine recovery from anesthetic, restoration of swallowing ability, and ability to swallow without aspiration; also to determine adequacy of nutritional intake.
	Consult swallowing therapist or dietitian if necessary.	If nursing assessment shows impaired swallowing, a more complete evaluation, including videofluoroscopy, may be indicated to determine problem area.
	Provide soft diet; encourage patient to cut food into small pieces.	If esophagoscopy with or without removal of a foreign body was performed, some edema of the esophagus is expected; soft food and small, well-chewed pieces of food pass easily through the esophagus.
Impaired verbal communication related to edema and surgical procedure	Encourage patient to rest her voice.	To minimize edema and allow vocal cords to heal without irritation.
	Instruct patient to avoid whispering.	Whispering involves approximating the vocal cords, which will irritate the cords and increase swelling.

→ > >

NURSING DIAGNOSIS	NURSING INTERVENTIONS	RATIONALE
	Elevate head of bed.	To minimize edema.
	Force fluids; administer humidified air by mask or bedside humidifier.	To thin secretions and provide comfort.
	Provide alternative methods of communication (paper and pen, magic slate, communication board).	To encourage patient to rest her voice while allowing nonverbal communication.
	Anticipate patient's needs.	To reduce need to speak.
	If patient is a smoker, instruct her not to smoke and to avoid second hand smoke if possible.	Cigarette smoke can irritate surgical site and mucous membranes.

5　EVALUATE

PATIENT OUTCOME	DATA INDICATING THAT OUTCOME IS REACHED
Patient has recovered from surgery without impaired breathing or infection.	Temperature and WBC are normal; chest x-ray is clear.
Patient's nutritional status is good.	Patient can swallow without aspiration and has maintained her body weight.
Patient can speak.	Speaking voice is normal; pain and edema have begun to subside.

PATIENT TEACHING

1. Instruct the patient to rest her voice for 5 to 7 days and to avoid voice abuse.
2. If the patient smokes, refer her to a smoking cessation clinic.
3. Encourage the patient to use a bedside humidifier and to increase fluids or force fluids to thin secretions.
4. Encourage the patient to eat soft foods, to chew well, and to cut food into small pieces until esophageal edema is gone.
5. Review the Heimlich maneuver with the patient and family.
6. *If laryngoscopy was performed:* instruct the patient to notify her physician if fever, pain, voice changes, or breathing difficulty occurs.
7. *If esophagoscopy was performed:* instruct the patient to notify her physician if fever, back pain, crackling under skin, or rapid pulse develops, since these may indicate perforation of the esophagus.
8. Recommend follow-up sessions with a speech therapist, and encourage the patient to continue any exercises the therapist may recommend.

Treatment of Vocal Cord Paralysis

Once a patient has been diagnosed with vocal cord paralysis and a thorough evaluation has been done to determine possible causes, the patient is kept under observation. If spontaneous recovery occurs, it will be within 6 to 12 months, and treatment of the paralysis usually is delayed for that time. If the patient develops complications associated with the paralysis, such as inability to speak; pulmonary complications arising from aspiration (e.g., pneumonia, tracheobronchitis, or lung abscess); or nutritional deficits resulting from inability to swallow, immediate interventions must be considered.

VOCAL CORD INJECTION

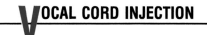

With unilateral vocal cord paralysis, the vocal cord usually is in the paramedian or abducted position. In time the vocalis muscle will atrophy. Patients who require immediate use of their voice or who have chronic aspiration may benefit from injection of an alloplastic material such as absorbable gelatin (Gelfoam) or Teflon; this increases the intrafold mass, allowing the moving cord to approximate the paralyzed cord. Because Gelfoam is reabsorbed within 4 to 6 weeks, it is used as a temporary measure, since the benefits are relatively short-lived. Teflon is a permanent substance, and it has become the standard treatment for patients in whom function is not expected to return. Vocal cord injection is done with the patient awake. Mild sedation can be used in addition to the local anesthetic to improve the patient's comfort and reduce the gag reflex. A laryngoscope and microscope are used for this procedure to adequately visualize the vocal cord. The patient is instructed to phonate during the procedure so that the amount of material to be injected can be determined. Possible sequelae of vocal cord injection are inconsistent results and late granulomatous reactions on the vocal cord.

INDICATIONS
Vocal cord paralysis

CONTRAINDICATIONS
Vocal cord paralysis under 6 months duration unless no spontaneous recovery is expected

COMPLICATIONS

Inconsistent results
Migration of Teflon
Airway compromise
Infection

THYROPLASTY

Thyroplasty is a surgical procedure in which the paralyzed vocal cord is moved into a midline position. Before undergoing this procedure, the patient should be thoroughly evaluated to assess the potential results. Speech recordings, videostroboscopy, and manual compression of the thyroid ala at the level of the vocal cord to determine movement of the vocal cord and potential improvement are done before the procedure is scheduled. Thyroplasty is performed using local anesthesia with sedation to allow the patient to phonate on request. An incision is made in the skin over the thyroid cartilage, and the area of the vocal cord is identified. A small window is created in the thyroid cartilage, and pressure is applied to the cartilage to move the vocal cord. While this pressure is applied, the patient is instructed to phonate, and the physician observes the movement of the vocal cord to determine the correct position. A silicone shim, or plug, is placed through the window to move the vocal cord to the midline position. Hemostasis is achieved, and the wound is closed. A small dressing is put over the incision in the skin to prevent formation of a hematoma or seroma. Dyspnea or stridor may occur for up to 1 month. In addition, poor hemostasis may result in the formation of a hematoma or seroma, causing airway distress and requiring evacuation and possibly a tracheotomy. The skin incision may become infected if meticulous aseptic technique has not been carried out.

1 ASSESS

ASSESSMENT	OBSERVATIONS
Respiration	Increased respirations, shortness of breath, dyspnea, decreased oxygen saturation, restlessness, decreased breath sounds
Infection	Fever, elevated WBC, malaise, bronchorrhea
Communication	Difficulty speaking

2 DIAGNOSE

NURSING DIAGNOSIS	SUBJECTIVE FINDINGS	OBJECTIVE FINDINGS
Impaired breathing pattern related to edema	Complains of struggling to breathe, shortness of breath, and noisy breathing; appears anxious	Dyspnea, increased respirations, tachycardia, stridor, decreased breath sounds, oxygen level via pulse oximetry <90%
Potential risk for infection related to surgical procedure	Complains of redness, discomfort, and purulent drainage from incision	Elevated temperature and WBC; incision shows signs of inflammation, including redness, purulent drainage, and edema
Impaired verbal communication related to postoperative edema	Complains of continued difficulty speaking	Dysphonia

3 PLAN

Patient goals

1. The patient will recover from surgery without complications.
2. The patient will be able to clear secretions from his tracheobronchial tree.

3. The patient will be able to communicate verbally.

4 IMPLEMENT

NURSING DIAGNOSIS	NURSING INTERVENTIONS	RATIONALE
Impaired breathing pattern related to edema	Monitor respiratory rate and depth, pattern of breathing and stridor; auscultate chest for breath sounds; obtain pulse oximetry measurements as ordered.	To monitor breathing pattern and detect early breathing impairment.
	Elevate head of bed.	To minimize edema.
	Administer humidified oxygen or air as ordered.	To maintain oxygen saturation; moisten secretions and provide comfort.

NURSING DIAGNOSIS	NURSING INTERVENTIONS	RATIONALE
Potential risk for infection related to surgical procedure	Clean surgical incision with hydrogen peroxide and water or saline, and apply sterile dressing.	Aseptic technique is necessary to prevent infection.
	Observe area of incision for color, temperature, and drainage; record and report any change.	Changes in incision may indicate infection.
	Evaluate patient's temperature, pulse rate, and blood parameters (especially WBC).	To detect infection.
	Monitor breath sounds, and notify physician of rales, rhonchi, or decreased breath sounds.	To detect aspiration pneumonia.
	Instruct patient in proper deep-breathing and coughing techniques.	To rid lungs of accumulated secretions, to promote oxygenation, and to prevent improper coughing technique, which may irritate vocal cords.
	Evaluate any complaints of pain.	Discomfort is expected from intubation and surgical procedure.
	Observe secretions for color and consistency.	Bronchorrhea, purulent secretions, and odor may indicate infection.
	Administer antibiotics as ordered.	Antibiotics may be used to prevent or treat infection.
Impaired verbal communication related to postoperative edema	Encourage patient to rest her voice.	To minimize edema and allow vocal cords to heal without irritation.
	Instruct patient to avoid whispering.	Whispering involves approximating the vocal cords, which will irritate the cords and increase swelling.
	Elevate head of bed.	To minimize edema.
	Force fluids; administer humidified air by mask or bedside humidifier.	To thin secretions and provide comfort.
	Provide alternative methods of communication (paper and pen, magic slate, communication board).	To encourage patient to rest her voice while allowing nonverbal communication.
	Anticipate patient's needs.	To reduce need to speak.
	If patient is a smoker, instruct her not to smoke.	Cigarette smoke can irritate surgical site and mucous membranes.

→ 〉 〉

5 EVALUATE

PATIENT OUTCOME	DATA INDICATING THAT OUTCOME IS REACHED
Patient has recovered from procedure without impaired breathing or infection.	Temperature and WBC are normal; chest x-ray is clear and shows no evidence of pneumonia
Patient can clear secretions from his tracheobronchial tree.	Patient can swallow without aspiration and maintains his body weight.
Patient can communicate verbally.	Patient's voice has increased in volume; voice does not fatigue with use.

PATIENT TEACHING ▪▪▪▪▪▪▪▪▪▪▪▪▪▪▪▪▪▪▪▪▪▪▪▪▪▪▪▪▪▪▪▪▪

1. Instruct the patient to rest his voice rest for 5 to 7 and days to avoid voice abuse.
2. If the patient smokes, refer him to a smoking cessation clinic.
3. Encourage the patient to use a bedside humidifier and to increase fluids to thin secretions.
4. Instruct the patient to notify his physician if fever, pain, voice changes, or breathing difficulty occurs.
5. Recommend follow-up sessions with a speech therapist, and encourage the patient to continue any exercises recommended by the therapist.

Cricopharyngeal Myotomy and Surgery for Zenker's Diverticulum

Whether a patient with a Zenker's diverticulum should undergo surgery for the condition depends on the size of the diverticulum and the severity of the patient's symptoms (see Chapter 9). Surgery may involve excision of the diverticulum with cricopharyngeal myotomy or suspension of the diverticulum with cricopharyngeal myotomy. The procedure is performed using a general anesthetic. An incision is made in the left side of the neck so that the esophagus can be entered in the area of the diverticulum. The neck of the diverticulum is clamped and excised for diverticulectomy or inverted and suspended for a smaller diverticulum. The transverse fibers of the cricopharyngeus muscle are cut, and the area is closed. If the diverticulum was excised, a nasogastric (N/G) tube and drain are kept in place for 24 to 48 hours and the patient is given nothing by mouth (NPO). If the diverticulum was suspended, the patient may eat by mouth once she has recovered from the anesthetic. If there is no evidence of fistula formation, the N/G tube and drain are removed and the patient is started on a clear liquid diet, which is advanced as tolerated.

INDICATIONS

Zenker's diverticulum with aspiration

CONTRAINDICATIONS

None

COMPLICATIONS

Mediastinitis (caused by leakage at the resection site)
Hematoma (caused by poor hemostasis)
Fistula (caused by poor healing of the suture line)
Infection

---

1 ASSESS

ASSESSMENT	OBSERVATIONS
Nutrition	Inadequate fluid intake, presence of N/G tube
Skin	Neck incision with Penrose drain or drainage catheters connected to closed suction device; dressing over incision

2 DIAGNOSE

NURSING DIAGNOSIS	SUBJECTIVE FINDINGS	OBJECTIVE FINDINGS
Nutrition: less than body requirements related to surgical procedure	Complains of inability to swallow saliva, sore throat, and swelling of neck and throat	N/G tube, edema of pharynx, pooling of saliva
High risk for infection related to surgery	Complains of redness and soreness of incision, fever, and increased drainage from drain onto dressing	Elevated temperature, WBC, and pulse rate; increased erythema of incision; increased drainage from drain; increased edema around incision

3 PLAN

Patient goals

1. The patient will recover from surgery without complications.
2. The patient will maintain her nutritional status.
3. The patient will not develop an infection.

➔ ➤ ➤

4   IMPLEMENT

NURSING DIAGNOSIS	NURSING INTERVENTIONS	RATIONALE
Nutrition: less than body requirements related to surgical procedure	Maintain NPO status.	To allow mucosal suture line to begin healing before introducing food and fluids.
	Maintain IV line.	To maintain hydration until bowel sounds return and N/G tube feedings begin.
	Administer N/G tube feedings as ordered once bowel sounds are present (see page 000).	To maintain nutritional status before oral diet is begun.
	Weigh patient daily and record; record intake and output.	To monitor weight and nutritional status.
High risk for infection related to surgery	Monitor vital signs, especially temperature and pulse rate.	Elevated temperature and tachycardia may indicate infection.
	Observe dressing for tightness and increased drainage.	Increased drainage may indicate infection at mucosal suture line; tight dressing may indicate edema.
	Observe characteristics of drainage (e.g., color, type).	Hematoma formation is noted by an increase in bloody drainage; seroma formation is noted by an increase in serous drainage; saliva may indicate a fistula at mucosal incision line; purulent drainage indicates infection.
	Notify physician of possibility of infection, seroma, hematoma, or fistula.	If a hematoma or seroma has developed, the incision may be reopened, the hematoma or seroma evacuated, and hemostasis achieved.
	Administer antibiotics as ordered; maintain NPO status.	If infection or a salivary fistula develops, the patient will receive IV antibiotics to treat the infection and will be kept NPO to allow the mucosal incision to heal.
	Change neck dressing as needed using aseptic techniques.	Aseptic technique is necessary to prevent further contamination of the wound and cross-contamination.

5   EVALUATE

PATIENT OUTCOME	DATA INDICATING THAT OUTCOME IS REACHED
Patient has recovered from surgery without complications.	Temperature and pulse are normal; no hematoma or seroma has formed.

PATIENT OUTCOME	DATA INDICATING THAT OUTCOME IS REACHED
Patient maintains her nutritional status.	Patient can swallow regular diet without discomfort or aspiration; patient has maintained her body weight.
Patient has not developed an infection.	Incision line shows no erythema, drainage, or edema.

PATIENT TEACHING

1. Instruct the patient to notify her physician if she has difficulty swallowing, fever, increased swelling around the incision, or increased drainage from the incision.

2. Instruct the patient and family to add foods gradually to the patient's diet. Suggest a consultation with a dietitian if the patient is losing weight for advice on maintaining the patient's caloric and nutritional intake.

CHAPTER 11

Tumors of the Head and Neck

Tumors of the Nose, Nasopharynx, and Paranasal Sinuses

> Tumors of the head and neck can be classified as benign or malignant neoplasms. Although only a biopsy of the mass can produce a definitive diagnosis of the type of tumor, a detailed history and physical examination help provide the differential diagnosis.

JUVENILE NASOPHARYNGEAL ANGIOFIBROMA

Juvenile nasopharyngeal angiofibroma is a tumor composed of fibrous stroma and a rich vascular network that arises in the nasopharynx.

PATHOPHYSIOLOGY

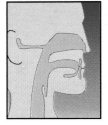

Although a nasopharyngeal angiofibroma originates in the nasopharynx, it can expand to fill the nasal cavity, displacing the septum, and can put pressure on the bone of the posterior wall of the maxillary sinus, the sphenoid sinus, the infratemporal fossa, and the dura of the middle fossa. Juvenile nasopharyngeal angiofibroma is a slow-growing tumor that predominantly affects young men, usually before puberty. The blood supply to the tumor is from the internal maxillary artery.

CLINICAL MANIFESTATIONS

The patient usually complains of a history of intermittent nosebleeds and nasal obstruction. Examination includes assessment of nasal obstruction, a mass in the nasopharynx, and/or mouth breathing.

Once the diagnosis of juvenile nasopharyngeal angiofibroma has been made, an angiogram with embolization may be done. The angiogram identifies the blood supply to the tumor, and embolization with a substance to occlude the vessels may decrease potential bleeding during subsequent excision of the tumor. Excision usually is scheduled 2 days after embolization to allow inflammation to decrease and any procedural sequelae to subside.

COMPLICATIONS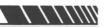

Nasal bleeding
Cerebrospinal fluid leak
Incomplete tumor removal

DIAGNOSTIC STUDIES AND FINDINGS

Diagnostic test	Findings
Computed tomography	Vascular mass in posterior nasal cavity or nasopharynx; bowing of posterior wall of maxillary sinus
Angiography	Identifies major blood supply to tumor

MEDICAL MANAGEMENT

SURGERY

Embolization of tumor: To decrease blood supply to tumor.

Excision of tumor: Removal of tumor by way of an incision along the lateral nasal wall to enter the posterior nasal cavity and nasopharynx; palate may be split to increase visibility and access to tumor.

NURSING CARE

See pages 218 to 222.

Inverting Papilloma

Inverting papilloma is a tumor of the nasal cavity and paranasal sinuses characterized by polyps with fingerlike projections.

PATHOPHYSIOLOGY

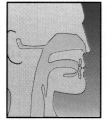

Inverting papillomas differ from nasal polyps under microscopic analysis. Inverting papillomas are characterized by a proliferation of fingerlike inversions of the covering epithelium that invade the underlying stroma. These tumors usually originate from the lateral nasal wall and secondarily may involve the ethmoid and/or maxillary sinus. Inverting papillomas may arise simultaneously with squamous cell carcinoma or may undergo malignant transformation if left untreated.

CLINICAL MANIFESTATIONS

The symptoms of inverting papilloma are similar to those of other obstructive lesions of the nasal cavity: unilateral nasal obstruction, a polypoid mass in the nose, and intermittent epistaxis; many patients with inverting papilloma also have a long history of nasal polyps and nasal polypectomy.

COMPLICATIONS

Chronic nasal crusting.

DIAGNOSTIC STUDIES AND FINDINGS

Diagnostic test	Findings
Computed tomography	Bone destruction or erosion

MEDICAL MANAGEMENT

SURGERY

The treatment for both juvenile nasopharyngeal angiofibroma and inverting papilloma is excision of the tumor. Although small angiofibromas may be excised using a transpalatal approach, a lateral rhinotomy incision may be used in treating both angiofibromas and inverting papillomas. A lateral rhinotomy is an incision along the side of the nose; it can be extended to split the upper lip or across the margin of the lower eyelid to increase exposure. A lateral rhinotomy incision allows access to the internal nose, the ethmoid, maxillary, and sphenoid sinuses, and the nasopharynx. Excision of a juvenile nasopharyngeal angiofibroma should be preceded by embolization of the tumor to decrease bleeding during the surgery. The internal maxillary artery is identified and ligated, and the tumor mass is removed. If the incision has been used to remove an inverting papilloma, an en bloc resection of the lateral nasal wall (medial maxillectomy) may be performed; this involves removing the nasal turbinates and the contents of the ethmoid, sphenoid, and maxillary sinuses. A lateral rhinotomy with medial maxillectomy produces minimal facial deformity. However, removal of the turbinates and lateral nasal wall produces an abnormal internal nasal cavity and changes in air flow and velocity.

NURSING CARE

See pages 218 to 222.

Malignant Tumors of the Paranasal Sinuses

Malignant tumors of the paranasal sinuses are cancerous growths arising in one or more of the sinus cavities.

Approximately 2% of head and neck tumors originate in the paranasal sinuses. Approximately 80% of sinus tumors are found in the maxillary sinus, and fewer than 20% are found in the ethmoid sinuses. Malignant tumors are rare in the sphenoid and frontal sinuses. Tumors of the sinuses affect men more than women and are found primarily among older people, usually those over 60 years of age.

PATHOPHYSIOLOGY

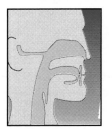

Approximately 80% of paranasal sinus tumors are squamous cell carcinomas. Adenocarcinoma, adenoid cystic carcinoma, and mucoepidermoid carcinoma account for approximately 20% of tumors. Some types of tumors are believed to arise from exposure to carcinogens. For example, the incidence of adenocarcinoma is higher in woodworkers and is believed to be related to the inhalation of wood dust. Nickel and other metal workers have a higher incidence of carcinoma of the maxillary sinus. Some research is being done on the possibility of a relationship between chronic sinusitis and carcinoma of the maxillary sinus. This may be related to metaplasia of the respiratory epithelium caused by chronic infection.

CLINICAL MANIFESTATIONS

The symptoms of paranasal sinus obstruction are similar, regardless of the cause of obstruction. Because tumors of the paranasal sinus may mimic sinus disease, the patient may be treated symptomatically for a long time before the neoplasm is diagnosed. The symptoms of tumors of the maxillary sinus depend on the location of the tumor. Tumors on the lateral wall or nasal wall of the sinus produce unilateral nasal obstruction, unilateral nasal bleeding, and drainage. Superior wall tumors put pressure on the orbital floor, resulting in diplopia, proptosis, or loss of vision. Inferior wall tumors affect the palate and alveolar ridge, resulting in a tumor mass that can be palpated on the palate, loosening of the maxillary teeth, or an ill-fitting denture. Anterior wall tumors may attach the tumor to the skin of the face, resulting in asymmetry of the face or edema of the cheek. Posterior wall tumors, involving the infratemporal fossa, may result in paresthesia overlying the sinus from involvement of the infraorbital branch of the trigeminal nerve. Other symptoms may include trismus from invasion of the pterygoid muscles; mental numbness from involvement of the mandibular branch of the trigeminal nerve; otitis media as a result of nasopharyngeal extension; and facial and dental pain.

The tumor, node, metastasis (TNM) staging system is used to classify malignant tumors of the paranasal sinuses. Ohngren's line is also used to help determine the prognosis. Ohngren's line is a line drawn on a lateral x-ray film from the inner canthus of the eye to the angle of the mandible, dividing the maxillary sinus into the posterosuperior and inferior maxillary cavities. Tumors in the posterosuperior portion, the area above Ohngren's line, are associated with a poor prognosis because of later presentation and the proximity of the tumor to the orbit, cribriform plate, pterygoid muscles, and central nervous system.

COMPLICATIONS

Bleeding, leakage of cerebrospinal fluid (CSF), infection, epiphora.

DIAGNOSTIC STUDIES AND FINDINGS

Diagnostic test	Findings
Computed tomography (CT)	Tumor mass, bone erosion, soft tissue involvement
Magnetic resonance imaging (MRI)	Swelling

MEDICAL MANAGEMENT

Treatment of sinus tumors combines radiation therapy and surgical excision.

RADIATION THERAPY

Preoperative versus postoperative radiation therapy continues to be a controversial decision. Preoperative radiation therapy lasts approximately 6 weeks, and surgery is performed 4 to 6 weeks after the therapy is completed. Advocates of this form of therapy believe that the increased oxygen supply to the tumor results in increased radiosensitivity. However, there is concern that patients who have had preoperative radiation therapy may have difficulty with wound healing after surgery. Radiation therapy may be given after surgical excision.

Complications: Complications include dental caries, xerostomia, mucositis/esophagitis, taste changes.

SURGERY

Surgical intervention for tumors of the maxillary sinus may involve subtotal maxillectomy, total maxillectomy with or without orbital exenteration, or craniofacial resection. The surgical procedure, which is determined by the results of the computed tomography (CT) scan, reflects the extent of disease. If the soft tissue of the orbit is involved, an orbital exenteration usually is done. If the anterior and middle cranial fossae are involved, a craniofacial resection may be performed. A total maxillectomy involves removal of the maxilla, nasal bone, ethmoid sinus, and pterygoid plates. A lateral rhinotomy incision is used to enter the maxillary sinus cavity. The incision is extended to remove the inferior margin of the maxillary sinus, which is the hard palate. After the tumor has been resected, the cheek flap is lined with a split-thickness skin graft. A

Continued.

MEDICAL MANAGEMENT—cont'd

bolus packing of xeroform gauze is inserted to prevent seroma or hematoma formation under the skin graft, and a surgical prosthesis is inserted and sutured into place. The bolus packing and surgical prosthesis restore oral-nasal separation, allowing the patient to maintain the ability to swallow and speak. Nasal packing may also be used at the completion of the procedure.

A craniofacial resection usually is performed jointly by a neurosurgeon and an otolaryngologist. A bicoronal incision, as well as the lateral rhinotomy incision, is used to approach the anterior skull base and the pterygoid plates. Each surgical procedure is tailored to meet the specifics of the tumor.

Tumors that involve the orbital apex or nasopharynx and deeply infiltrating tumors may be classified as inoperable. However, with the current advances in skull base surgery, many large tumors may be surgically removed.

POSTOPERATIVE NURSING CARE

1 ASSESS

ASSESSMENT	OBSERVATIONS
Respiratory	Crusting of sinus and nasal cavities, nasal drainage
Infection	WBC and temperature elevation; CSF leak; malodorous drainage
Sensory	Decreased vision, trismus, diplopia, epiphora, facial paresthesia, pain
Body image	Incision on face, removal of sinus, facial disfigurement, anxiety

2 DIAGNOSE

NURSING DIAGNOSIS	SUBJECTIVE FINDINGS	OBJECTIVE FINDINGS
Pain (acute) related to surgical procedure	Complains of pain or discomfort of face/eye/oral cavity or skin graft donor site	Guards site, grimaces, requests pain medication
Impaired skin integrity and high risk for infection related to incisions, surgical defect, skin graft donor and recipient sites, CSF leak	Complains of fever, increased drainage with foul odor, headache, fatigue	Incisions, surgical defect, skin graft donor and recipient sites; redness; increased drainage from incision or defect; elevated temperature; elevated white blood count (WBC); malaise; halo pattern of drainage on pillow; clear fluid draining from nose and ears

NURSING DIAGNOSIS	SUBJECTIVE FINDINGS	OBJECTIVE FINDINGS
Anxiety related to diagnosis, hospitalization, surgical procedure	Crying, withdrawn, restless, limited attention span	Pacing, wringing hands; increased pulse and respirations; diaphoresis; misunderstands instructions
Body image disturbance related to surgical incisions and associated changes in appearance	Expresses fear of rejection; refuses to look at defect; refuses to leave room; will not perform activities of daily living (ADLs)	Patient isolates himself; expresses anger about change in appearance; shows decreased communication

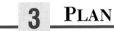

3 PLAN

Patient goals

1. The patient's pain will be controlled.
2. The surgical incisions will heal without complications.
3. The patient will be able to discuss his concerns, thereby lessening his anxiety.
4. The patient will adjust to changes in his body image.

4 IMPLEMENT

NURSING DIAGNOSIS	NURSING INTERVENTIONS	RATIONALE
Pain (acute) related to surgical procedure	Assess patient's pain status (intensity, location, characteristics, factors that increase or decrease pain).	To determine need for intervention.
	Identify methods useful in controlling pain (relaxation, movement and positioning).	Increased pain may be related to discomfort from tubes and dressings as well as from anxiety. Additional pain relief may accompany changes in position and use of relaxation.
	Administer pain medication as ordered, and evaluate effectiveness.	To determine pain relief and need for alternative measures.
	Encourage patient to use pain-relief measures *before* planned activities.	If patient is in pain, ambulation and participation in self-care activities or instruction will be ineffective.
Impaired skin integrity and high risk for infection related to incisions, surgical defect, skin graft donor and recipient sites, CSF leak	Assess incisions, surgical defect, skin graft sites for encrustation, drainage, and odor; observe color of mucosa.	To determine whether healing is progressing satisfactorily.
	Cleanse incisions with half-strength hydrogen peroxide in water or saline; apply antibiotic ointment.	To remove crusting and drainage and promote wound healing.

→ > >

NURSING DIAGNOSIS	NURSING INTERVENTIONS	RATIONALE
	Begin nasal and/or oral cavity care when bolus packing is removed or as ordered by physician.	The bolus usually remains in place for 5 days to promote hemostasis and to apply pressure to skin graft recipient site in order to prevent accumulation of blood or serum between graft and flap. Once the bolus has been removed, oral/nasal irrigations remove dry secretions and debris and promote healing.
	Observe skin graft donor site for bleeding, drainage, and increased pain. The split-thickness skin graft donor site may be covered with Opsite, a medicated mesh gauze, or nonadhering dressing, depending on physician's preference and institutional policy. Minimal drainage followed by drying is to be expected.	To determine whether healing is progressing satisfactorily.
	Allow split-thickness skin graft donor site to be exposed; avoid pressure from bed linens or pajamas.	Donor site is sensitive, because only a thin layer of skin is removed, leaving nerve fibers present. Pressure increases discomfort.
	Expose donor site to air; apply heat lamp, if ordered.	To promote healing by drying of serous secretions.
	Once donor site is dry and covered with eschar, instruct patient to soak the leg in bathtub.	To remove eschar without disturbing healing tissue.
	Observe nasal drainage for CSF leak by testing for glucose with test strips; beta-2 transferrin. Notify physician if CSF leak is suspected.	To detect CSF leakage. Immediate attention is mandatory to prevent meningitis.
	Monitor temperature and report elevation; monitor laboratory data, especially WBC, and report abnormalities.	Elevated temperature and WBC may indicate infection.
	Administer antibiotics as ordered.	To prevent infection (perioperative antibiotics may be prescribed, beginning before surgery).
	Instruct patient in removal, cleaning, and reinsertion of obturator, if present.	If maxillary prosthesis is used, it must be cleaned and reinserted as a denture to prevent odor and infection.
Anxiety related to diagnosis, hospitalization, surgical procedure	Assess degree of anxiety (ability to concentrate, comprehend, and communicate).	To determine patient's ability to perform ADLs.
	Explain all procedures, and provide information about the disease, hospital procedures, and medical and nursing interventions.	To reduce anxiety related to fear of unknown and to correct any misconceptions.

NURSING DIAGNOSIS	NURSING INTERVENTIONS	RATIONALE
Body image disturbance related to surgical incisions and associated changes in appearance	Assess patient's perception of body image by asking how patient feels about changes resulting from surgery, what changes patient perceives, and what impact patient feels these changes will have on his life.	To determine patient's baseline body image and how he perceives changes.
	Evaluate patient's ability to look at surgical defect and incisions. Discuss and describe changes in appearance caused by surgery; encourage patient to express his concerns and fears and ask questions.	Patient must be ready to see changes in appearance to be able to cope with alterations.
	Help patient to recall effective coping behaviors used in the past and to develop new ones.	Using previous coping behavior allows patient to deal with current changes.
	Begin instructions for self-care, viewing defect as soon as possible after recovery from anesthesia.	To encourage acceptance of and coping with defect.
	Remain with patient during initial viewing of defect.	To provide emotional support.
	Encourage patient to continue self-care through discharge.	To allow patient to feel secure in care before discharge.
	Encourage patient to use techniques to improve body image (e.g., bathing, combing hair, shaving, using makeup).	To emphasize positive body image rather than focusing on defect.
	Discuss possible experiences patient may have with those who are not health care workers; encourage patient to discuss feelings or concerns.	Health care workers do not view surgical incisions and defects as abnormal; therefore, the patient may develop a false sense of security.
	If patient cannot look at defect or express concerns and fears, refer to counseling service or community agencies such as American Cancer Society and support groups.	Although body image disturbance is an expected nursing diagnosis, prolonged inability to cope with the surgical changes may require multidisciplinary interventions to support coping skills.

5   EVALUATE

PATIENT OUTCOME	DATA INDICATING THAT OUTCOME IS REACHED
Patient's pain is under control.	Patient uses a variety of pain-control measures, depending on severity of symptoms; he has returned to normal activities and states that pain is under control.
Surgical incisions have healed without complications.	Temperature and WBC are within normal limits; incision has healed without dehiscence, erythema, or increased drainage; no CSF is present in nasal drainage.

→ > >

PATIENT OUTCOME	DATA INDICATING THAT OUTCOME IS REACHED
Patient's anxiety has been reduced.	Patient recognizes signs of anxiety and can initiate appropriate coping skills; he can also discuss causes of anxiety.
Patient has adjusted to changes in body image.	Patient performs self-care activities, socializes with staff, family, and others, is able to discuss change in appearance, and uses resources to help in coping with changes.

PATIENT TEACHING

1. Teach the patient to cleanse suture lines with hydrogen peroxide and saline/water and apply antibiotic ointment.
2. Instruct the patient in the proper techniques for removing the palate obturator, cleansing it with peroxide and water, denture cleaner, or toothpaste, and replacing it after each meal and at bedtime.
3. Teach the patient how to perform irrigation of a nasal or surgical defect (see page 266).
4. Instruct the patient to notify the physician at any sign of infection (e.g., increased drainage, foul odor, elevated temperature, bleeding, change in pain).
5. Help patient find ways to camouflage defect (e.g., eye patch, makeup).
6. Encourage the patient to participate in a support group.
7. See Patient Teaching following nasal surgery on page 170.

Malignant Tumors of the Oral Cavity and Oropharynx

Malignant tumors of the oral cavity are neoplasms arising in the mouth.

The oral cavity and oropharynx are considered separately because of their embryologic development and lymphatic drainage systems; these differences account for a difference in presentation and treatment of tumors. The oral cavity consists of the lips, buccal mucosa, gingivae, alveolar ridges, retromolar trigone, floor of the mouth, anterior two thirds of the tongue, and the hard palate. The oropharynx consists of the soft palate, tonsillar pillars and tonsils, base of the tongue, and posterior oropharyngeal wall. The lymphatic drainage from the oral cavity flows to the submental, submandibular, and upper deep jugular chains. Lymphatic drainage from the oropharynx flows primarily to the jugular digastric region of the upper jugular chain and the retropharyngeal and parapharyngeal lymph nodes.

PATHOPHYSIOLOGY

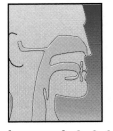

Squamous cell carcinoma accounts for 90% to 95% of all oral cavity and oropharyngeal tumors. Although unusual, mucoepidermoid carcinoma, adenocarcinoma, adenoid cystic carcinoma, and lymphomas may also be found in the oral cavity and oropharynx. A combination of tobacco and alcohol use is the leading etiologic factor in the development of squamous cell carcinoma. Smoking and the use of smokeless tobacco create morphologic changes in the lining mucosa. Cigarette smoking may cause general changes in the upper aerodigestive tract, whereas smokeless tobacco creates changes in the mucosa according to the placement of the tobacco. Alcohol is a direct irritant to the lining membranes of the upper aerodigestive tract. Alcohol may act as a cocarcinogen or have a synergistic effect with tobacco, resulting in squamous cell carcinoma. Other factors associated with malignant tumors of the oral cavity and oropharynx are poor oral hygiene, resulting in chronic irritation from poor dental condition or ill-fitting dentures; dietary deficiencies, especially riboflavin and iron deficiency anemias, such as Plummer-Vinson syndrome; herpes virus; and inhalation or ingestion of chemicals.

CLINICAL MANIFESTATIONS

The first symptom of a tumor of the oral cavity or oropharynx is an ulcer or mass that fails to heal. However, tumors of the oral cavity and oropharynx may not be diagnosed until they are large enough to interfere with tongue movement, resulting in a speech or swallowing dysfunction or pain. Pain associated with tumors of the oral cavity and oropharynx may be local pain or referred pain to the ear (otalgia). Lesions of the oral cavity that infiltrate the lingual nerve may radiate to the ipsilateral ear, because the lingual nerve is a branch of the mandibular nerve, which provides sensation to the external auditory meatus, the tympanic membrane, and the temporomandibular joint through the auriculotemporal nerve. Tumors of the oropharynx may cause referred ear pain by way of the glossopharyngeal nerve, which provides sensory innervation to the middle ear.

Premalignant changes in the oral cavity that have a potential for malignant degeneration include leukoplakia, erythroplakia, and lichen planus. Leukoplakia are white patches caused by chronic irritation that results in tissue proliferation. Erythroplakia are red lesions generally described as raised, granular lesions that bleeds easily. Erythroplakia have a higher malignant potential than do leukoplakia. Lichen planus is a white,

---

CHARACTERISTICS OF TUMORS OF THE ORAL CAVITY AND OROPHARYNX
Exophytic   Superficial tumors that grow outward and have late metastatic spread   *Ulcerative*   Ulcers that bleed easily   *Infiltrative*   Tumors that extend into the musculature of the oral cavity or oropharynx   *Verrucous*   Wartlike, bulky, elevated lesions that do not invade or metastasize

filmy lesion with a lace pattern. Its potential for transformation is questionable.

The prognosis for tumors of the oral cavity and oropharynx depends on the size of the tumor, its location, involvement of adjacent structures, histologic differentiation, and regional lymph node metastasis. In addition, 15% to 20% of patients who have a tumor of the head and neck may have a second primary tumor of the upper aerodigestive tract. These multiple primary tumors may be *synchronous* (appearing at the same time or within 6 months of the original tumor diagnosis) or *metachronous* (appearing in a separate location 6 months or longer after the original diagnosis).

Tumors of the oral cavity and oropharynx are staged according to the tumor, node, metastasis (TNM) system (see Chapter 2). As with all staging methods, the TNM system is used to help determine the proper treatment, to standardize reporting of end results, and to compare the effectiveness of treatments.

NURSING CARE

See pages 225 to 230.

RESECTION OF TUMORS OF THE ORAL CAVITY AND OROPHARYNX

In resecting tumors of the oral cavity and oropharynx, the goals are to remove the tumor, restore function, and preserve the patient's appearance as much as possible.

Tumors of the floor of the mouth and the tongue can be resected transorally or transcervically. The tumor and a margin of normal tissue are removed. If diagnostic evaluation has revealed that the tumor approaches the mandible, a marginal mandibulectomy may be performed, in which a partial thickness of bone is removed while mandibular continuity is preserved. However, if

the tumor involves the mandible, a segmental resection is necessary. Segmental resection of the lateral mandible is not a disabling procedure. Prosthetic rehabilitation to prevent movement of the mandible to the side of the defect may be all that is needed to restore function. If the anterior mandible must be resected, the patient will have an incompetent oral commissure, resulting in drooling, speech and swallowing dysfunction, and cosmetic deformity. Consideration should be given to immediate reconstruction after anterior mandibular resection. Reconstruction of defects of the floor of the mouth and the tongue can involve (1) primary closure, or suturing the wound closed if sufficient tissue remains; (2) creating local flaps of tissue from adjacent areas; or (3) using a split-thickness skin graft (usually taken from the thigh). If a larger resection is necessary to ensure removal of the tumor or if the mandible is involved in the resection, a distant flap or microvascular free tissue transfer may be required. A pectoralis major myocutaneous flap, which uses the skin and underlying subcutaneous tissue of the pectoralis muscle, is a versatile flap that is frequently used in oral cavity reconstructions to provide bulk and soft tissue coverage. Microvascular free flaps for the oral cavity are used primarily when a resection of the mandible or removal of the entire tongue was necessary. The radius, fibula, and scapula are currently the most common areas for harvesting free flaps, because there is little functional deformity of the donor site. These distant flaps are revascularized by anastomosing the vascular pedicle of the flap to recipient vessels in the neck.

Resection of the anterior floor of the mouth and of the lateral tongue produces minimal long-term disability. Once the initial healing phase has been completed, most patients have normal swallowing and minimal change in articulation. However, subtotal or total glossectomy for large tumors of the tongue may result in a substantial swallowing dysfunction and severe problems with articulation.

The patient's pulmonary function must be thoroughly evaluated before surgery to determine his ability to produce an effective cough, which is necessary to prevent complications from aspiration. Because of the high risk of aspiration, some surgeons perform a total laryngectomy or laryngeal separation with resection of the base of the tongue, or a total glossectomy. Others suggest inserting a gastrostomy tube at the time of resection to ensure adequate intake.

Because tumors of the oral cavity and oropharynx show a high rate of metastasis to the regional cervical lymph nodes, neck dissection may be done in conjunction with resection of the oral cavity. In patients with no clinical evidence of palpable lymph nodes, the decision on neck dissection depends on the size and location of the primary tumor and the rate of metastatic spread.

COMPLICATIONS

Fistula, delayed wound healing, persistent or recurrent tumor, metastasis.

DIAGNOSTIC STUDIES AND FINDINGS

Diagnostic test	Findings
Examination and palpation	Exophytic, ulcerative, infiltrative or verrucous lesion in oral cavity or oropharynx
Computed tomography (CT)	Abnormal area with involvement of adjacent structures
Magnetic resonance imaging (MRI) better for evaluating tumors of the tongue	Abnormal area with involvement of adjacent structures
Endoscopy and biopsy	Synchronous primary tumors in upper aerodigestive tract or malignant tumor

MEDICAL MANAGEMENT

Once a patient has been diagnosed as having a malignant tumor of the oral cavity or oropharynx, different treatments are discussed. For small lesions (T_1 and T_2), surgery and radiation therapy are equally effective in controlling the tumor. The decision on which to use depends on the extent and location of the tumor, the patient's medical status, and the patient's preference. Because second primary tumors are quite common in the upper aerodigestive tract, most head and neck surgeons encourage surgical removal of small lesions of the oral cavity and oropharynx, reserving radiation therapy for later treatment of second primary tumors.

SURGERY

Transoral excision of floor of mouth with or without marginal mandibulectomy

Partial glossectomy

MEDICAL MANAGEMENT—cont'd

Base of tongue resection

Total glossectomy

Composite resection

RADIATION THERAPY

External beam radiation

Brachytherapy

CHEMOTHERAPY

POSTOPERATIVE NURSING CARE

1 ASSESS

ASSESSMENT	OBSERVATIONS
Respiratory	Edema of the oral cavity or oropharynx, causing airway obstruction; tracheotomy
Nutrition	Decreased intake, edema of the tongue and the floor of the mouth, decreased sensation, pain, aspiration on swallowing
Mucous membrane	Altered oral cavity or oropharynx; graft or flap at defect
Speech	Altered speech

2 DIAGNOSE

NURSING DIAGNOSIS	SUBJECTIVE FINDINGS	OBJECTIVE FINDINGS
Ineffective airway clearance related to postoperative edema	Complains of difficulty breathing, increased secretions, fear of not being able to breathe, restlessness	Abnormal blood gases or pulse oximetry reading; decreased breath sounds, rales or rhonchi on auscultation; increased mucus production; increased pulse rate and respirations; tracheotomy tube present
High risk for aspiration related to resection of oral cavity, injury to hypoglossal nerve, presence of tracheotomy	Complains of inability to swallow saliva, inability to move tongue; coughing when swallowing; increased mucus	Pooling of saliva in oral cavity; immobile tongue; edema of oral cavity; aspirates when attempting to swallow; tracheotomy tube present

NURSING DIAGNOSIS	SUBJECTIVE FINDINGS	OBJECTIVE FINDINGS
Altered oral mucous membrane related to surgical treatment	Complains of decreased sensation in mouth; swelling of tongue, throat; discomfort or pain in mouth; can feel sutures, flap, or graft in mouth	Unable to feel touch in oral cavity; edema of tongue; sutures, graft or flap in oral cavity
Impaired skin integrity related to surgical incisions; **high risk for altered peripheral tissue perfusion** related to occlusion of blood vessel supplying flap used for reconstruction	Complains of increased swelling, change in sensation in oral cavity, increased pain, blood in oral cavity	Increased edema, hematoma or seroma at graft or flap site, decreased or altered Doppler signals, increased bleeding of graft or flap, altered color of graft or flap
Impaired verbal communication related to presence of tracheotomy	Complains of difficulty communicating needs	Tracheotomy; unable to speak
Impaired swallowing related to surgical resection	Complains of swelling in mouth, inability to move tongue, inability to swallow saliva, and weakness	Loss of weight; pooling of saliva in oral cavity; decreased or absent tongue movement; presence of surgical incisions, flap or graft in oral cavity; abnormal serum laboratory values; presence of tracheotomy
Pain (acute) related to surgical incisions, tubes, and dressings	Complains of pain or discomfort in mouth and throat; appears restless; has decreased ability to concentrate	Requests pain medication; increased blood pressure, pulse, respirations; decreased attention span; refuses to participate in self-care
Body image disturbance related to surgical procedure	Expresses concern over appearance, other people's reaction to appearance; feels depressed	Refuses to look in mirror, participate in self-care; cries easily; refuses to leave room
Fear related to diagnosis of cancer and treatment	Expresses fear of cancer, treatment, disfigurement, death; feels out of control of life	Appears withdrawn, cries easily, displays anger, expresses need to regain control

3 PLAN

Patient goals

1. The patient will maintain a patent airway.
2. The patient will not aspirate or develop aspiration-related complications.
3. The patient will maintain nutrition and hydration.
4. The patient's pain and discomfort will be controlled.
5. The patient will recover from the surgical procedure without infection or complications.
6. The patient will communicate effectively; speech intelligibility will improve.
7. The patient will be able to discuss fears and accept change in body image.

4 IMPLEMENT

NURSING DIAGNOSIS	NURSING INTERVENTIONS	RATIONALE
Ineffective airway clearance related to postoperative edema	Place patient in high Fowler's position.	To decrease postoperative edema, facilitate chest expansion, and improve patient's comfort.
	Monitor rate and depth of respiration.	To evaluate breathing.
	Auscultate lungs to assess breath sounds for rales, rhonchi, and changes in sounds.	To determine changes in lungs.
	Encourage coughing and deep breathing.	To promote expansion of lungs and prevent accumulation of secretions.
	Suction oral cavity.	To remove secretions.
	Monitor arterial blood gases (ABGs) and pulse oximetry as ordered.	To determine changes in oxygen level.
	Administer humidified oxygen as ordered.	To provide supplemental oxygen and prevent drying of airway membranes.
	Monitor for passage of air through nose and mouth and for airway distress.	To determine need for tracheotomy (if was not performed prophylactically during surgery).
	See Postoperative Nursing Care for Tracheotomy, page 253.	
High risk for aspiration related to resection of oral cavity, injury to hypoglossal nerve, presence of tracheotomy	Maintain nothing by mouth (NPO) status until patient can swallow saliva, tracheotomy is removed, and tongue movement is restored.	To prevent aspiration of food and fluids into tracheobronchial tree.
	Suction oral cavity as needed.	To remove secretions.
	Elevate head of bed.	To reduce postoperative edema and minimize aspiration.
	Monitor patient for signs of aspiration such as coughing, increased production of mucus, altered breath sounds.	To determine need for further intervention.
	See Postoperative Nursing Care for Tracheotomy, page 254.	
Altered oral mucous membrane related to surgical treatment	Assess oral cavity for wound healing and collection of serum or blood under skin graft.	To assess healing and potential for complications.

NURSING DIAGNOSIS	NURSING INTERVENTIONS	RATIONALE
Impaired skin integrity related to surgical incisions; **high risk for altered peripheral tissue perfusion** related to occlusion of blood vessel supplying flap used for reconstruction	Assess flap viability (color, warmth, and drainage; blanch and refill with digital pressure [see box on page 231]). Document any changes.	To assess healing of flap.
	Provide gentle oral cavity care as ordered after bolus dressing is removed, using oral rinses, oral swabs, catheter and syringe, or power spray.	To remove secretions and debris from intraoral suture lines, promoting healing and preventing infection.
	Provide gentle oral suction using soft catheter or tonsil suction.	To remove intraoral secretions.
	Clean exposed suture line.	To remove drainage.
	Monitor flap viability with electronic monitoring devices, if available; notify physician immediately of any change in electronic monitoring results, and in color, blanching, and temperature of flap.	To detect changes in tissue perfusion of flap (changes in flap viability can result in death of flap if immediate intervention is not taken).
	Change patient's position frequently.	To avoid pressure on flaps and development of pressure areas.
	Assess skin graft donor site (see the box on page 231).	To evaluate healing.
	Encourage ambulation.	To decrease muscle spasm associated with skin graft donor site.
	Avoid pressure on donor site (avoid heavy bed covers, pajama bottoms).	To decrease discomfort.
Impaired verbal communication related to presence of tracheotomy	See Postoperative Nursing Care for Tracheotomy, pages 252 to 256.	
Impaired swallowing related to surgical resection	Administer tube feedings as ordered (see box on page 231).	To maintain nutritional and hydration status.
	Assess tongue mobility.	To determine decrease in oral cavity edema, movement of tongue, and ability to swallow.
	Assess gag and cough reflexes.	To determine patient's ability to protect airway and restore swallowing.
	Monitor and document intake and output.	To determine hydration status.
	Evaluate laboratory values, especially serum albumin, serum ferritin, electrolytes, glucose, and WBC.	To monitor hydration and nutritional status.

NURSING DIAGNOSIS	NURSING INTERVENTIONS	RATIONALE
	Initiate oral feedings as ordered (see box on page 231).	Once postoperative edema has subsided, aspiration has decreased, and gag reflex has returned, oral feedings can resume.
	Advance diet as tolerated.	To return patient to normal diet as soon as possible.
	Perform calorie count.	To determine adequate nutrition.
	Inspect oral cavity and provide mouth care after meals.	To cleanse oral cavity and remove accumulated food.
Pain (acute) related to surgical incisions, tubes, and dressings	Assess location, characteristics, and intensity of pain.	To determine what pain-relief measures are needed.
	Elevate head of bed, and help patient assume a comfortable position.	Pain after head and neck surgery usually is related to incisions and placement of tubes and dressings. Changing patient's position relieves pressure and reduces discomfort.
	Administer analgesics as ordered, and evaluate their effectiveness.	To reduce pain and determine need to adjust dosage.
	Instruct patient in relaxation techniques.	To provide comfort through nonpharmacologic methods.
Body image disturbance related to surgical procedure	Encourage patient to discuss concerns.	To identify problem areas.
	Identify coping mechanisms used successfully in the past.	To determine coping strategies that may be used.
	Assess patient's readiness to participate in self-care.	Usually the first acknowledgment of acceptance of change.
	Reinforce instructions and descriptions during nursing care.	To begin preparing patient for changes.
	Remain with patient during initial viewing of defects and first attempts at self-care.	To provide support.
	Explore potential responses by other people. Encourage social interaction with staff, other patients, family, and visitors.	To help prepare patient for possible reactions after leaving hospital.
	Encourage referrals to other team members, including social worker and psychiatric liaison, if depression is prolonged.	To help patient cope with changes in body image.
Fear related to diagnosis of cancer and treatment	Teach patient about type of cancer, treatment, and procedure, and involve him in treatment planning.	To reduce fear of the unknown and foster a sense of control.

NURSING DIAGNOSIS	NURSING INTERVENTIONS	RATIONALE
	Encourage patient to talk about fears and concerns.	To allow patient to acknowledge fears and develop a plan to allay them.
	Consult with social worker or therapist.	To provide additional therapeutic interventions.

5   EVALUATE

PATIENT OUTCOME	DATA INDICATING THAT OUTCOME IS REACHED
Patient demonstrates normal breathing.	ABGs and pulse oximetry are normal for patient; patient can resume ADLs without dyspnea; respirations are regular.
Patient can swallow without aspirating.	Patient's weight is stable; there is no evidence of aspiration on swallowing.
Patient's pain is under control.	Patient requires minimal use of analgesics, effectively uses relaxation techniques.
Wounds have healed without infection or complications.	There are no signs of infection; skin grafts and flaps show good color and no drainage; there is no wound dehiscence.
Patient can communicate intelligibly.	Tracheotomy has been removed, speech can be understood.
Patient can talk about fears and accepts changes in body image.	Patient discusses concerns, is developing coping skills, socializes, and performs self-care.

PATIENT TEACHING ▪▪▪▪▪▪▪▪▪▪▪▪▪▪▪▪▪▪▪▪▪▪▪▪▪▪▪▪▪▪▪▪▪▪

1. Instruct the patient in the technique for oral cavity assessment to evaluate healing and detect signs of recurrence or of a new tumor.
2. Teach the patient the signs and symptoms of infection (fever, increased, foul-smelling drainage, change in characteristics of pain).
3. Teach the patient and significant other ways to increase the patient's calorie and protein intake (e.g., adding foods to diet as tolerated, choosing foods high in calories and protein, using dietary supplements). Instruct patient to notify physician if weight loss or change in ability to swallow occurs.
4. Reinforce self-care instructions on oral hygiene (e.g., use of oral care appliance such as Water Pik, catheter and syringe, oral swabs; removal of debris from flap or graft site).
5. Instruct the patient in the care of the donor site.
6. See Patient Teaching for Tracheotomy on page 256.

CARE OF THE SKIN FLAP

Maintain continuous suction and patency of wound drainage catheters at the flap donor site to promote healing. Jackson Pratt or Hemovac drains are inserted in the incision during surgery to remove blood and serum and thus prevent the formation of a hematoma or seroma.

Aspirate drains, using sterile technique, to remove clots from drainage catheters, which will minimize the flow and the effects of suctioning.

Eliminate any pressure on the flap (e.g., from dressings, tracheotomy ties, or the elastic on the tracheotomy oxygen mask) to avoid compromising circulation to the flap.

CARE OF THE SKIN GRAFT DONOR SITE

Keep an outer protective dressing on the site for 24 hours to provide protection and absorb drainage. Maintain the inner covering over the donor site for protection.

Once the area has dried (7 to 10 days), soak donor site in bathtub to remove dressing without disturbing healing.

If donor site has not dried, use a heat lamp to promote drying.

Avoid pressure on the donor site (avoid heavy bed covers and pajama bottoms) to decrease discomfort.

TUBE FEEDING

- Assess proper placement of feeding tube by x-ray evaluation when tube is first placed; thereafter aspirate gastric contents, or instill air into the tube and auscultate over epigastric region.
- Assess for residual feedings by aspirating gastric contents.
- Place patient in high Fowler's position to prevent early satiety and aspiration of feeding by reflux.
- Begin each feeding with water to determine patency of tube.
- Administer feeding at room temperature to prevent cramping and discomfort.
- End each feeding with water to rinse tube and maintain patency.
- Document patient's tolerance of feeding.

INITIATING ORAL FEEDINGS

Consult with dietitian and swallowing therapist when oral feedings begin. These team members can assist with determining the proper food consistency, compensatory techniques for swallowing, and with placement of food in the mouth.

After anterior oral cavity resection

Begin with liquids and foods of thin consistency, because these foods are easily moved to the posterior oral cavity to initiate swallowing.

After base of tongue resection or total glossectomy

Begin with foods of thick consistency, because thin foods move too quickly if patient faces risk of aspiration. Thicker foods can be manipulated.

Mechanics of oral feeding

Place food on unaffected side. The patient will have better movement and sensation on this side, permitting movement in the oral cavity.

Instruct the patient to place small amounts of food in his mouth, to experiment with placement of food, and to try tools such as a long-handled spoon, shot glass, and syringe and catheter to help move the food to the posterior oral cavity.

Tumors of the Larynx

Cancer of the larynx is a malignant tumor of the larynx including the supraglottic larynx, glottic larynx, or subglottic larynx.

Tumors of the larynx account for approximately 2% of all cancers. Laryngeal carcinoma is second in incidence only to carcinoma of the oral cavity among all tumors of the head and neck.

The main etiologic agent in cancer of the larynx is heavy cigarette smoking. As with other head and neck cancers, alcohol appears to play a synergistic role in the development of laryngeal tumors. Cancer of the larynx affects men more than women and generally is seen after age 60. However, with the increased number of younger cigarette smokers, the age at which cancer of the larynx develops appears to be decreasing.

PATHOPHYSIOLOGY

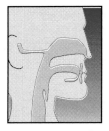 Because the larynx is lined with ciliated columnar squamous epithelium, it produces the most common cell type of squamous cell carcinoma. Tumors of the larynx may be ulcerative, infiltrative, or exophytic, and submucosal invasion of adjacent areas is common.

As was explained in Chapter 1, the larynx is divided into three areas: (1) the supraglottic larynx, an area of rich lymphatic drainage into the jugular digastric lymph nodes, which comprises the epiglottis, the false vocal cords, the ventricle, the aryepiglottic folds, and the arytenoids; (2) the glottic larynx, an area of sparse lymphatic vessels that is defined as the area of the true vocal cords; and (3) the subglottic (or infraglottic) larynx, the area below the true vocal cords.

CLINICAL MANIFESTATIONS

The symptoms of tumors of the supraglottic larynx usually are related at first to swallowing. The patient may complain of dysphagia (difficulty swallowing), odynophagia (pain on swallowing), aspiration on swallowing, or a foreign body sensation. Unilateral sore throat and referred pain to the ear (otalgia) are other symptoms. The symptoms of tumors of the glottic larynx include hoarseness or voice change, unilateral sore throat and otalgia. Respiratory distress may develop if the tumor is large and obstructive. Because of the location of the subglottic larynx, diagnosis of subglottic tumors usually is delayed for lack of symptoms. By the time the diagnosis is made, the tumor may be large enough to cause the patient to complain of a lump in the neck, difficulty breathing, and airway compromise.

COMPLICATIONS

Poor wound healing, bleeding, pharyngocutaneous fistula, pharyngeal stricture.

DIAGNOSTIC STUDIES AND FINDINGS

Diagnostic test	Findings
Laryngoscopy (direct and indirect)	Lesion of the larynx, decreased mobility of vocal cord, inadequate airway; tissue diagnosis of carcinoma, second primary tumor
Chest x-ray	Metastatic disease, second primary tumor, chronic obstructive lung disease
Barium swallow	Tumor extent, second primary tumor in esophagus
Computed tomography (CT)	Lymph node metastases, involvement of adjacent structures

MEDICAL MANAGEMENT

SURGERY

Surgery for tumors of the larynx depends on the size and location of the primary tumor and the patient's needs. Initial treatment of small tumors (T_{IS}, T_1) may involve vocal cord stripping with or without the use of a laser. Malignant and dysplastic tissue is removed from the vocal cord, and the epithelium is allowed to re-

MEDICAL MANAGEMENT—cont'd

generate. This procedure usually is repeated until no tumor or dysplastic tissue is present. Treatment of larger tumors of the vocal cord (T_2) may require a vertical partial hemilaryngectomy. Hemilaryngectomy involves removing a vocal cord or part of a vocal cord and reconstructing the area with local tissue, creating a pseudocord. Treatment of T_3 and T_4 tumors of the larynx usually involves total laryngectomy with or without radiation therapy and chemotherapy.

Tumors of the supraglottic larynx may be treated with a horizontal partial laryngectomy (also called supraglottic laryngectomy). A supraglottic laryngectomy is performed only on certain patients whose tumors are limited to the supraglottic larynx. The epiglottis is removed in this procedure, and these patients aspirate on swallowing after the surgery. Because of this chronic aspiration, only patients with good pulmonary reserve and an adequate general medical condition are eligible for this procedure.

Because tumors of the subglottic larynx usually are diagnosed so late in their course, total laryngectomy is the standard treatment. Radiation therapy and chemotherapy may be added before or after the surgical procedure to improve the prospect of a cure.

Regardless of the type of treatment selected, removal of the cancer and rehabilitation of function are the treatment objectives. To achieve the latter goal, a tracheoesophageal puncture may be done during the total laryngectomy or several weeks or months later. This procedure creates a small fistula from the superior wall of the tracheal stoma into the proximal wall of the esophagus. A red rubber catheter (no. 14 Fr) is inserted through the fistula and secured to the patient's neck to maintain the opening. Once this area has healed, the catheter is removed and a small, silicone voice prosthesis with a one-way valve is inserted. The prosthesis allows air to pass from the patient's lung by way of the tracheal stoma into the esophagus, allowing the patient to use structures of the upper aerodigestive tract to articulate words. Because the prosthesis has a one-way valve, food and saliva from the esophagus do not enter the tracheostoma.

NURSING CARE

See pages 234 to 239.

Tumors of the Hypopharynx

Tumors of the hypopharynx include malignant growths of the pyriform sinus, pharyngeal walls, and posterior cricoid area of the larynx.

PATHOPHYSIOLOGY

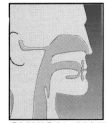

Most hypopharyngeal lesions are of squamous cell origin. Tumors of the hypopharynx have the same epidemiology as other head and neck cancers. The prognosis for patients with tumors of the hypopharynx is poor.

CLINICAL MANIFESTATIONS

The symptoms of hypopharyngeal tumors usually arise late and may include a mass in the neck; dysphagia and odynophagia, with resultant weight loss; unilateral sore throat and otalgia; hoarseness and other voice changes; and a foul odor from superficial infection of the tumor.

COMPLICATIONS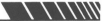

Fistula formation, local infection, stricture, dysphagia from stricture, free flap necrosis due to thrombosis of the microvascular anastomosis, small bowel obstruction and wound dehiscence from the abdominal surgery.

DIAGNOSTIC STUDIES AND FINDINGS

Diagnostic test	Findings
Laryngoscopy (direct and indirect)	Lesion of the hypopharynx, decreased mobility of vocal cord, inadequate airway; tissue diagnosis of carcinoma, second primary tumor
Chest x-ray	Metastatic disease, second primary tumor, chronic obstructive lung disease
Barium swallow	Tumor extent, second primary tumor in esophagus
Computed tomography (CT)	Lymph node metastases, involvement of adjacent structures

MEDICAL MANAGEMENT

SURGERY

Treatment for tumors of the hypopharynx usually involves a pharyngectomy with or without total laryngectomy, depending on the location and size of the primary tumor. Radiation therapy and chemotherapy often are used as adjuvant treatments because of the size and location of the primary tumor.

Reconstruction after surgical extirpation of hypopharyngeal tumors is of primary concern. The reconstructive technique used to close the surgical defect depends on the size of the primary tumor. Small tumors with substantial tissue remaining after resection may be closed primarily or with local tissue flaps. Larger defects in the pharyngoesophageal area may require a regional pedicle flap or a free flap. When tumor resection requires total esophagectomy with total laryngectomy, the surgeon may choose to reconstruct the defect by mobilizing the stomach and doing a gastric "pull-up," in which the stomach is pulled up into the neck and sutured to the residual tongue and pharynx. If the whole pharynx and larynx must be removed but the esophagus can be preserved, an alternative reconstructive technique is a free jejunal graft. Microvascular techniques are required to connect arteries and veins to support this graft. An implantable Doppler probe may be placed on the artery supplying the tissue transfer to provide an auditory and graphic signal of the blood flow in the anastomosed vessels. Sentinel loops, which are small pieces of jejunum brought through the skin, may also be used to monitor the viability of the jejunal free flap.

The nursing care of these patients after surgery is the same as that for a patient who has had a total laryngectomy. Maintaining the viability of the jejunal free flap and the use of a needle catheter jejunostomy feeding tube are the major differences.

POSTOPERATIVE NURSING CARE

1 ASSESS

ASSESSMENT	OBSERVATIONS
Respiratory	Increased mucus, ineffective cough, decreased breath sounds, dry or bloody secretions, abnormal ABG and pulse oximetry readings
Skin	Incisions; tracheostoma; neck drainage catheters

ASSESSMENT	OBSERVATIONS
Infection	Erythema of skin; increased drainage; saliva or purulent drainage in neck catheters; elevated temperature and WBC
Nutrition	Inability or decreased ability to swallow due to edema, aspiration on swallowing
Speech	Absence of normal speaking voice
Anxiety	Tension, apprehension, restlessness

2   DIAGNOSE

NURSING DIAGNOSIS	SUBJECTIVE FINDINGS	OBJECTIVE FINDINGS
Ineffective airway clearance related to aspiration of mucus and body fluids; increased mucus production; decreased ability or inability to cough effectively; obstruction of stoma or tracheotomy tube	Complains of inability to cough up secretions, increased mucus, difficulty breathing, blood in mucus	Increased secretions in oral cavity or tracheotomy tube; ineffective cough; dyspnea; decrease in pulse oximetry and ABGs; decreased breath sounds
Impaired skin integrity related to surgical incisions; **high risk for infection** related to surgical incisions	Complains of irritation at incision site; discomfort of dressings and tubes Complains of increased drainage; fever	Surgical incision, neck drainage catheters, tracheostoma Increased erythema, drainage from surgical incisions and drains; elevated temperature and WBC; saliva in neck drains or incision line
Impaired verbal communication related to surgical removal of larynx	Complains of inability to speak	Unable to speak; has tracheotomy tube
Pain (acute) related to surgical incisions; presence of tubes and dressings	Complains of pain and awkwardness of tubes and dressings	Requests pain medication; movement is decreased
Impaired swallowing related to surgery of larynx	Complains of pain; unable to swallow	Increased oral secretions, aspiration on swallowing
Body image disturbance related to surgical incisions; presence of stoma; altered communication	Expresses concern about appearance, presence of breathing hole in neck; uncommunicative	Refuses to look in mirror or participate in self-care, stays in bed, does not socialize, refuses to use alternate communication devices

→ > >

3 PLAN

Patient goals

1. The patient will maintain a patent airway.
2. The patient's incisions and stoma will heal without infection.
3. The patient will communicate effectively.
4. The patient will have minimal pain and discomfort.
5. The patient will maintain his nutritional status.
6. The patient will adapt to changes in structure and function.

4 IMPLEMENT

NURSING DIAGNOSIS	NURSING INTERVENTIONS	RATIONALE
Ineffective airway clearance related to aspiration of mucus and body fluids; increased mucus production; decreased ability or inability to cough effectively; obstruction of stoma or tracheotomy tube	See Postoperative Nursing Care for Tracheotomy, pages 252 to 256.	
	Assess patient's airway for signs of mucus plug: whistling sound, blood in mucus, dry mucus, decrease in passage of air through tracheotomy tube.	Dry air is inhaled directly into the trachea through the stoma, bypassing the normal humidification system of the nose and mouth. This may result in drying of the mucous secretions, which can obstruct the opening of the tracheotomy tube.
	Remove mucus plug (see the box on page 240).	To remedy airway obstruction.
	Change tube daily once cuffed tube is removed.	To allow adequate cleaning of stoma and to provide a clean tube.
	Instruct patient in proper technique for changing the tube (see the box on page 258).	To familiarize patient with procedure to prepare for discharge.
	Assess stoma size.	The stoma is created by suturing the cut end of the trachea to the skin. A circle heals smaller if not properly stented. The tracheotomy tube maintains the size of the stoma.
Impaired skin integrity related to surgical incisions; **high risk for infection** related to surgical incisions	Assess surgical incision for increased erythema, edema, and drainage (especially evidence of purulent drainage or saliva), and odor.	To detect infection.
	Evaluate integrity of surgical incision.	Separation of incision may indicate hematoma, seroma, or infection under skin flap.
	Using sterile technique, cleanse incision with hydrogen peroxide and rinse with water or saline; apply antibiotic ointment.	To remove drainage, promote healing, and prevent superficial infection; ointment also keeps secretions soft.
	Maintain patency of closed-suction wound drainage catheters.	To prevent accumulation of blood and serum under skin flaps.
	Evaluate vital signs; monitor elevated temperature and WBC.	To detect infection.

NURSING DIAGNOSIS	NURSING INTERVENTIONS	RATIONALE
	Monitor Doppler signal and sentinel loops and notify physician of any changes.	To determine adequacy of microvascular anastomosis. If alteration in blood supply is detected, immediate surgical intervention is required to prevent loss of free flap.
	Avoid constricting articles around flap (e.g., tracheotomy ties, elastic ties on oxygen mask, compressive dressings).	To avoid compromising circulation to free flap.
Impaired verbal communication related to surgical removal of larynx	See Postoperative Nursing Care for Tracheotomy, pages 252 to 256.	
	Encourage use of alternative communication; reinforce instruction given by speech therapist for use of speech device (Figures 11-1 and 11-2).	To allow patient to express needs, concerns, and fears.
	Instruct patient in use of tracheoesophageal puncture; technique to insert red rubber catheter into puncture site (Figure 11-2).	To maintain puncture until tract forms, catheter should be inserted within a few hours to prevent closure of opening.
	Reinforce care to avoid accidental removal of catheter before tract forms (hold in place with tape).	To prevent accidental removal.
	Tie distal end of catheter before taping.	To prevent reflux of gastric contents through catheter.
	Reinforce technique for using tracheo-esophageal speech (occluding tracheostoma).	To shunt air from lungs through airflow port and out one-way valve into esophagus to produce vibration; other articulating areas form words.
	Reinforce instructions given by speech therapist for care of speech prosthesis.	To ensure longevity of speech prosthesis.
Pain (acute) related to surgical incisions; presence of tubes and dressings	Evaluate alternative positions to improve comfort.	The neck incisions used for head and neck surgery sever the sensory nerve supply, resulting in numbness of the surgical area. Much of the discomfort expressed by the patient is related to pressure dressings, tracheotomy tube, and drains. Changing positions can relieve this discomfort.
	Assess and document location and intensity of pain.	To evaluate need for analgesics.
	Evaluate response to analgesics.	To determine need for change in analgesic.
Impaired swallowing related to surgery of larynx	Attach nasogastric tube, if present, to low, continuous suction.	To prevent emesis, which would cause high-pressure gastric contents to disrupt the pharyngeal suture line, resulting in dehiscence, infection, and/or fistula.

NURSING DIAGNOSIS	NURSING INTERVENTIONS	RATIONALE
	Institute tube feedings as ordered once bowel sounds return.	Tube feedings are not started until bowel sounds return to prevent obstruction.
	Begin with clear liquids, advance to high-calorie, high-protein diet by tube as ordered or directed by institutional protocol. Administer tube feedings by bolus or drip technique. Administer jejunostomy tube feedings if jejunal free flap is present (see the box on tube feeding, page 231).	Diet is advanced according to patient's tolerance.
	Begin oral diet as ordered for hemilaryngectomy or total laryngectomy. Usually begin clear liquids on day 7-10, and advance diet as tolerated (see the box on page 240 for supraglottic laryngectomy feeding).	Liquids are best tolerated initially to avoid stress on suture line and are more easily swallowed with residual edema.
	Consult with dietitian to determine high-calorie, high-protein diet.	To promote wound healing and maintain nutrition.
	Encourage patient to eat small, frequent meals, to choose soft foods, and to cut food into small pieces.	To prevent food obstruction caused by persistent edema, which may result in nasal regurgitation.
	Consult with speech and swallowing therapists.	These team members can assist with modified barium swallow, evaluating patient's ability to swallow, determining types and consistency of foods best tolerated, and helping patient with institution of swallowing.
Body image disturbance related to surgical incisions; presence of stoma; altered communication	See body image disturbance for Resection of Tumors of the Oral Cavity (page 229) and for Tracheotomy (page 255).	

5 EVALUATE

PATIENT OUTCOME	DATA INDICATING THAT OUTCOME IS REACHED
Patient has patent airway.	ABG and pulse oximetry readings are within normal limits for patient; no dyspnea or stridor is present; patient has effective cough and clear breath sounds bilaterally.
Skin incisions and stoma have healed without evidence of infection.	Skin edges of incision approximate; there is no drainage; temperature and WBC are within normal limits; no fistula is present.

PATIENT OUTCOME	DATA INDICATING THAT OUTCOME IS REACHED
Patient communicates effectively.	Patient uses alternative communication device.
Patient's pain is minimal.	Patient ambulates and requires minimal use of analgesics.
Patient maintains adequate nutrition.	Patient maintains his weight, swallows without aspiration, and has resumed a general diet.
Patient has adapted to change in body image.	Patient performs self-care, socializes, uses effective coping strategies, and participates in support groups.

PATIENT TEACHING

1. See Patient Teaching for Tracheotomy, page 256.
2. Instruct patient in care of tracheoesophageal puncture.
3. Provide nutritional instruction (reinforce supraglottic swallow, provide diet plan for high-calorie, high-protein diet).
4. Refer to support groups (International Laryngectomy Association, Lost Cord Club, American Cancer Society, Home Health Nursing, Alcoholics Anonymous, smoking cessation program).
5. Provide information on obtaining supplies.
6. Encourage coughing and deep breathing rather than suctioning of stoma.
7. Review emergency measures (mouth-to-stoma resuscitation, removal of mucus plug, use of tube or button to maintain size of stoma).
8. Review signs of infection, and encourage patient to notify physician if problems occur.
9. Encourage follow-up visits with physician, speech therapist, and support groups.

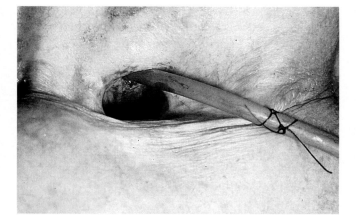

FIGURE 11-1
Speech valve in place.

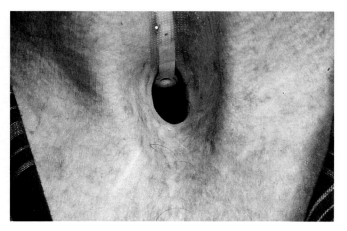

FIGURE 11-2
Red rubber catheter inserted in tracheoesophageal puncture site.

REMOVING A MUCUS PLUG

When a mucus plug is discovered, it must be removed immediately to prevent obstruction of the airway.

1. Remove the tracheotomy tube to provide more space through which to expel the mucus plug.
2. Instill 3 to 5 ml of normal saline into the stoma to loosen dry secretions and stimulate coughing.
3. Suction the trachea, repeating until the plug is expelled. The tracheal lining is fragile, and the plug must be loosened before it can be removed.
4. Gently remove the plug with forceps, avoiding trauma, to prevent bleeding.

SUPRAGLOTTIC SWALLOW

Action	Effect
Take deep breath	To aerate lungs
Perform Valsalva maneuver (bear down)	To approximate vocal cords
Place food in mouth and swallow	Some food will enter airway and remain on top of closed vocal cords
Cough	To remove food from top of vocal cords
Swallow	To swallow food moved from top of vocal cords
Breathe	Restoring breathing before the cough-swallow sequence would result in aspiration of food collected by vocal cords

FEEDING A PATIENT WHO HAS HAD A SUPRAGLOTTIC LARYNGECTOMY

After a supraglottic laryngectomy, the patient is at risk for aspiration. There are various schools of thought on how to institute an oral diet for these patients. Some advocate oral feeding while the tracheotomy is in place, to maintain the ability to suction the tracheobronchial tree. Others believe that an effective cough cannot be achieved while the tracheotomy is open; therefore an oral diet should not be started until decannulation is complete and the stoma is closed. This provides the patient with the ability to approximate the vocal cords and produces increased subglottic pressure, resulting in an effective cough and a protected airway.

When it is time to institute oral feedings, follow these guidelines:

- Begin feedings with nonpourable, pureed foods; this gives the patient more control over placement and movement of the food.
- Avoid thin liquids, because they move quickly to the posterior oral cavity, causing aspiration.
- Gradually introduce liquids, beginning with carbonated ones. Their effervescence provides a clue to the liquid's position.
- Reinforce the "supraglottic swallow" (see facing box), a technique that allows the patient to swallow with minimal aspiration.

Masses of the Neck

Masses of the neck may be congenital or neoplastic (benign or malignant). The patient's age and history and the location of the mass are evaluated for possible differential diagnoses. Most malignant tumors of the neck are metastatic from the upper aerodigestive tract rather than from below the clavicle. Primary malignant tumors of the neck are unusual except for lymphomas and tumors of the salivary glands and thyroid gland.

CONGENITAL NECK MASSES

Branchial cleft cysts are inflammatory masses that develop in a remnant of the branchial system of embryologic life.

Branchial cleft cysts are remnants of the branchial apparatus and may be classified as first, second, or third cleft anomalies. These cysts usually are lined with squamous or columnar epithelium. Second branchial cleft cysts, the most common type, are found along the sternocleidomastoid muscle.

Branchial cleft cysts can occur at any age but usually become evident in children or young adults. Inflammation of a branchial cleft cyst usually is associated with an upper respiratory infection, which causes the inflammation and possibly formation of an abscess.

For Diagnostic Studies and Findings and Nursing Care, see pages 244 to 249.

COMPLICATIONS

Wound infection

MEDICAL MANAGEMENT

Branchial cleft cysts initially are treated with antibiotics to resolve the inflammation and/or abscess.

SURGERY

Complete excision of the branchial cleft cyst is the treatment of choice once the inflammation has subsided. A horizontal neck incision is made, and the cyst and any sinus tract that may be attached are removed.

For a picture of a thyroglossal duct cyst, see the color plate on page xiii.

THYROGLOSSAL DUCT CYST

Thyroglossal duct cyst is an anomaly arising from the duct through which the thyroid gland descends during embryologic life.

Thyroglossal duct cysts are anomalies that arise from a remnant of the duct through which the thyroid gland descends during embryologic life. The duct extends from the foramen cecum in the midline of the base of the tongue to the thyroid gland overlying the trachea. Normally the thyroglossal duct disappears during fetal life once the thyroid gland has descended completely. Because the thyroglossal duct is lined with squamous respiratory epithelium, inflammation usually follows an upper respiratory infection.

Thyroglossal duct cysts may occur in children or adults. The cyst usually is located in the midline of the neck at the level of the hyoid bone and characteristically moves up and down with swallowing.

COMPLICATIONS

Wound infection

For Diagnostic Studies and Findings and Nursing-Care, see pages 244 to 249.

MEDICAL MANAGEMENT

An infected thyroglossal duct cyst is treated with antibiotics. Because these cysts have been known to contain malignant cells, surgical excision is recommended once the infection has subsided.

SURGERY

Surgery for a thyroglossal duct cyst involves excising the cyst and the duct (tracking the duct up to the base of the tongue) and removing the central portion of the hyoid bone. This surgery is also known as the Sistrunk operation. The cyst and corresponding duct must be completely removed to prevent recurrence.

GLOMUS TUMORS

Glomus tumors are neoplasms arising from chemoreceptor tissue associated with the great vessels.

Glomus tumors, also known as paragangliomas, arise from the chemoreceptor tissue associated with the great vessels. The most common paragangliomas originate at the carotid bifurcation and are known as carotid body tumors, or chemodectomas. The patient has a neck mass at the carotid bifurcation, and a bruit is audible on auscultation. Tumors that arise at the jugular bulb are known as glomus jugulare. A patient with a glomus jugulare shows lower cranial nerve deficits such as hoarseness, dysphasia, and unilateral tongue atrophy with deviation of the tongue to the side of the tumor. Glomus tumors may also develop along the course of the vagus nerve and may be associated with vocal cord paralysis. Glomus tympanicum occurs in the middle ear space; these patients have pulsatile tinnitus and conductive hearing loss. A bluish mass may be visible behind the tympanic membrane, and when pressure from a pneumatic otoscope is applied, the tumor mass blanches (positive Brown's sign).

Glomus tumors usually are benign, but they may exhibit local invasion and destruction and may extend to the base of the skull. Malignant glomus tumors are diagnosed only by the presence of metastasis. Occasionally, patients with glomus tumors have a family history of these lesions.

For Diagnostic Studies and Findings and Nursing Care, see pages 244 to 249.

COMPLICATIONS

Cranial nerve deficits (swallowing dysfunction, facial nerve paralysis, hearing loss), leakage of cerebrospinal fluid (CSF),

MEDICAL MANAGEMENT

SURGERY

Surgical excision is the recommended treatment for glomus tumors. Glomus tympanicum requires a postauricular incision to enter the middle ear space (nursing care of patients with glomus tympanicum can be found under Nursing Care for Ear Surgery, pages 108-111).

Surgical excision of carotid body tumors, glomus vagale, and glomus jugulare is approached through a neck incision; the nursing care of these patients appears at the end of this section.

TUMORS OF THE PAROTID GLAND

Tumors of the parotid gland are benign or malignant neoplasms arising in the largest of the major salivary glands.

The parotid gland, the largest of the salivary glands, is divided by the facial nerve into a superficial and a deep component. The superficial component is adjacent to the masseter muscle, and the deep component extends toward the pharyngeal wall (parapharyngeal space). Saliva produced by the parotid gland passes into the oral cavity by way of Stensen's duct, which opens near the upper second molar.

The arterial blood supply to the parotid gland is provided by the external carotid artery by way of the internal maxillary and the superficial temporal arteries. Venous drainage is through the superficial temporal vein, which joins the internal maxillary vein and the posterior facial vein into the jugular veins.

Cranial nerve VII (the facial nerve) supplies the motor function to the face. It exits the base of the skull by way of the stylomastoid foramen. The main nerve trunk enters the posterior border of the parotid and divides into five branches: the temporal branch, which supplies the temporal region of the head; the zygomatic branch, which supplies the lateral orbit; the buccal branch, which supplies the nose and mouth; the marginal mandibular branch, which supplies the lower lip and chin; and the cervical branch, which supplies the platysma muscle. The greater auricular nerve of the cervical plexus supplies sensation to the ear and earlobe, and the auricular temporal nerve and parasympathetic fibers stimulate gland secretion.

The parotid gland contains many lymph nodes. These nodes receive drainage from the external auditory canal, auricle, skin of the face and scalp, eyelids, lacrimal gland, and the parotid gland.

Most growths, or neoplasms, of the parotid are benign. The main symptom of a benign tumor is a slow-growing, asymptomatic mass in the region of the parotid gland. Pleomorphic adenomas (benign mixed tumors) are the most common benign tumors of the parotid gland. A small percentage of benign mixed tumors may undergo malignant change. Warthin's tumor is the second most common benign tumor of the parotid gland. Malignant tumors of the parotid gland are unusual and have the same symptom of benign tumors (slow-growing, asymptomatic mass). As malignant tumors enlarge, pain becomes a major feature and facial nerve paralysis may ensue. Mucoepidermoid carcinoma is the most common malignant tumor of the parotid gland. Other types of malignant tumors that develop are adenoid cystic carcinoma, carcinoma expleomorphic adenoma (malignant mixed tumor, malignant pleomorphic adenoma), primary or metastatic squamous cell carcinoma, and melanoma.

COMPLICATIONS

Facial nerve paralysis, Frey's syndrome (gustatory sweating), salivary fistula, infection, hematoma.

For Diagnostic Studies and Findings and Nursing Care, see pages 244 to 249.

MEDICAL MANAGEMENT

SURGERY

Treatment of parotid tumors involves complete excision of the tumor with a cuff of normal tissue, most commonly accomplished by means of a superficial parotidectomy. An incision is made around the ear and into a skin crease in the neck. The facial nerve must be identified and preserved. The risk of injury to this nerve during surgery is considerably reduced if the surgeon uses a microscope and a nerve stimulator to determine nerve functioning.

Surgical excision of malignant parotid gland tumors involves removing both the superficial and the deep lobe of the gland. Preservation of the facial nerve depends on the type of tumor and nerve involvement.

TUMORS OF THE THYROID GLAND

Tumors of the thyroid gland are benign or malignant neoplasms arising in the thyroid gland.

The most common thyroid tumor is a benign adenoma. Such tumors most often are an incidental finding discovered on palpation of the thyroid gland during a routine physical examination. A thyroid scan usually is ordered, and a *hot* or *cold* nodule may be diagnosed. A hot nodule is an area in the thyroid gland that takes up the radioactive iodine. These functioning nodules usually are benign adenomas. Cold nodules do not take up the radioactive iodine and are considered nonfunctioning nodules. Cold nodules usually are benign, but they have a higher incidence of malignancy than do hot nodules; therefore a cold nodule is not diagnostic.

Malignant tumors that can affect the thyroid gland include papillary, follicular, medullary, and anaplastic carcinoma, and lymphomas. Papillary carcinoma is the most common malignant tumor of the thyroid gland. It is a low-grade tumor that occurs most often in young adults and is more common in women than in men. Medullary carcinoma may be a familial form of thyroid carcinoma and may be associated with pheochromocytoma. Anaplastic carcinoma is an extremely malignant thyroid carcinoma that affects older people.

COMPLICATIONS

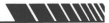

Injury to the recurrent laryngeal nerve, hypocalcemia, infection, hematoma.

For Diagnostic Studies and Findings and Nursing Care, see pages 244 to 249.

MEDICAL MANAGEMENT

Except for benign nodules, surgery is the primary treatment choice for thyroid tumors. Fine needle aspiration biopsy may identify patients with malignant disease. Initially suppression may be attempted by administering exogenous thyroid hormone to decrease or eliminate the nodule. If this does not eliminate the tumor, surgical intervention will be suggested.

SURGERY

Surgical excision of benign tumors involves removing the thyroid lobe containing the nodule. Malignant tumors are most often treated with a total thyroidectomy followed by radioactive iodine to ablate any remaining thyroid tissue. For this procedure, an incision is made in a skin line above the sternal notch that is cosmetically acceptable. The recurrent laryngeal nerve is identified (it lies 1 to 2 cm lateral to the trachea near the lower pole of the thyroid). The blood vessels are identified, and the thyroid gland is removed. The parathyroid glands are identified and preserved if possible. After the thyroid gland has been removed and hemostasis has been achieved, the incision is closed. Small-wound drainage catheters may be placed to prevent the formation of a hematoma or seroma during the postoperative period.

LYMPH NODE METASTASIS

Cervical lymph node metastases are tumors in the regional lymph nodes containing metastatic deposits from tumors in another area of the body.

Malignant tumors of the lymph nodes, other than lymphomas, are caused by metastatic spread from primary tumors that may be in the upper aerodigestive tract or areas below the clavicle. By reviewing the lymphatic drainage channels from the aerodigestive tract, the examiner generally can locate the site of the primary tumor. If a primary tumor cannot be located, biopsies of the tonsils, base of the tongue, and pharynx must be done to find an occult tumor. If no primary tumor is found, an open biopsy of the node may be done with frozen-section diagnosis. If metastatic squamous cell carcinoma is diagnosed by frozen section, neck dissection is performed immediately to prevent tumor seeding.

COMPLICATIONS

Infection, fistula, wound dehiscence, chylous fistula, hematoma or seroma formation, shoulder disability, airway compromise.

DIAGNOSTIC STUDIES AND FINDINGS

Diagnostic test	Findings
Endoscopy	Mucosal tumor causing neck mass (metastasis)
Radionuclide scan	Abnormality of thyroid gland
Arteriography	Vascular tumor, tumor attached to carotid artery
Sialography	Abnormality of salivary gland
Computed tomography (CT)	Mucosal tumor, location of lymph node involvement, cystic or solid mass
Biopsy	
Fine needle aspiration biopsy	To determine tumor type
Open biopsy with frozen section	Done only if other evaluation techniques fail to provide diagnosis; plans should be made to proceed with neck dissection after frozen-section confirmation

MEDICAL MANAGEMENT

Treatment of the cervical lymph nodes depends on the potential for metastasis from the primary tumor, the size of the primary tumor, and the size and location of enlarged cervical lymph nodes.

SURGERY

An incision is made from the mandible to the clavicle to the midline of the neck to allow maximum exposure of the vital structures. Surgical removal of the lymph nodes can involve a radical neck dissection, modified neck dissection, or selective neck dissection. A radical neck dissection removes all the lymph nodes from the clavicle to the mandible, the sternocleidomastoid muscle, the submandibular gland, the internal jugular vein, and the spinal accessory nerve. A modified neck dissection spares the spinal accessory nerve, and a selective neck dissection removes only lymph node groups that drain the primary site (Zones I-V).

Disability after neck dissection depends on whether the spinal accessory nerve, which innervates the upper trapezius muscle, is sacrificed. Radical neck dissection may cause increased pain, shoulder drooping with forward displacement, winging of the scapulae, and decreased range of motion and muscle strength in the shoulder and arm. The modified and selective neck dissections remove less tissue and spare the spinal accessory nerve, thereby producing less disability. Nevertheless, stiffness, osteoarthritis, and adhesive capsulitis may occur, producing some shoulder dysfunction if no rehabilitative efforts are made.

RADIATION THERAPY

The results of the histologic evaluation of the lymph nodes after removal help determine whether adjuvant therapy is required. Extracapsular spread of the tumor or involvement of the capsule of the lymph node or soft tissues indicates a greater potential for recurrence of the tumor, and radiation therapy and possibly chemotherapy may be recommended.

Radiation therapy may be used to treat the N_O neck in a patient who has a primary tumor with potential for metastasis to the regional lymph nodes. The choice between elective neck dissection and radiation therapy depends on the physician's preference. Under either circumstance, the patient must be closely monitored for tumor recurrence.

POSTOPERATIVE NURSING CARE

1 ASSESS

ASSESSMENT	OBSERVATIONS
Respiratory	Dyspnea, incisional edema, pressure dressing, cough when swallowing, inability to clear airway of secretions, breathy quality to voice
Infection	Erythema, increased drainage, fever
Nutrition	Aspiration on swallowing; weight loss; pain when swallowing
Sensory perception/ body image	Hypocalcemia, numbness, facial paralysis, pain

→ > >

2　DIAGNOSE

NURSING DIAGNOSIS	SUBJECTIVE FINDINGS	OBJECTIVE FINDINGS
Ineffective airway clearance related to postoperative edema	Complains of shortness of breath, tight dressing, compression or tightness around neck	Dyspnea; inability to clear secretions; rales, rhonchi on auscultation; decreased respiratory rate and depth
High risk for infection related to surgical incision	Complains of fever, drainage from incision, swelling of surgical site	Elevated temperature and WBC, increased erythema, edema, and drainage from surgical site
Impaired swallowing related to postoperative edema; injury to recurrent laryngeal nerve	Complains of pain on swallowing, difficulty swallowing or inability to swallow	Aspiration, decreased oral intake, facial grimacing, cough when swallowing
Pain (acute) related to surgery	Complains of pain	Requests pain medication, exhibits diaphoresis, has increased pulse and shallow respirations, splints incision and arm
Altered sensory perception related to surgical incision; facial nerve paralysis; hypocalcemia	Complains of numbness around surgical incision; weakness of face; inability to close eye; numbness of fingers, toes, lips; general weakness	Decreased sensation around surgical incision, facial paralysis, circumoral pallor, positive Chvostek's and Trousseau's signs
Body image disturbance related to facial paralysis; neck and facial incisions	Expresses concern over appearance, appears depressed	Refuses to look in mirror, isolates self, refuses to participate in self-care, cries easily

3　PLAN

Patient goals

1. The patient's breathing will be normal.
2. The patient will show no signs of infection.
3. The patient will be able to maintain body weight.
4. The patient will have minimal pain.
5. The patient will understand reason for altered sensory perception and will be able to adapt to changes in sensation.
6. The patient will be able to cope well with body image changes.

4　IMPLEMENT

NURSING DIAGNOSIS	NURSING INTERVENTIONS	RATIONALE
Ineffective airway clearance related to postoperative edema	Elevate head of bed.	To reduce edema and promote lung expansion.
	Assess rate and depth of respirations; assess for stridor or any difficulty breathing; auscultate breath sounds.	To detect breathing problems for prompt intervention.

NURSING DIAGNOSIS	NURSING INTERVENTIONS	RATIONALE
	Encourage deep breathing and coughing.	To mobilize secretions.
	Maintain pressure dressing; assess for dressing tightness, increased edema above incision, hematoma.	To assess for external compression, which would compromise airway.
	Assess patient's ability to speak, cough, and swallow (postoperative thyroidectomy).	To determine injury to vagus nerve or recurrent laryngeal nerve.
	See ineffective airway clearance and ineffective breathing pattern, pages 227, 253.	
High risk for infection related to surgical incision	Maintain pressure dressing and neck drains (see the box on page 249).	To prevent seroma or hematoma formation.
	Clean suture line with hydrogen peroxide and rinse with saline or water; apply antibiotic ointment to incision.	To remove accumulated secretions, promote healing, prevent superficial infection, and keep secretions soft.
	Monitor integrity of suture line.	To detect wound separation.
	Monitor vital signs, WBC.	To detect infection.
Impaired swallowing related to postoperative edema; injury to recurrent laryngeal nerve	Monitor oral intake, consistency of foods, and caloric intake.	To maintain weight and ensure proper wound healing.
	Assess patient for dysphagia and aspiration.	Dysphagia may be related to presence of endotracheal tube during surgery and may be alleviated with analgesics and a change in the consistency of food. Aspiration may be related to vocal cord paralysis caused by injury to the vagus nerve or recurrent laryngeal nerve.
Pain (acute) related to surgery	Evaluate intensity and location of pain.	To determine need for intervention.
	Help patient assume a position of comfort.	High Fowler's position with splinting by pillows may decrease discomfort caused by tubes and dressings.
	Administer analgesics as ordered, and evaluate effectiveness.	To relieve pain and determine need for alternative pain-control measures.
	After neck dissection, support affected arm with pillows and sling; do not allow arm to dangle.	To prevent stretching of muscle, which can result in muscle spasm.
	Begin postoperative exercises as ordered (passive range of motion to neck and affected arm beginning on postoperative day 2 or 3, active range of motion and muscle strengthening after removal of neck drains).	To reduce pain (acute and chronic) and restore range of motion and muscle strength.

➔ ❯ ❯ ❯

NURSING DIAGNOSIS	NURSING INTERVENTIONS	RATIONALE
	Encourage patient to continue exercises.	To prevent adhesive capsulitis, osteoarthritis, and decrease in range of motion and muscle strength.
Altered sensory perception related to surgical incision; facial nerve paralysis; hypocalcemia*	Observe patient for facial nerve paralysis (postoperative parotidectomy).	Temporary or permanent facial paralysis is caused by trauma to or resection of the facial nerve.
	Provide eye care (administer artificial tears, apply eye shield to affected eye, apply ointment to eye at bedtime, tape eye at bedtime).	To prevent corneal dryness, irritation, and abrasion resulting from patient's inability to close eye.
	Provide mouth care (instruct patient to place food on unaffected side of mouth; teach patient to manually remove food from affected side; rinse mouth with hydrogen peroxide and water or normal saline).	Patient will have drooping of affected side and will be unable to feel presence of food and debris in affected side of mouth (facial paralysis).
	Instruct patient to exercise muscles of face as ordered by circle massage of muscle groups innervated by facial nerve.	To maintain muscle tone.
	Caution patient about effects of numbness of face and ear (avoid extreme heat or cold; use electric razor to avoid cutting the skin).	Patient cannot feel temperature extremes or injury to skin that can result in tissue trauma (e.g., cuts, burns, frostbite).
Body image disturbance related to facial paralysis; neck and facial incisions	See body image disturbance, pages 221, 229	

5 EVALUATE

PATIENT OUTCOME	DATA INDICATING THAT OUTCOME IS REACHED
Airway is patent.	Breath sounds are clear bilaterally; respiratory rate and depth are within normal limits; no dyspnea is observed.
Incision has healed without infection.	There are no signs of erythema or drainage; temperature and WBC count are within normal limits.
Body weight is maintained.	Patient does not aspirate on swallowing and shows no weight loss.
Patient's pain is minimal.	Patient requires minimal use of analgesics and effectively uses exercise to prevent or minimize pain.

*Assess the patient for signs of hypocalcemia (see the facing page).

PATIENT OUTCOME	DATA INDICATING THAT OUTCOME IS REACHED
Patient has adapted to altered sensory perception.	Patient understands appropriate safety measures and knows signs of hypocalcemia.
Patient has adapted to changes in body image.	Patient participates in self-care, socializes with others, and participates in support groups.

PATIENT TEACHING

1. Reinforce range-of-motion, muscle strengthening, and facial exercises.
2. Instruct the patient to notify her physician of any signs of an infection or seroma, such as fever, increased drainage, increased inflammation or swelling, pain.
3. Encourage the patient to eat a high-calorie, high-protein diet and to increase her intake of calcium and vitamin D for hypocalcemia.
4. Instruct the patient in the administration, dosage, and side effects of thyroid replacement drugs.
5. If the patient is undergoing radioactive iodine therapy after surgery and thus is not taking a thyroid replacement drug, encourage energy-saving activities and frequent rest periods. Encourage her to walk with assistance if muscle weakness occurs.
6. Instruct the patient to notify her physician if signs of hypocalcemia occur (i.e., numbness or tingling of lips, fingers, and toes; circumoral pallor; weakness; muscle irritability).
7. Reinforce safety measures for altered sensory perception (e.g., use caution with heat-producing appliances such as hair dryer, hot rollers, and heating pad; increase protective covering over areas of decreased sensation in cold weather to prevent frostbite; use electric razor to avoid cutting skin).

CARE OF NECK DRAINS AFTER NECK SURGERY

Monitor the amount and consistency of drainage. Drainage will gradually decrease. Initially 100 to 150 ml of sanguineous drainage can be expected after neck dissection. Other neck procedures produce less drainage. An increase in bloody drainage may indicate bleeding or hematoma. By postoperative day 2, drainage from removal of a congenital cyst, parotidectomy, or thyroidectomy should be minimal and the drains usually are removed. Following neck dissection, the drainage is serosanguineous by postoperative day 2 and gradually becomes serous. An increase in serous drainage may indicate seroma formation. Observe any change in the consistency of the drainage, especially after ingestion of food. Appearance of opaque, milky-colored drainage may indicate a chylous fistula resulting from injury to the thoracic duct.

ASSESSING THE PATIENT FOR SIGNS OF HYPOCALCEMIA

During a total thyroidectomy, the parathyroid glands may be injured or removed. This could result in hypocalcemia, because these glands are responsible for calcium metabolism. Hypocalcemia can cause neuromuscular irritability with symptoms of paresthesia, weakness, cardiac dysfunction, tetany, and seizures.
Evaluate the patient for signs of hypocalcemia as follows:
1. Monitor serum calcium levels.
2. Check Chvostek's and Trousseau's signs.
3. Observe the patient for circumoral pallor.
4. Instruct the patient to notify the nurse of signs of numbness or tingling in her face, fingers, or toes.
5. Assess the patient's ability to ambulate with and without assistance.
6. Administer calcium supplements and vitamin D as ordered.
7. Consult with a dietitian to instruct the patient in a diet high in calcium and vitamin D.

Tracheotomy

A tracheotomy is an incision into the trachea with insertion of a cannula. **Tracheostomy** is the creation of an opening into the trachea through the neck. The two terms may be used interchangeably in most situations. The term tracheotomy will be used in this chapter.

The trachea is a cylindric tube that extends inferiorly from the larynx into the thorax, where it divides into the two mainstem bronchi. The trachea is made up of a series of C-shaped cartilages joined by connective tissue. The major blood supply is by way of the inferior thyroid artery, and the nerve supply is by way of branches of the vagus nerve. The thyroid gland lies lateral to the trachea, with the thyroid isthmus overlying the trachea between the second and fifth tracheal rings.

INDICATIONS

Possible or actual upper airway obstruction
Ventilatory assistance
To protect airway and provide pulmonary suctioning

Preoperative assessment for a tracheotomy may reveal the following observations:

- Signs of airway obstruction (dyspnea, abnormal ABG and pulse oximetry values, stridor, suprasternal retraction, restlessness)
- Ineffective cough
- High risk for airway obstruction related to surgical intervention
- Chronic aspiration

Ideally a tracheotomy is performed in the operating room. The patient is placed in a supine position, and a roll is placed under the shoulders to hyperextend the neck. A head ring may be placed under the head to stabilize the position and help make the patient more comfortable. In patients with acute airway distress or in a patient whose neck cannot be hyperextended, a tracheotomy may be performed in a sitting or semisitting position. Either local or general anesthesia may be used for a tracheotomy. Local anesthesia is preferred, because intubation is not required to secure the airway before beginning the tracheotomy. A tracheotomy is performed between the second and third or third and fourth tracheal rings. A transverse or vertical incision may be used to enter the trachea. The anterior portion of the tracheal ring may be removed to create a window, which prevents false passage of the cannula and allows for easier reinsertion of a tracheotomy tube. Traction sutures, long sutures inserted above and be-

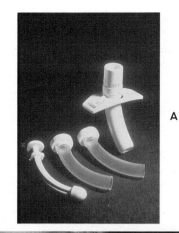

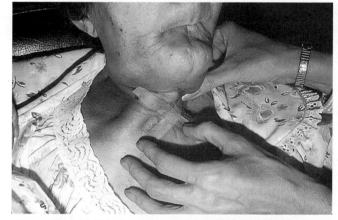

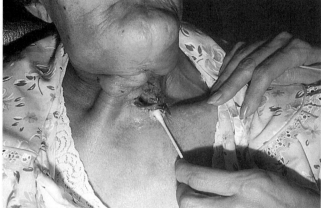

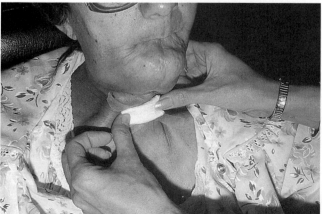

A, Tracheotomy tube. **B** to **D,** Closing the Stoma. **B,** Cleaning stoma. **C,** Taping stoma. **D,** Applying occlusive dressing to stoma.

low the window, may be used to open the stoma in case of accidental decannulation. Traction sutures are taped to the skin above and below the opening (Figure 11-3). In case of accidental decannulation, these sutures can be pulled to reopen the window. The tracheotomy tube may be sutured or tied in place. If tracheotomy ties are used, they should be tied tightly enough that only one finger can be inserted between the patient's skin and the tracheotomy ties.

A cuffed tracheotomy tube usually is used in the immediate postoperative period. A cuffed tracheotomy tube minimizes aspiration and creates a seal around the tube during ventilatory assistance. A low-pressure cuff should be used to prevent pressure necrosis on the tracheal wall. The recommended cuff pressure for tracheotomy tubes is 20 to 30 cm of water. Cuff pressure may be evaluated by using a manometer. The minimal leak technique (inflating and then deflating the cuff until movement of air is felt through the nose and mouth) is not recommended for patients who have had head and neck surgery. These patients have had a tracheotomy because of upper airway obstruction, usually caused by edema from the surgical procedure, and air cannot pass through the nose and mouth.

DIAGNOSTIC STUDIES AND FINDINGS

Diagnostic test	Findings
Laryngoscopy (direct or indirect)	Airway abnormality
Blood gases	May or may not reflect decrease in oxygen level

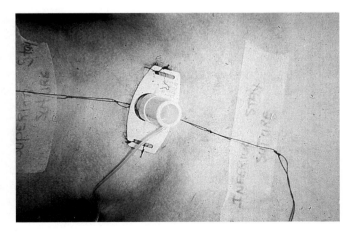

FIGURE 11-3
Position of tracheotomy sutures with tracheotomy tube in place.

COMPLICATIONS OF SURGERY

Bleeding: Postoperative bleeding may occur in a patient taking anticoagulant drugs or who has coagulation defects. Hemostasis should be ensured after a tracheotomy. Bleeding from the innominate artery may occur with aberrant positioning of the innominate artery or if a low tracheotomy was performed. This can be detected by pulsating of the tracheotomy tube after insertion.

Subcutaneous emphysema: Subcutaneous emphysema develops when air is trapped between the trachea and the subcutaneous tissues. The patient has crepitus at the tracheotomy site. A cuffed tracheotomy tube is used, and subcutaneous emphysema resolves spontaneously.

Tracheoesophageal (TE) fistula: A TE fistula is created if the anterior wall of the esophagus is cut during the tracheotomy, creating an opening between the trachea and the esophagus.

Pneumothorax: A pneumothorax may be identified if a false passage is created between the anterior tracheal wall and the anterior mediastinum. This may occur more frequently in patients who are restless or show increased activity after placement of the tracheotomy tube. A chest x-ray is taken to ensure correct placement of the tracheotomy tube and to detect a pneumothorax.

Displaced tracheotomy tube: If the tracheotomy tube is accidentally removed before a tract has formed, reinsertion may be difficult. The tracheotomy tube may be inserted into a false passage created in the subcutaneous tissue. This will be noted by obstruction to breathing, decreased passage of air through the tracheotomy tube, or inability to pass a suction catheter. The tracheotomy tube must be put in the correct position immediately (see box on page 257).

Cardiopulmonary arrest: Cardiopulmonary arrest may be caused by improper placement or displacement of the tracheotomy tube into a false passage or by loss of the respiratory drive in patients with chronic obstructive pulmonary disease. These patients may lose their hypoxic stimulus on the chemoreceptive centers, decreasing the ability to breathe.

POSTOPERATIVE NURSING CARE

1 ASSESS

ASSESSMENT	OBSERVATIONS
Respiratory	Presence of tracheotomy; adequate passage of air through tracheotomy, ABGs and pulse oximetry below normal limits for patient, increased mucus production, clear breath sounds
Nutrition	Pain on swallowing, inability to swallow (edema, aspiration, mucosal incisions)
Verbal communication	No verbal communication until edema subsides
Skin	Presence of tracheotomy; secretions around stoma
Pain	Complains of discomfort
Body image	Cries easily; does not perform self-care

2 DIAGNOSE

NURSING DIAGNOSIS	SUBJECTIVE FINDINGS	OBJECTIVE FINDINGS
Ineffective airway clearance related to increased mucus production; aspiration of secretions; ineffective cough; tracheotomy tube obstruction	Complains of increased mucus, difficulty breathing, increased coughing, fear	Rales and rhonchi in lungs on auscultation, requires frequent suctioning, ABGs and pulse oximetry below normal for patient, restlessness
Impaired swallowing related to presence of tracheotomy tube	Complains of inability to swallow saliva, pain on swallowing, coughing when swallowing	Aspirates when swallows, minimal laryngeal movement when swallowing, saliva pools in oral cavity
Impaired verbal communication related to tracheotomy	Complains of inability to speak	Inability to speak, tracheotomy
Impaired skin integrity related to tracheotomy skin incision	Complains of incision in neck; has drainage and mucus around stoma	Tracheotomy, drainage around stoma
Pain (acute) related to surgical incision	Complains of pain at surgical site; is restless	Requests pain medication; increased blood pressure, pulse, and respirations; restless; unable to participate in care
Body image disturbance related to presence of tracheotomy	Expresses fear, refuses to look in mirror, refuses to leave room, expresses concern over appearance and other people's reaction to appearance	Refuses to look in mirror or participate in self-care, cries and isolates herself

NURSING DIAGNOSIS	SUBJECTIVE FINDINGS	OBJECTIVE FINDINGS
Impaired home maintenance management related to care of tracheotomy	Reports that she is unable to care for herself at home	Finds excuses to delay hospital discharge; lacks resources (significant other, equipment, money)

3 PLAN

Patient goals

1. The patient will maintain a patent airway.
2. The patient will swallow without aspiration and be able to maintain body weight.
3. The patient will effectively use alternative communication methods.
4. The tracheotomy site will heal with minimal drainage and erythema and without infection.
5. The patient will have relief of pain.
6. The patient will show acceptance of change in body image.
7. The patient will demonstrate ability to care for tracheotomy tube or incisions if decannulated before discharge from the hospital.

4 IMPLEMENT

NURSING DIAGNOSIS	NURSING INTERVENTIONS	RATIONALE
Ineffective airway clearance related to increased mucus production; aspiration of secretions; ineffective cough; tracheotomy tube obstruction	Assess respirations (rate, rhythm, depth), auscultate lung fields, and monitor ABGs and pulse oximetry.	To monitor airway, oxygen levels, and need for suctioning.
	Encourage coughing and deep breathing.	To promote expansion of lungs and mobilize secretions.
	Place in semi-Fowler's or high Fowler's position.	To reduce edema, facilitate chest expansion, and ensure comfort.
	Assess for complications: bleeding (increased blood in mucus); pneumothorax (difficulty breathing, absent breath sounds); subcutaneous emphysema (crepitus).	To ensure proper healing.
	Suction tracheotomy as needed (see the box on page 257).	To remove secretions and maintain a patent airway.
	Supply supplemental humidification (see the box on page 257).	To thin secretions and allow for their easier removal, to prevent crusting and obstruction, and to maintain a patent airway.
	Ensure patient receives chest physiotherapy and intermittent positive-pressure breathing treatments as ordered.	To mobilize secretions.

→ > >

NURSING DIAGNOSIS	NURSING INTERVENTIONS	RATIONALE
	Maintain cuff pressure at 20 to 30 cm of water if cuffed tracheotomy tube is used.	To prevent overinflation of cuff, which may result in pressure on tracheal wall, ischemia of tracheal wall, and stenosis at cuff site.
	Deflate cuff as directed by institutional protocol (see box on page 258).	To remove secretions that may accumulate above cuff.
	Change tracheotomy tube as ordered (temporary tracheotomy tubes are not changed until tract has formed [5 to 7 days]; permanent tracheotomy tubes [laryngectomy] are changed on postoperative day 5) (see the box on page 258).	To facilitate decannulation process, to change tube size, and to begin patient teaching.
	Assess patient's readiness for decannulation.	When pathologic conditions necessitating tracheotomy have resolved, the tracheotomy tube can be safely removed (see the box on page 258).
Impaired swallowing related to presence of tracheotomy tube	Assess patient's ability to swallow without aspiration.	To discontinue oral feedings if aspiration is noted.
	Evaluate consistency of food patient can swallow without aspiration.	Some foods of thicker consistency may be better tolerated, since patient has more control over movement and initiation of swallowing.
	Maintain inflation of cuff during oral feedings and for 1 hour after meals.	To minimize aspiration of food or fluids into tracheobronchial tree.
	Instruct patient to eat in a sitting position and to stay in this position for 1 hour after meals.	To decrease aspiration and to prevent reflux and subsequent aspiration of food and fluids.
	Monitor weight; perform calorie count.	To determine need for alternate feeding technique.
	Maintain NPO status if tracheotomy has been performed with a surgical procedure using mucosal suture lines or if patient aspirates when swallowing.	To prevent disruption or contamination of mucosal suture lines and to prevent pulmonary complications.
	Administer tube feedings per institutional protocol (see the box on page 240).	To maintain body weight and promote wound healing.
Impaired verbal communication related to tracheotomy	Assess patient's understanding of altered communication.	To allay anxiety.
	Evaluate patient's ability to read and write.	Communication after tracheotomy initially is by writing.
	Explore alternative methods of communication (flash cards, picture communication boards).	To be used by patients who cannot write.

NURSING DIAGNOSIS	NURSING INTERVENTIONS	RATIONALE
	Provide patient with tools needed for alternative communication (magic slate, paper and pencil, communication board, flash cards, computer-generated devices).	To provide patient with the ability to communicate.
	Encourage patient to communicate by providing adequate time; sit with patient.	To allow patient to communicate.
	Consult with speech therapist to use other devices (electrolarynx, Passey-Muir valve,* fenestrated tracheotomy tube,* plugging tube with finger*). (*Requires physician's order.)	If tracheotomy will be present for an extended time, alternative devices may provide verbal communication.
	Observe patient for nonverbal cues.	To enhance understanding of patient's communication.
Impaired skin integrity related to tracheotomy skin incision	Cleanse tracheotomy site, tube, and under neckplate of tube.	To remove drainage and crusts.
	Assess stoma for bleeding and drainage.	To detect infection.
	Change tracheotomy ties as needed to maintain cleanliness and dryness.	Soiled, wet tracheotomy ties may excoriate skin and may stretch to alter security of tube.
	Apply unlined gauze sponge under neckplate of tracheotomy tube.	To prevent pressure on skin around incision from neckplate (unlined gauze is used to prevent inhalation of fibers in lining).
	Change wet or soiled gauze sponge.	To prevent excoriation of skin.
Pain (acute) related to surgical incision	Assess location, characteristics, and intensity of pain.	To determine interventions needed.
	Administer analgesics as ordered, and evaluate effectiveness.	To reduce pain.
	Help patient assume a comfortable position (e.g., elevate head of bed).	To improve comfort.
Body image disturbance related to presence of tracheotomy	Encourage patient to discuss concerns.	To identify problems.
	Identify past coping mechanisms used by patient.	To identify possible coping strategies.
	Assess patient's readiness to participate in self-care.	May be acknowledgment of acceptance.
	Remain with patient during self-care.	To provide support.

→ > >

NURSING DIAGNOSIS	NURSING INTERVENTIONS	RATIONALE
Impaired home maintenance management related to care of tracheotomy	Reinforce all self-care instruction (tracheotomy care, incision care, humidification technique).	To ensure that patient and significant other can perform all care in the home.
	Arrange for equipment to be available in the home.	To decrease patient's anxiety about making her own arrangements and her fear of obtaining incorrect equipment.
	Arrange home health nursing visits after discharge if ordered.	To facilitate transition from hospital to home.

5 EVALUATE

PATIENT OUTCOME	DATA INDICATING THAT OUTCOME IS REACHED
Airway is patent.	ABGs and pulse oximetry results are within normal limits for patient; patient has no dyspnea; secretions are minimal, and coughing is effective in removing secretions.
Patient maintains weight and swallows without aspiration.	Body weight is stable; intake of calories and proteins is adequate; patient can swallow without aspiration, or if unable to swallow, can administer tube feedings.
Patient communicates effectively.	Patient can communicate using alternative devices or verbally if decannulation is complete.
Wounds have healed without infection.	Temperature and WBC are within normal limits; there is no purulent drainage, blood, or odor associated with tracheal secretions; stoma is closed (if decannulation is complete).
Patient's pain has been relieved.	Patient does not complain of pain.
Patient has accepted change in body image.	Patient performs self-care, socializes with others, and communicates concerns.
Patient anticipates hospital discharge.	Patient expresses desire to return home, and arrangements have been made for equipment and home health nurse.

PATIENT TEACHING

1. Reinforce patient teaching about location of tracheotomy at level below vocal cords and why the patient cannot breathe through her nose or mouth or cannot speak.
2. Review self-care procedures associated with tracheotomy.
3. Emphasize the need for supplemental humidification.
4. If the tracheotomy tube has been removed, teach the patient how to tape the stoma and put on an occlusive dressing. Stress the importance of splinting the stoma site with the fingers when speaking or coughing.
5. Inform the patient of the signs of infection and the need to notify her physician.
6. Arrange for home health nursing visits and equipment to be used in the home.
7. Encourage the patient to participate in support groups.

SUCTIONING A TRACHEOTOMY PATIENT*

- Assemble equipment:
  Gloves
  Source of negative pressure
  Suction catheter (no larger than half the diameter of the tracheotomy tube)
  Basins for hydrogen peroxide and water
  Oxygen, Ambu-bag
  Tracheotomy brush
- Put on gloves.
- Connect suction catheter, and fill basins with hydrogen peroxide and water.
- Remove inner cannula, and place in basin with hydrogen peroxide to loosen secretions.
- Administer oxygen or use Ambu-bag to hyperoxygenate patient.
- Insert catheter, without suction, to minimize oxygen removal.
- Use suction during withdrawal of catheter to remove secretions.
- Suction only for 5 to 10 seconds to minimize oxygen removal.
- Administer oxygen or use Ambu-bag to replace oxygen.
- Repeat procedure until airway is clear.
- Clean inner cannula with tracheotomy brush to remove accumulated secretions.
- Rinse inner cannula in basin containing water to remove hydrogen peroxide.
- Reinsert inner cannula.
- Apply humidified oxygen collar to thin secretions.

*Author's Note: It is this author's belief that suctioning and tracheotomy care performed by a nurse should be done using strict aseptic technique. Once the patient assumes care of the tracheotomy, a clean technique may be used.

ACCIDENTAL DECANNULATION OF TRACHEOSTOMY TUBE

If tube becomes displaced or is prematurely removed:
- Release traction sutures
- Pull top suture upward and outward
- Pull lower suture downward and outward
- Replace tube in opening
- Secure tube with ties
- Assess tube placement

Alternate method:
- Insert suction catheter to allow passage of air and to serve as a guide for insertion
- Thread tracheotomy tube over catheter
- Insert tube over suction catheter
- Remove suction catheter
- Secure tube with ties
- Assess tube placement

SUPPLEMENTAL HUMIDIFICATION

A tracheotomy patient requires additional humidity in the environment because the upper airway, where humidification normally occurs, is bypassed, permitting dry air to enter the trachea. This air will dry the mucous membranes lining the trachea, resulting in crusting of secretions. When these crusts are removed by coughing, superficial blood vessels are exposed, causing bleeding. The patient can increase environmental humidity by (1) applying warm, humidified oxygen via tracheotomy collar (2) using a bedside humidifier, (3) instilling 3 to 5 ml of normal saline into the tracheotomy to moisten and loosen secretions and stimulate coughing, (4) sitting in a steam-filled bathroom, and (5) wearing a moist covering over the tracheotomy site.

CARE OF THE INNER CANNULA

Clean or change the inner cannula at least once per shift to maintain tube patency.

Conventional inner cannula

Apply gloves
Remove inner cannula
Soak inner cannula in basin with hydrogen peroxide to loosen secretions
Use a tracheotomy brush to remove secretions
Rinse with water to remove the hydrogen peroxide
Reinsert the inner cannula

Disposable inner cannula

Apply gloves
Remove inner cannula and discard
Replace new inner cannula

DECANNULATION PROCEDURE

- Deflate the cuff to determine the patient's ability to handle secretions without aspiration.
- Change to a smaller, uncuffed tube if no aspiration is observed; this will determine the patient's ability to breathe around the tube and through the nose and mouth.
- Occlude the opening of the tracheotomy tube for 24 hours to ensure the patient can breathe through her nose and mouth.
- If the patient tolerates this process, complete decannulation by removing the tracheotomy tube.
- Apply an occlusive dressing to the stoma to promote healing. (see figure on page 250).

CHANGING THE TRACHEOTOMY TUBE

- Put on gloves.
- Assemble equipment:
  Tracheotomy tube with outer cannula, inner cannula, and obturator
  Tracheotomy ties (twill tape, plastic IV tubing, commercial Velcro ties)
  Water-soluble lubricant
- Insert ties into neck plate of tracheotomy tube.
- Place obturator into outer cannula.
- Apply thin layer of water-soluble lubricant.
- Remove tube from stoma by cutting ties.
- Cleanse stoma with hydrogen peroxide on cotton-tipped applicators, and rinse with water or saline.
- Instruct patient to tip head back slightly and take a deep breath.
- Insert tracheotomy tube gently, using obturator to guide tube into trachea.
- Remove obturator.
- Tie tube securely, allowing one finger to be inserted between ties on neck.
- Insert inner cannula.
- Clean tube with hydrogen peroxide, and rinse with water. Tube may be placed in boiling water for 15 to 20 minutes, then dried and stored until the next change.

DEFLATING THE TRACHEOTOMY CUFF

- Suction tracheotomy tube and mouth to remove secretions that may be aspirated during deflation.
- Deflate cuff during exhalation to prevent aspiration of secretions into the tracheobronchial tree.*
- Instruct patient to cough, or suction patient during deflation so that accumulated secretions are expelled.
- Remain with patient while cuff is deflated, because she is at higher risk for aspiration.
- Reinflate cuff during inspiration to make patient more comfortable.

*The use of tracheotomy tubes with low-pressure cuffs has eliminated the need for routine cuff deflation. (Cuff deflation was used to restore circulation to the tracheal wall, thus preventing ischemia and the possibility of long-term stenosis at the cuff site.) However, cuff deflation is still required to remove accumulated secretions.

RADIATION THERAPY

Radiation therapy may be used as a curative treatment for small tumors (T_1 and T_2), as an adjuvant treatment for larger tumors, or as a palliative measure for patients with inoperable or recurrent tumors.

Most small lesions respond equally to radiation therapy or surgery, depending on the tumor's location. Proximity to bone and cartilage may make lesions relatively radioresistant. External beam radiation to the head and neck usually requires 5,000 to 7,000 rad delivered in fractions of 200 rad/day for 5 to 7 weeks. Small laryngeal lesions require a small treatment portal over the larynx and rarely show significant side effects. However, radiation therapy to the oral cavity, nasopharynx, oropharynx, hypopharynx, or neck may result in substantial side effects, making surgery a better choice for these tumors because it is easier to tolerate, less time is involved in the treatment, and function can be restored without side effects.

Adjuvant radiation may be given before or after surgery. Preoperative radiation may be used for large tumors considered unresectable. Some current protocols combine chemotherapy and radiation therapy, with chemotherapy used as a radiation sensitizer and radiation therapy used to decrease the tumor's mass. A maximum of 4,000 to 5,500 rad usually is recommended as a preoperative dose to prevent tissue damage, which can affect the healing process. Postoperative radiation therapy usually is preferred. A full dose can be given after surgery, depending on the tumor's size and location and on lymph node involvement. Postoperative radiation should begin within 6 to 8 weeks after surgery; the treatment portal usually includes the primary site and present or potential lymph node metastases.

Palliative radiation may use external beam therapy or brachytherapy (radiation placed into or adjacent to the tumor mass). Radiation implants can supply a high dose of radiation to a small area, sparing normal tissue. Brachytherapy catheters may be placed at the time of surgery if positive margins or residual tumor is anticipated. Loading of the catheters can take place once the patient has stabilized after surgery. The radioactive seeds are placed in the hollow catheter at the patient's bedside. The patient is kept in a radiation-safe environment during the time the radioactive seeds are in place. After the appropriate radiation dose has been delivered, the catheters are removed and the patient is sent home.

RADIATION SIDE EFFECTS

Dental caries

A decrease in saliva production causes plaque buildup and removes the protective enzymes that prevent dental caries. Because fluoride helps combat dental caries, the patient should wear a fluoride carrier that is made from impressions of his teeth to apply topical fluoride treatments each day. Other steps the patient can take to prevent dental caries are to brush with a soft bristled brush, floss his teeth, and avoid use of commercial mouthwashes that contain alcohol.

Xerostomia

Radiation therapy to the head and neck also affects salivary production, causing a dry mouth. The decrease in saliva that begins within the first few weeks of treatment may last for several weeks or may be a permanent condition. Steps to overcome xerostomia include: increasing fluid intake; using artificial saliva preparations; increasing humidity in the environment; and sucking on sugarless candy or chewing sugarless gum.

Mucositis/esophagitis

Inflammation of the mucous membranes of the oral cavity, pharynx, and esophagus is caused by a combination of the radiation effects, xerostomia, and secondary bacterial or fungal infections. The oral cavity should be examined for infection. The patient should be provided with a mixture of equal parts of viscous Xylocaine, liquid antacid, and Benadryl elixir for topical relief of ulcerative areas. Other steps the patient can take to combat the inflammation include eating soft, bland foods; avoiding spicy and citrus foods; avoiding temperature extremes; using mild saline rinses; avoiding tobacco and alcohol; and increasing intake of yogurt.

Taste changes

The patient will also experience taste changes that result from the destruction of taste buds during radiation therapy. The amount of change in taste depends on the dosage and radiation fields used. To minimize taste changes the patient should experiment to determine which foods are still palatable. He should eat small, frequent meals, including finger foods and snacks, and use dietary supplements. These steps will help increase calorie and protein intake.

CHEMOTHERAPY

Chemotherapy also may be used to treat tumors of the head and neck. Chemotherapy may be used before surgery to decrease the tumor's mass; it may be used in conjunction with radiation therapy as a sensitizer so that simultaneous therapy can increase tumor destruction; and it may be used as a palliative treatment for persistent, recurrent, or inoperable tumors. Adjuvant therapy after the standard treatment of surgery and radiation is also being used in an attempt to increase the disease-free interval in patients with extracapsular spread in the histologic specimen after radical neck dissection. Extracapsular spread has been found to be a poor prognostic sign, and it increases the possibility both of recurrence in the neck and of distant metastasis.

Most chemotherapy regimens are considered investigational in the head and neck and are not used as primary therapy. The drugs that have shown effectiveness in the head and neck are bleomycin, cisplatin, methotrexate, and 5-fluorouracil. Biologic response modifiers such as the interleukins and interferon are also being used in investigational trials.

The side effects of the drugs used in the head and neck must be managed while the patient is in the hospital and after discharge. Bleomycin has not been used much in the past few years because of the pulmonary fibrosis associated with its use. Various combinations of the other drugs are currently being studied.

CHAPTER 12

Patient Teaching Guides

Patient education about ear, nose, and throat disorders, diagnostic tests, treatment procedures, and ongoing care needs is vital to the patient's health. While the patient may be the focus of the teaching/learning activities, certainly the inclusion of the patient's family members and significant others is important and necessary to the supportive or caregiver role each may have. Each member of the professional team caring for the patient has a responsibility to participate in the educational process. Often the same information needs to be shared numerous times and using various teaching methods in order for the patient to adequately learn necessary self-care skills. While some educational encounters may be more formal than others, the opportunity to teach the patient at any appropriate moment should be seized. Written teaching guides, such as those included in this chapter, provide the learner with information and the sequence of procedural steps that can be referred to during both the teaching session and later to refresh one's memory or share with others. Written material should always be reviewed with the patient.

The first step in patient teaching is a thorough assessment of the learner(s) and the situation that requires teaching/learning. Learner attributes include cognitive and physical capabilities; educational level; degree of coping with current health crisis; awareness of own knowledge deficit/readiness to learn; fears and anxieties concerning own abilities; and general feelings about prior learning experiences. A situation/environment assessment includes identification of skills and information to be learned; physical needs of the learner that must first be met; educational resources available; staff teaching skills; and necessary modifications of the environment so it is conducive to learning.

The evaluation of learning is ongoing during the teaching process, since modification of teaching methods and adaptation of techniques are an ongoing process. Adequate time must be set aside for uninterrupted teaching sessions. While the learning of certain information and skills is necessary before a safe home visit or before actual discharge, it is important to remember that new learning needs emerge after discharge. A plan to address these new needs should be a part of subsequent discharge referrals and follow-up visits.

As with all aspects of the nursing process, documentation of the teaching-learning process is necessary. This not only documents the care of a specific patient but also permits the evaluation of an overall educational program. Patient teaching guides that follow may be copied and used.

PATIENT TEACHING GUIDE

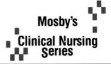

Instructions for use of Ear Wash and Drops

You have been given a prescription that you should have filled at your own drugstore. You will also need a 2- or 3- ounce ear syringe, which you can buy at a drugstore if you do not have one.

Someone Else Should Wash Your Ear for You

You cannot do it as well yourself. The instructions below should be followed very carefully.

1. Wash hands before and after this procedure.
2. Fill the ear syringe with the solution.
3. The solution must be at body temperature. If the solution is too warm or too cool, you will feel dizzy. Warm the solution by placing the syringe in a pan of hot water. Do *not* warm the solution on the stove.
4. Lie down with the ear to be washed facing up and pull up and out on the external ear. Place the tip of the ear syringe into the ear canal. Do not be afraid to push it down into the ear. However, you should get a return flow. If you do not, you have it in too far. Pull the syringe out slightly.
5. Pump the warmed solution from the syringe back and forth into the ear by squeezing and releasing the bulb of the syringe. Do this very vigorously and repeatedly. The ear wash must be forced back and forth, in and out of the ear canal.
6. Lean over the side and let the solution run out of the ear.
7. Pull the ear up, back, and out to straighten the ear canal.
8. Put three to five warmed drops into the ear.
9. If the solution burns too much at first, you may dilute the solution. Mix two ounces of water with two ounces of the solution. Later, decrease the amount of water used with each irrigation.
10. Use the solution and drops twice a day for 2 weeks and then until the ear stops running or becomes dry. If you are not sure that the ear is dry, check it by putting a cotton swab down into the ear canal. If the cotton swab comes out dry, stop using the solution and drops. If the cotton swab is wet or there is an odor, continue using the solution and drops for 4 days.
11. Do not use the solution and drops as long as the ear remains dry and is not running, and as long as there is no odor. Should the ear start to run after being dry for a period of time, start using the ear solution and drops until the ear is dry again.
12. **Do not get any water in your ears.** You should not go swimming until you are told you may do so. Whenever there is a chance of getting water in your ears, such as when you shower or wash your hair, use cotton in the ear. First, place a dry piece of cotton in the ear and then a second piece that has been saturated with petroleum jelly.
13. If you have any questions, call your doctor.

Cleaning Your Ears

Ear wax, also called cerumen, is made by wax glands in the skin of the ear canal. Ear wax is healthy and serves to clean the ear. Since ear wax is sticky, it catches foreign material. Most of the time, ear canals are self-cleaning due to migration of the wax.

Sometimes ear wax must be removed—when the ear looks dirty or the wax blocks the ear canal, causing a hearing loss. Cleaning the outside of the ear is easy and is done when bathing. Ear wax in the ear canal is more difficult, and precautions are in order.

There are three ways for you to clean ear wax from your ears. The first is the careful use of a cotton swab. Only the cotton portion should be placed in your ear canal and turned. Caution is necessary because you can damage the ear drum if your arm is bumped. Also, cotton swabs sometimes push the wax into the ear canal, causing a wax impaction.

The second method is to use an ear canal irrigation with a rubber ear syringe. Use warm water to vigorously flush your ear either over the sink or in the shower. If the water is too warm or cold, you may experience a temporary dizziness. The biggest problem with an irrigation is causing an infection if a hole is present in the ear drum. If an irrigation causes pain, stop immediately.

The third method is to use ear drops that soften and remove the wax. Rarely, these ear drops for cleaning irritate the ear canal. A combination of cleaning ear drops and an ear canal irrigation may be necessary to remove an ear wax impaction.

If your ear is still blocked after using the above methods, see an ear doctor. Doctors use either microscopic techniques or increased pressure irrigations to finally remove the ear wax. Also see an ear doctor if your ear itches or hurts when you clean.

Prophylactically, use a cotton swab once a month after bathing to keep the ear wax from building up. If you use a dry cotton swab daily, you may irritate the tender skin of your ear canal. Placing an ointment on the cotton swab will lessen this problem.

Cleaning your ears is a logical, cautious process. **Don't use other objects in your ears—even if it feels good!**

PATIENT TEACHING GUIDE

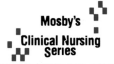

Protecting Your Ears From Noise

Loud noises, or noise over a long period of time, can cause a permanent hearing loss. Noises also cause a temporary hearing loss, but over the years a permanent high-tone hearing loss develops. Protecting your ears from noise is necessary to keep normal hearing.

The best way to protect your ears is to avoid loud noise. Most of us don't have a choice; but if you are around loud noise, pay attention to your hearing. One way to monitor the presence of a hearing loss from noise is to listen for a ringing in your ears. If your ears ring, there is ear damage and possibly a hearing loss. A hearing loss from noise is permanent.

Any ear protection (also called noise defenders) is better than none at all. The best noise defender is one that is comfortable to wear. Different noise defenders are available, made from various materials, including sponge rubber, soft rubber, dense cotton, and molded materials. Try several noise protectors to find the one most comfortable for you—so you will wear it. If your ears ring after noise exposure while wearing a noise defender, change the type of defender you are using or wear an ear muff.

When around very loud noises, ear muffs are the only defender that will protect your ears. Ear muffs also vary in type. Under rare circumstances, both an ear canal noise defender and an ear muff must be worn to protect the ears.

Government regulations exist in the workplace that make it mandatory to use ear protection. But equally loud noises exist in the home and with hobbies. If you hear loud noises that hurt your ears, cause ringing, or cause you to shout to be heard—wear a noise defender!

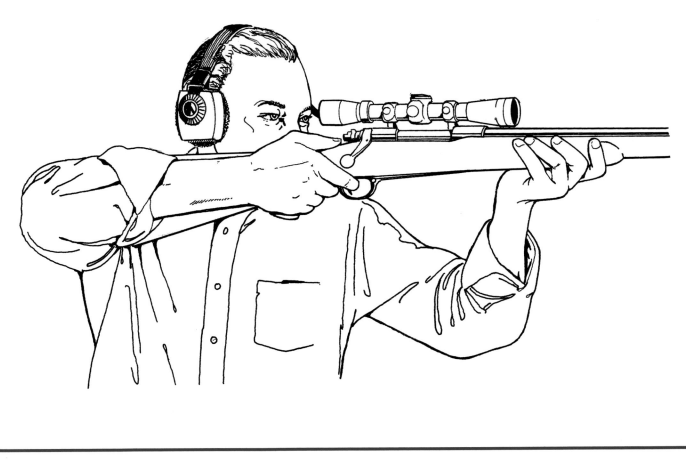

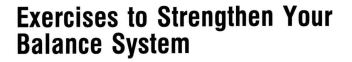
Exercises to Strengthen Your Balance System

Balance exercises decrease dizziness, and have been prescribed for you. Although the exercises are accomplished by turning your head and neck, the exercises are performed to help the brain compensate for the injury to the balance system.

The balance exercises are done while sitting with your feet on the floor for stability. These balance exercises may make you dizzy. If dizziness occurs, allow the dizziness to subside, but then continue with the exercises.

The head is turned quickly in six different directions. A "sequence" consists of quickly jerking the head right; left; up; down; tilt right; and tilt left. The distance that the head is turned is unimportant. An inch in each direction is sufficient as long as the head is stopped suddenly. After each position, return your head to the midline before beginning the next position. The entire sequence should be repeated ten times, twice per day. The diagrams illustrate how these balance system exercises should be done. Over a period of months, these will help the balance system to compensate. Remember to turn your head quickly and stop your head suddenly.

Any physical activity or movement that causes dizziness should be repeated several times. For example, if turning quickly to the right or looking up causes dizziness, these maneuvers should be repeated often. Instead of avoiding certain situations or positions that cause dizziness, repeat them. These repetitions will hasten the recovery process. While avoiding dizziness is more comfortable for most patients, the only way to regain complete balance function is to use your balance system. The goal of these exercises is to improve compensation over the next several months.

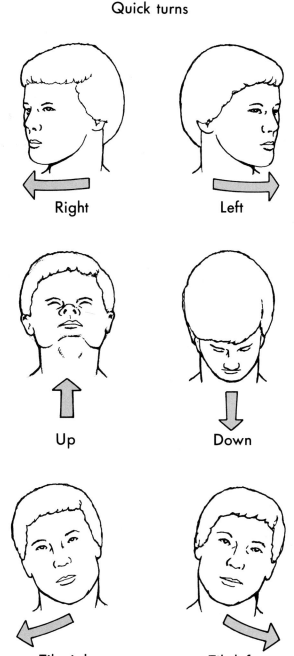

Quick turns

Right

Left

Up

Down

Tilt right

Tilt left

PATIENT TEACHING GUIDE

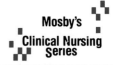

Eye Care for Facial Nerve Weakness

1. Wash hands.
2. Remove drainage, crusts, and oils from eye and lashes.
3. Use a mirror, or have someone instill the drops or ointment for you.
4. Tilt face upward and head back.
5. Look up.
6. Gently pull down lower lid exposing the conjunctiva (the white background of the eye). Do not apply pressure to the eyeball.

During the day or while awake:
7. Squeeze 3 drops into the lower lid at least every hour or when the eye feels dry or irritated (Figure A).
8. Keep medicine bottles clean and sterile. Do not reuse if dropped on the floor. Avoiding touching eye dropper or tube to the eyeball or skin

At bedtime or when napping:
7. Squeeze ointment onto the lid margin for ¼ or ½ inch. Blinking and body temperature will distribute and melt the ointment (Figure B).
8. Tape the eye closed when sleeping (naps and bedtime). It's important to tape top and bottom, smoothing out all wrinkles and skin folds as you go. Skin must be clean and dry, otherwise the tape will not stick (Figure C).

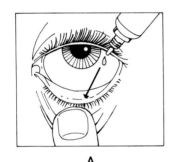
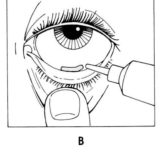
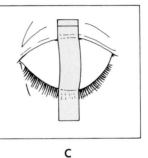

A   B   C

Eye Sling for Facial Nerve Weakness

An eye sling is simply a piece of tape used to hold the lower eyelid in alignment.

With facial nerve weakness (resulting from surgery, Bell's palsy, trauma, virus, etc.), the lower eyelid may droop causing a pooling of tears and a dryness and irritation of the eye (Figure A).

The sling is made of ¼-transpore tape. The tape is placed midway underneath the lower lid and lashes. The end is drawn up and secured to the outer angle of the eye (Figure B).

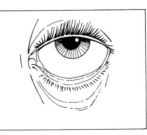
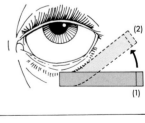

A   B

Mosby's
Clinical Nursing
Series

Nasal Irrigations

1. Purchase an "ear syringe" (small rubber bulb syringe) from the drugstore.
2. Mix solution:
   Normal Saline:
   1 teaspoon salt
   1 quart water (boiled)   Store in clean bottle
3. Squeeze bulb of syringe to withdraw solution.
4. Leaning over a sink, insert tip of syringe about 1½ to 2 inches into nostril.
5. Gently squeeze bulb to irrigate nose.
6. Blow nose gently after first irrigation.
7. Repeat the irrigation with second syringeful.
Note: The normal saline solution can be placed in a nasal spray bottle for moisturizing the nasal mucosa.

Irrigations Using Water Pik

1. Mix solution as above
2. Set irrigator to lowest pressure setting.
3. Insert irrigator tip into nose or oral cavity.
4. Leaning over a sink, irrigate nose or sinus through oral cavity defect. Keep your mouth open as some solution will come out through the mouth.
5. Repeat the irrigation.

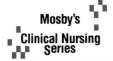
Care of the Tracheoesophageal Puncture

An opening (fistula) has been created between the tracheostoma (windpipe) and esophagus (food passage) in order to place a speech valve (prosthesis). Temporarily, a red rubber catheter will stent the fistula open. Once healing has taken place, a speech prosthesis will replace the catheter.

If the Prosthesis Comes Out

1. Insert a red rubber catheter (10, 12, 14 Fr) into fistula approximately 6-8 inches.
2. Tie a knot in the external end of the catheter to prevent passage of stomach contents.
3. Tape external end of catheter to skin of chest.
4. If catheter cannot be inserted, contact your physician or speech therapist immediately. This may indicate closure of the fistula.

Replacing the Prosthesis

1. Remove prosthesis.
2. Cleanse neck and stoma.
3. Using inserter that is supplied with prosthesis, reinsert clean prosthesis into fistula.
4. Tape in place.
5. Clean prosthesis with hydrogen peroxide and water. Rinse well.
6. The voice prosthesis will last from 2 weeks to several months between changes. The length of time a prosthesis remains in place is dependent upon you. If food or fluid leaks around the prosthesis, it should be changed. If leakage continues, contact your speech therapist for a new size or length of prosthesis.

To Use the Prosthesis

1. Cover your stoma with your thumb. This will allow air from your lungs to pass through the opening of the prosthesis into the esophagus. The walls of your throat and the structures in your mouth will form the words for speech.

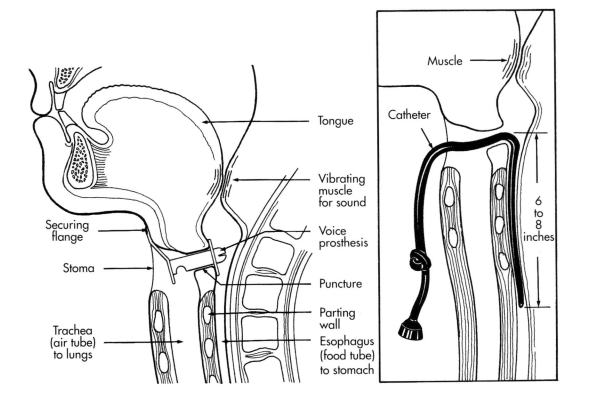

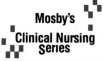
Exercises After Neck Dissection

The following exercises have been developed to increase the movement and strength in your neck, arms, and shoulders.

Neck Range of Motion

1. Bring chin to chest in a relaxed way and then let it fall gently backwards so a stretch on the neck muscles is felt.
2. Slowly turn head as far as possible to one side as if attempting to look over that shoulder. Do the same to the other side.
3. Bend the head toward the shoulder on the unaffected side. A stretching will be felt on the operated side.

Shoulder Mobility

1. Standing with shoulders relaxed and head facing forward, let arm on the affected side hang freely. Make circles with the shoulder by moving it:
   a) forward
   b) upward
   c) backward
   d) downward
2. With a wand or cane in front of body and shoulders and arms relaxed, raise wand as high as possible keeping elbows extended. After you are able to raise it directly overhead, slowly lower it behind the neck. Raise wand overhead and return it to starting position.
3. Stand facing a wall with your feet a few inches from it. Slide the hand on your affected side up the wall as far as possible, using the wall for support. Perform the same exercise with your affected side facing the wall. Repeat the motion of sliding your hand up the wall but do not turn your body when doing this exercise.

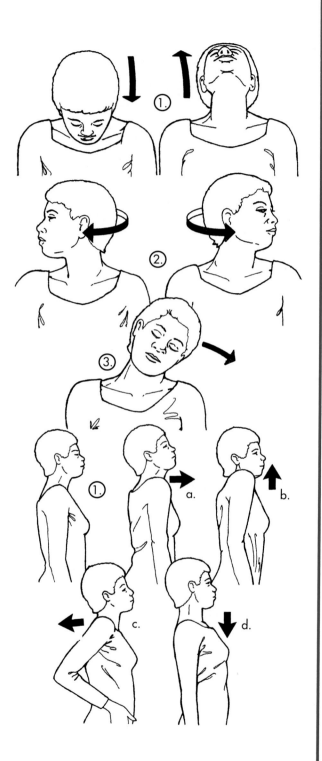

CHAPTER 13

Ear, Nose, and Throat Drug Therapy

The variety of drugs used to treat ear, nose, and throat disorders reflects the evolution of this specialty. Ear, nose, and throat (otorhinolaryngology) once was part of the specialty known as eye, ear, nose, and throat. It became its own specialty of otolaryngology, and later head and neck surgery was added to the name. Currently the specialty known as otolaryngology–head and neck surgery encompasses many subspecialties with a wide range of treatment modalities requiring a variety of drug therapies.

ANTIINFECTIVE DRUGS

Each organ and infection demands specific consideration. Although ideally treatment is based on cultures, most treatment is empiric at the onset, with cultures used for treatment failures.

EAR

Acute infections usually are caused by *Streptococcus pneumoniae* and, in younger patients, *Haemophilus influenzae.*

Chronic suppurative infections are mixed infections caused by aerobic and anaerobic organisms. The most common aerobic organisms are the *Pseudomonas* and *Staphylococcus* species. *Bacteroides fragilis* is the most common anaerobic organism.

External ear infections usually are caused by *Pseudomonas aeruginosa*, sometimes complicated by the fungus *Aspergillus niger.* Under certain circumstances a malignant form of infection warrants aggressive intravenous therapy.

Central nervous system infections are a rare but important complication of mastoid infections.

NOSE AND SINUS

Acute sinusitis is caused by the same organisms as acute ear infections. Sinusitis that develops secondary to indwelling nasal catheters or nasal packing often is caused by mixed organisms.

Chronic sinusitis is caused by the same organisms as the acute type but shows a greater incidence of *Staphylococcus aureus*. Sinusitis associated with cystic fibrosis and acquired immunodeficiency syndrome (AIDS) may also involve *Pseudomonas* organisms and fungi.

THROAT (HEAD AND NECK)
Tonsil and Adenoid Infection

The most common organism causing tonsil and adenoid infection is *Streptococcus pyogenes*. With chronic infection, *Staphylococcus aureus* may be found. Infections accompanied by an exudate may be caused by infectious mononucleosis or some other such illness.

Pharyngitis

Throat infections are also caused primarily by *Streptococcus pyogenes*. Other organisms usually cultured are the same as those found in tonsil and adenoid infections. Pharyngitis left untreated is a concern because of the risk of rheumatic fever.

ANTIINFECTIVE AGENTS COMMONLY USED TO TREAT EAR INFECTIONS

Acute infection

Amoxicillin
Erythromycin plus sulfonamide
Cephalosporins

Chronic infection

Neomycin plus polymyxin B with hydrocortisone otic drops
Ear irrigations
Ciprofloxacin plus metronidazole

External ear infection

Neomycin plus polymyxin B with hydrocortisone otic drops
Gentamicin drops
Intravenous aztreonam plus clindamycin (malignant external otitis)
Mild acid and alcohol drops (antifungal)
Ear irrigations

ANTIINFECTIVE DRUGS COMMONLY USED TO TREAT HEAD AND NECK INFECTIONS

Tonsil and adenoid infection

Penicillin G or V
Clindamycin
Cephalosporins

Pharyngitis

Penicillin G or V
Erythromycin
Cephalosporins
Acyclovir

Laryngitis

Viral: symptomatic care
Bacterial: erythromycin plus sulfonamide

Epiglottitis

Amoxicillin plus clavulanate
Erythromycin plus sulfonamide
Cephalosporins
Ampicillin plus sulbactam

Head and neck infections

Culture-sensitive drugs

ANTIBIOTIC COMBINATIONS

Augmentin: amoxicillin and clavulanate
Timentin (IV): ticarcillin and clavulanate
Unasyn (IV): ampicillin and sulbactam
Primaxin: imipenem and cilastatin
Pediazole: erythromycin and sulfisoxazole

ANTIINFECTIVE DRUGS COMMONLY USED TO TREAT NOSE INFECTIONS

Acute rhinitis and sinusitis

Amoxicillin
Erythromycin plus sulfonamide
Amoxicillin plus clavulanate (Augmentin)
Trimethoprim/sulfamethoxazole (Bactrim, Septra)

Chronic sinusitis

Antistaphylococcal penicillin
Augmented penicillin
Cephalosporins

DRUG TRADE NAMES

Amoxicillin: Amoxil, Polymox, Robamox, others
Amoxicillin/clavulanate: Augmentin
Antistaphylococcal drug: Penicillin—Cloxapen, Dynapen
Augmented penicillin: Augmentin
Ampicillin/sulbactam: Unasyn
Aztreonam: Azactam
Cephalosporins: Keflex, Ceclor, Suprax
Ciprofloxacin: Cipro
Metronidazole: Flagyl
Clindamycin: Cleocin
Erythromycin: E-Mycin, Ilosone, E.E.S., Erythrocin
Erythromycin plus sulfisoxazole: Pediazole
Gentamicin drops: Gentamicin Ophthalmic Drops
Neomycin: Polymyxin B hydrocortisone
Otic drops: Cortisporin Otic Solution, Otocort
Penicillin: Penicillin G or V
Ticarcillin/clavulanate: Timentin

Laryngitis

Infection of the larynx is caused by viruses, most likely rhinoviruses, respiratory syncytial viruses, adenoviruses, or group A streptococcus. With prolonged infection, a secondary bacterial invasion is possible. Treatment is symptomatic for viral laryngitis.

Epiglottitis

Epiglottitis, also known as croup in children, is caused by *Haemophilus influenzae or group A streptococcus.* Early treatment is necessary to preclude the need for a tracheotomy. Croup in the respiratory tree is usually a viral infection.

HEAD AND NECK ABSCESSES

Deep infections, or abscesses, of the head and neck are most commonly mixed infections. Therefore culturing should be done to determine which antibiotic should be used.

HEAD AND NECK INFECTIONS

Infections of the head and neck include stomatitis (which has several causes), facial cellulitis, salivary gland infections, and cervical lymphadenopathy.

I RRIGANTS

In many cases the ear canals and nasal cavity must be cleaned prior to therapy to remove exudate for treatment to be effectrive. Procedures for ear and nasal irrigations are demonstrated to the patient so she can perform them at home (see the Patient Teaching Guides on pages 261, 262, and 266).

Nasal irrigations with normal saline solution can be used to clean and moisten the nasal cavity.

The ear canal is irrigated with a variety of solutions both to clean cerumen and debris and to treat a disorder.

D ECONGESTANTS

Decongestants are sympathomimetic amines that stimulate adrenergic receptors on blood vessels to relieve nasal edema and rhinorrhea. Constriction of the mucous membranes improves breathing, promotes drainage, and relieves nasal congestion.

Decongestants are administered systemically or topically to the mucous membranes. Some of these drugs are available without a prescription, but most decongestants, with or without an antihistamine, require a physician's order.

Topical decongestants are best for immediate action, but overuse produces a rebound congestion. Topical decongestants should be used for short time periods. For long-term treatment the oral decongestants should be used (see the box below).

A NTIHISTAMINES

Antihistamines are available both by prescription and over the counter. Antihistamines are the most commonly prescribed and purchased drugs (see the box below).

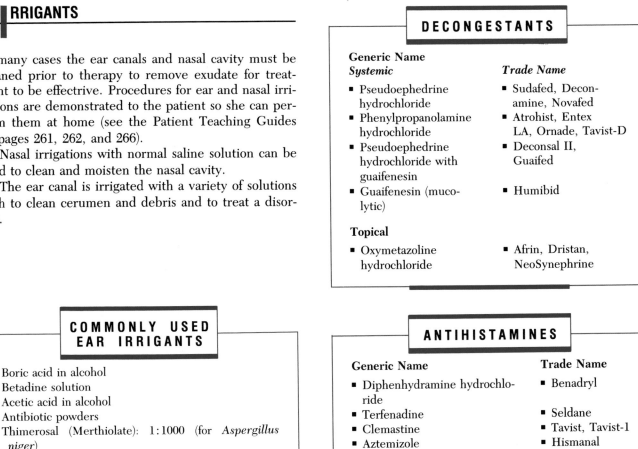

DECONGESTANTS	
Generic Name	
Systemic	*Trade Name*
▪ Pseudoephedrine hydrochloride	▪ Sudafed, Deconamine, Novafed
▪ Phenylpropanolamine hydrochloride	▪ Atrohist, Entex LA, Ornade, Tavist-D
▪ Pseudoephedrine hydrochloride with guaifenesin	▪ Deconsal II, Guaifed
▪ Guaifenesin (mucolytic)	▪ Humibid
Topical	
▪ Oxymetazoline hydrochloride	▪ Afrin, Dristan, NeoSynephrine

COMMONLY USED EAR IRRIGANTS
Boric acid in alcohol
Betadine solution
Acetic acid in alcohol
Antibiotic powders
Thimerosal (Merthiolate): 1:1000 (for *Aspergillus niger*)

ANTIHISTAMINES	
Generic Name	**Trade Name**
▪ Diphenhydramine hydrochloride	▪ Benadryl
▪ Terfenadine	▪ Seldane
▪ Clemastine	▪ Tavist, Tavist-1
▪ Aztemizole	▪ Hismanal

Histamine produces allergic symptoms, and antihistamines reduce histamine effects by competing for the receptor sites in the respiratory mucosa. Their primary action is to reduce allergic symptoms such as congestion, itching, sneezing, and secretions.

In the past antihistamines caused sedation and other central nervous system effects. Newer antihistamines have reduced side effects and also may decrease the production of histamine.

OTHER UPPER RESPIRATORY DRUGS

CORTICOSTEROIDS

The use of steroids in allergy and upper respiratory disorders is controversial. Compounding the problem is the fact that the precise action of steroids is unknown. Nevertheless, steroids are used to treat allergies, airway constriction, nasal obstruction, external otitis, perichondritis, sudden sensorineural hearing loss, and swellings of unknown cause. Corticosteroids are used both systemically and as nasal inhalants (see the box below).

CROMOLYN SODIUM

Cromolyn sodium is applied topically and is not absorbed. The mode of action is to stabilize mast cells, thus decreasing nasal congestion and secretions in the allergic patient.

ANTITUSSIVES

Antitussives relieve coughing. Both narcotic (codeine) and nonnarcotic antitussives are available. Most of the nonnarcotic antitussives are available over the counter, usually in combination with other drugs.

STEROID NASAL SPRAYS

Generic Name	Trade Name
• Beclomethazone dipropionate	• Beconase
• Dexamethasone sodium phosphate	• Vancenase
	• Decadron Phosphate Turbinaire
• Flunisolide	• Nasalide
• Triamcinolone acetonide	• Nasacort

DRUGS FOR DIZZINESS

Meclizine (Antivert, Bonine)

Meclizine, a labyrinthine suppressant, is the most commonly used drug in the treatment of dizziness. The site of action is the labyrinth.

Other, less effective agents for dizziness such as dimenhydrinate (Dramamine) and scopolamine have a central action site.

VASODILATORS

Vasodilators are prescribed on the theory that increasing the blood supply to the ear might be helpful in dizziness and hearing loss. This rationale points up the fact that drug therapy for dizziness is neither effective nor wide ranging. Also, the vasodilators usually chosen may have more of a placebo effect than a vasodilator effect. The most common vasodilators used are niacin and papaverine.

OTHER AGENTS

When dizziness is severe, nausea and vomiting occur and symptomatic treatment with antiemetics and sedatives becomes necessary. When the stress of the disease is evident, tranquilizers and antidepressants are used with caution. In Ménière's disease, diuretics are used to attempt to decrease ear fluids and lessen the attacks characteristic of this disease.

DRUGS FOR HEARING LOSS AND TINNITUS

Frustration with the lack of drug therapies for hearing loss and tinnitus, which are chronic symptoms, has fostered the production of numerous drugs, but none of them have shown a therapeutic effect. But they are still used, usually as a trial application.

ANTINEOPLASTIC DRUGS

Squamous cell carcinoma causes 90% of the malignant neoplasms found in the head and neck. Since surgery, radiation therapy, or a combination of both offer control of most neoplasms, chemotherapy often plays an ad-

DRUGS FOR THE TREATMENT OF HEARING LOSS AND TINNITUS

Treatment involves representative drugs from these categories:

Vasodilators	Sedatives
Steroids	Antidepressants
Vitamins	Sodium fluoride with calcium
Antibiotics	and vitamin D
Antihistamines	Treatments of 5% carbon di-
Tranquilizers	oxide and 95% oxygen

COMMON PROBLEMS IN DRUG THERAPY

1. Overuse of nasal drops and sprays
2. Inadequate ear cleaning before instilling ear drops
3. Incorrect antibiotic for the organism
4. Inappropriate use of antihistamines
5. Unjustified use of prophylactic antibiotics

OTOTOXIC DRUGS

Aminoglycoside antibiotics

Amikacin
Gentamicin
Kanamycin
Neomycin
Netilmicin
Streptomycin
Tobramycin

Other antibiotics

Colistin
Erythromycin (IV)
Minocycline
Polymyxin B
Vancomycin
Viomycin

Other drugs

Aspirin
Cisplatin
Diuretics (loop)
Quinidine
Quinine

The following factors affect the patient's response to chemotherapy:
Site of origin
Stage of disease
Previous therapy
Overall patient status
Nutritional status

junctive or a palliative role. Of course, chemotherapy is the primary therapy in patients with metastatic disease, although it is not curative. Chemotherapeutic techniques in the head and neck usually are systemic, either oral or intravenous.

Methotrexate

Methotrexate is commonly used to treat squamous cell carcinoma of the head and neck. This drug usually is administered intravenously, either weekly or biweekly. Methotrexate is a folate antagonist, inhibiting DNA synthesis and causing cell death. Because of this methotrexate must be given over a period of time to cover cell regeneration. The drug is excreted through the kidneys.

The toxicity of methotrexate is measured by blood and platelet counts. When the counts fall, therapy is suspended for at least a week.

Bleomycin

Bleomycin is an antibiotic that inhibits DNA synthesis. The drug is administered intravenously and shows significant skin and pulmonary toxicity. Because it is not a myelosuppressant, bleomycin usually is used in combination therapy.

Cisplatin

Cisplatin is a new alkylating new agent that is given intravenously and can cause nephrotoxicity, ototoxicity, and neuropathies. This toxicity can be reduced by diuresis. Cisplatin is used in combination therapies as well as before other treatment modalities to decrease tumor size and prevent early metastasis.

MISCELLANEOUS DRUGS

Symptomatic treatment in otolaryngology–head and neck surgery involves drugs for pain control, ointments for skin involvement, solutions for cerumen removal, and nutritional agents.

OTOTOXIC DRUGS

Some medicines can affect the cochlea, vestibular labyrinth, or cranial nerve VIII (the acoustic nerve) (see the box above). Individuals taking ototoxic drugs need to know the signs and symptoms of the side effects of these medicines to prevent loss of hearing or balance. If these symptoms (dizziness, decreasing hearing acuity, tinnitus) occur, the next dose of the drug should be omitted and the physician consulted. Audiometric and vestibular testing may be necessary.

SIGNIFICANT DRUG REACTIONS

Antibiotics

Hypersensitivity, rashes, gastrointestinal distress, tooth discoloration, ototoxicity, neurologic symptoms

Antihistamines

Drowsiness, sedation, dryness of mucous membranes, cardiac stimulation, decreased gastrointestinal and urinary tract motility

Decongestants

Rebound congestion (topical), CNS stimulation, cardiovascular symptoms

Corticosteroids

Nasal sprays: nasal dryness, perforations, ulcers, epistaxis, headaches, ocular hypertension; *systemic preparations:* gastrointestinal and cardiovascular symptoms

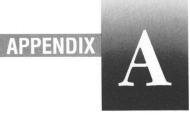

HEARING QUESTIONNAIRE

1. Do you have any problems with your hearing? _____
2. How long have you had a hearing loss in the

   right ear? _____Years
   left ear? _____Years

3. Which is your worse ear? (circle) R L
4. Have you had extensive ear drainage since childhood? _____
5. Who in your family was hard of hearing before age 50?
   Mother   Father   Brother   Sister
6. Did any of your blood relatives ever have ear surgery? If yes, who were the patient and the doctor? _____
7. Are you wearing hearing aids now?
   How old is the right aid? _____ Years
   How old is the left aid? _____ Years
8. Have you worked amid loud noise? _____
   If so, please indicate the number of years. _____ Years
9. Are you still working amid loud noise? _____
10. Were you in the military, and did you serve around loud noise there? _____
    How many rounds have you fired outside the service? _____
11. Do you have head noise or ringing? _____
12. Is dizziness or unsteadiness a major problem? _____
13. Have you had previous ear surgery? _____
14. If you have had previous ear surgery, please indicate which ear was operated on, the type of surgery, and the physician who performed the surgery.

Right Ear   19 _____ _____ _____
             19 _____ _____ _____
Left Ear   19 _____ _____ _____
             19 _____ _____ _____

15. If you are allergic to any medications, please list them here:
    _____
    _____

BALANCE QUESTIONNAIRE

A. Please answer these questions about your dizziness. "Dizziness" is a broad term used to define many sensations.

1. When did the dizziness first occur? _____

2. Did the dizziness start suddenly or gradually? _____

3. Describe your **first attack** of dizziness. _____
_____
_____

4. Is the dizziness constant, or does it come in "attacks"? _____

5. Overall, has the dizziness gotten better or worse since starting? _____

6. Describe the sensation without using the word "dizzy." _____
_____

7. Do any other symptoms occur simultaneously with the dizziness such as nausea, vomiting, or ear pressure? Please explain. _____
_____
_____

8. When was your last attack? _____

9. Describe your **last attack** of dizziness. _____
_____

10. How often do the attacks occur? _____

11. How long do the attacks last? _____

12. List anything that stops an attack of dizziness or makes it better. _____
_____

13. List anything that brings on an attack of dizziness or makes it worse. _____
_____

14. Are you completely free of dizziness between attacks? _____

15. Does the dizziness occur only in certain positions? _____
If yes, what positions? _____
_____

16. Does the dizziness occur only while standing or walking? _____

17. Does the dizziness affect your balance or make you walk abnormally? _____

18. Do you support yourself while standing or walking? _____

19. Have you ever fallen because of the dizziness? _____

20. Have you ever injured your head or neck? _____

21. Does stress have any relationship to the dizziness? _____

22. Do you faint, black out, or experience seizures with the dizziness? _____
_____

23. Are you prone to motion sickness? _____

B. Please answer these questions about your hearing.
    Check Yes or No, and circle which ear when necessary.

Yes No

☐   ☐   1. Do you have any **difficulty hearing?**   Right   Left   Both

               2. How long have you noticed the hearing loss?
                  Right ear _____
                  Left ear _____

☐   ☐   3. Do you have any difficulty understanding what you hear?
                  Right   Left   Both

               4. How long have you had **difficulty understanding?**
                  Right ear _____
                  Left ear _____

☐   ☐   5. Do you have any **noises** in your ears?   Right   Left   Both

☐   ☐   6. Is the noise constantly with you?

☐   ☐   7. Does the noise occur only with the dizziness?

☐   ☐   8. Have you worked in a noisy environment or been exposed to loud noise?

C. Please answer these questions about your ears.
    Check Yes or No, and circle which ear when necessary.

Yes No

☐   ☐   1. Do you have pain in your ears and/or drainage?   Right   Left   Both

☐   ☐   2. Have you had any surgery on your ears?   Right   Left   Both

               3. List the date of surgery, the reason, and the ear operated on.
               _____
               _____

D. Please check Yes or No, and circle the correct description of each symptom.

Yes No

☐   ☐   1. Blurred vision   Constant   In episodes

☐   ☐   2. Double vision   Constant   In episodes

☐   ☐   3. Numbness in hands or feet   Constant   In episodes

☐   ☐   4. Weakness in arms or legs   Constant   In episodes

☐   ☐   5. Numbness or tingling of mouth or face   Constant   In episodes

☐   ☐   6. Confusion or lack of coordination   Constant   In episodes

☐   ☐   7. Difficulty with speech   Constant   In episodes

☐   ☐   8. Difficulty swallowing   Constant   In episodes

☐   ☐   9. Do you get dizzy after heavy lifting, straining, exertion, or overwork?

☐   ☐   10. Did you get new glasses recently?

☐   ☐   11. Do you get dizzy if you have not eaten for a long time?

☐   ☐   12. For women: Is your dizziness connected with your menstrual cycle?

E. List all medications and the amounts that you are currently taking.
_____
_____
_____
_____

F. List any past injuries, operations, or chronic illnesses.
_____
_____
_____
_____
_____

G. Do any members of your immediate family (parents, brothers, and sisters) have any diseases of the ear or central nervous system (e.g., brain tumors, multiple sclerosis)?   Yes___ No ___

If Yes, please explain: _____

_____

_____

H. Personal History

Yes   No

☐   ☐   1. Married?

☐   ☐   2. Children?

☐   ☐   3. Employed?

☐   ☐   4. Are you physically active (e.g., exercise, sports)?

5. Habits:

☐   ☐   a. Do you use tobacco in any form? _____ If so, how much? _____

☐   ☐   b. Do you use alcohol? _____ If so, how much? _____

☐   ☐   c. Do you use caffeine? _____ If so, how much? _____

☐   ☐   d. Do you eat a well-balanced diet? _____

☐   ☐   6. Has the dizziness affected the quality of your life?

☐   ☐   7. Do you feel a lot of stress or tend to worry a lot?

☐   ☐   8. Have you ever seen a psychiatrist or psychologist for any reason?

REFERENCES

1. Adams R, Victor M: *Principles of neurology*, ed 3, New York, 1985, McGraw-Hill.
2. Alberti PM, Ruben RJ: *Otologic medicine and surgery*, 2 vols, New York, 1988, Churchill Livingstone.
2a. Barber HO, Sharpe JA: *Vestibular disorders*, Chicago, 1988, Mosby.
3. Belcher AE: *Cancer nursing*, St Louis, 1992, Mosby.
4. Blitzer A, Lawson W, Friedman WH: *Surgery of the paranasal sinuses*, ed 2, Philadelphia, 1991, WB Saunders.
5. Boring CC, Squires TS, Tong T: Cancer statistics 1993, *CA A Cancer Journal for Clinicians* 43(1):7-27, 1993.
6. Brandt B: What you should know about radiation implant therapy to the head and neck, *Oncology Nursing Forum* 16(4):579-582, 1989.
7. Bulechek GM, McCloskey JC: *Nursing interventions, treatments for nursing diagnoses*, Philadelphia, 1985, WB Saunders.
8. Campbell SL: Some sound advice for managing a hearing impaired patient, *Nursing '84* 14:46, 1984.
9. Chick K, Lacey D, Trelstad A: Nursing care of adults having craniofacial surgery, *Plastic Surgery Nursing* 9(1):16-20, 1989.
10. Chipps E, Clanin N, Campbell V: *Neurologic disorders*, St Louis, 1992, Mosby.
11. Coulthard SW et al: *Chemotherapy in head and neck oncology*, Alexandria, Va, 1985, American Academy of Otolaryngology–Head and Neck Surgery.
12. Counter RT: *Color atlas of temporal bone surgical anatomy*, London, 1980, Mosby.
13. Cummings CW et al: *Otolaryngology–head and neck surgery*, ed 2, St Louis, 1993, Mosby.
14. Cunningham MJ: The management of congenital neck masses, *American Journal of Otolaryngology* 13(2):78-93, 1992.
15. Curtin HD: The use of magnetic resonance imaging in otolaryngology–head and neck surgery, *Advances in Otolaryngology–Head and Neck Surgery* 5:71-107, 1991.
16. DeWeese DD, Sanders WH: *Textbook of otolaryngology–head and neck surgery*, ed 7, St Louis, 1988, Mosby.
17. Dropkin MJ: Coping with disfigurement and dysfunction after head and neck cancer surgery: a conceptual framework, *Seminars in Oncology Nursing* 5(3):213-219, 1989.
18. Droughton ML, Verbic M: Body image re-integration after head and neck surgery, *The Journal of the Society of Otorhinolaryngology and Head-Neck Nurses* 6(1):19-23, 1988.
19. Dudjak LA: Mouth care for mucositis due to radiation therapy, *Cancer Nursing* 10(3):131-140, 1987.
20. Fairbanks DNF: *Antimicrobial therapy in otolaryngology–head and neck surgery*, ed 6, Alexandria, Va, 1991, American Academy of Otolaryngology–Head and Neck Surgery.
21. Feldman JE, Baker KH: The psychodynamics of prolonged treatment in a patient with cancer of the hypopharynx, *Cancer Nursing* 11(6):362-367, 1988.
22. Gibbs L: Assessment and management of the allergic patient, *ORL–Head and Neck Nursing* 10(3):10-16, 1992.
22a. Glasscock ME, Stambaugh GE: *Surgery of the ear*, ed 4, Philadelphia, 1990, WB Saunders.
23. Goldstein JC, Kashima HK, Kooperman CF: *Geriatric otolaryngology*, Philadelphia, 1989, Mosby.
24. Hanawalt A, Troutman K: If your patient has a hearing aid, *AJN* 84:900, 1984.
25. Hawke M, Keene M, Alberti PW: *Clinical otoscopy*, New York, 1984, Churchill Livingstone.

26. Hughes GB: *Textbook of clinical otology*, New York, 1985, Thieme-Stratton.

27. Isshiki N: Laryngeal framework surgery, *Advances in Otolaryngology–Head and Neck Surgery* 5:37-57, 1991.

28. Jahn AF, Santos-Sacchi J: *Physiology of the ear*, New York, 1988, Raven.

29. Johnson JT: A surgeon looks at cervical lymph nodes, *Radiology* 175(3):607-610, 1990.

30. Johnson JT et al: Adjuvant chemotherapy for high-risk squamous cell carcinoma of the head and neck, *Journal of Clinical Oncology* (3):456-458, 1987.

31. Johnson JT et al: Cisplatin-5-fluorouracil chemotherapy for advanced inoperable squamous carcinoma of the head and neck, *Head and Neck Surgery* 336-340, 1987.

32. Johnson JT et al: The extracapsular spread of tumors in cervical node metastasis, *Archives of Otolaryngology* 107(12):725-729, 1981.

32a. Karb VK, Queener SF, Freeman JB: *Handbook of drugs for nursing practice*, St Louis, 1989, Mosby.

33. Kennedy SW, Zinreich SJ: Functional endoscopic surgery, *Advances in Otolaryngology–Head and Neck Surgery* 3:1-27, 1989.

34. Kim MJ, McFarland GK, McLane AM: *Pocket guide to nursing diagnosis*, St Louis, 1993, Mosby.

35. Lockhart JS, Bryce J: Restoring speech with tracheoesophageal puncture, *Nursing '93* (1):59-61, 1993.

36. Lockhart JS, Troff JL, Artim LS: Total laryngectomy and radical neck dissection, *AORN Journal* 55(2):458-479, 1992.

37. Mabry RL: A step-by-step case approach to the treatment of upper respiratory allergy, *Otolaryngology–Head and Neck Surgery* 107(6), 1992.

38. Mabry RL: Topical pharmacotherapy for allergic rhinitis: new agents, *Southern Medical Journal* 85(2):149-154, 1992.

39. Maksud DP: Nursing management of patients following combined free flap mandible reconstruction, *Plastic Surgical Nursing* 12(3):95-106, 1992.

40. Malkiewicz J: The fine art of giving a physical: how to assess the ears and test hearing acuity, *RN* 45(3):56-63, 1982.

41. Marsh BR: Foreign bodies in the air and food passages, *Advances in Otolaryngology–Head and Neck Surgery* 6:115-147, 1992.

42. McCall M: It killed George, or managing the peritonsillar abscess patient effectively, *ORL–Head and Neck Nursing*, 11(1):10-13, 1993.

43. McCance K, Huether SE: *Pathophysiology: the biologic basis for disease in adults and children*, St Louis, 1990, Mosby.

44. Meyerhoff WL, Rice DH: *Otolaryngology–head and neck surgery*, Philadelphia, 1992, WB Saunders.

45. Miller WE: The role of the outpatient nurse in endoscopic sinus surgery, *ORL–Head and Neck Nursing* 10(3):20-24, 1992.

45a. Mitchell VL: Cochlear implantation: a nursing perspective, *The Journal of the Society of Otorhinolaryngology and Head-Neck Nurses* 5(2):11-15, 1987.

46. Mulgrew B, Dropkin MJ: Coping with craniofacial resection: a case study, *The Journal of the Society of Otorhinolaryngology and Head-Neck Nurses* 9(3):8-19, 1991.

47. Myers EN, Stool SE, Johnson JT: *Tracheotomy*, New York, 1985, Churchill Livingstone.

48. Nathan MD: Protecting the elderly against drug-induced hearing loss, *Geriatrics* 36:96-98, 1981.

48a. Novak MA, Firszt JB, Meehan K: Cochlear implants in children, part I, *The Journal of the Society of Otorhinolaryngology and Head-Neck Nurses* 8(1):22-25, 1990.

48b. Novak MA, Firszt JB, Meehan K: Cochlear implants in children, part II, *The Journal of the Society of Otorhinolaryngology and Head-Neck Nurses* 8(2):12-18, 1990.

48c. Phipps WJ et al: *Medical–surgical nursing: concepts and clincal practice*, ed 4, St Louis, 1991, Mosby.

49. Programmed instruction: Patient assessment: examination of the ear, *AJN* 75(3):457-476, 1975.

50. Reiner A: *Manual of patient care standards*, Rockville, Md, 1988, Aspen.

51. Report of the task force on the National Strategic Research Plan of the National Institute on Deafness and Other Communication Disorders, Bethesda, Md, 1989, Institute of Health.

52. Rice DH, Spiro RH: *Current concepts in head and neck cancer*, Washington, DC, 1989, The American Cancer Society.

53. Riley, MAK: *Nursing care of the client with ear, nose, and throat disorders*, New York, 1987, Springer.

54. Rudy EB: *Advanced neurological and neurosurgical nursing*, St Louis, 1984, Mosby.

55. Schuring LT: Assessment of the ear. In Phipps WJ et al: *Medical-surgical nursing: concepts and clinical practice*, ed 4, St Louis, 1991, Mosby.

56. Schuring LT: Management of persons with problems of the ear. In Phipps WJ et al: *Medical-surgical nursing: concepts and clinical practice*, ed 4, St Louis, 1991, Mosby.

57. Seeley RR, Stephens TD, Tate P: *Anatomy and physiology*, ed 2, St Louis, 1992, Mosby.

58. Seidel HM et al: *Mosby's guide to physical examination*, ed 2, St Louis, 1991, Mosby.

59. Serra AM, Bailey CM, Jackson P: *Ear, nose, and throat nursing*, London, 1986, Blackwell.

60. Shestak KC, Myers EN: Reconstruction of the hypopharynx and cervical esophagus, *Advances in Otolaryngology–Head and Neck Surgery* 3:289-311, 1989.

61. Sievers AEF, Donald PJ: Staging system for head and neck cancer, *The Journal of the Society of Otorhinolaryngology and Head-Neck Nurses* 7(3):5-10, 1989.

62. Sigler BA: Nursing care of patients with laryngeal carcinoma, *Seminars in Oncology Nursing* 5(3):160-165, 1989.

63. Sigler BA: Nursing care of the head and neck cancer patient, *Oncology* 2(12):49-59, 1988.

64. Sigler BA: Nursing care for head and neck tumor patients. In Thawley SE, Panje WR, editors: *Comprehensive management of head and neck tumors*, Philadelphia, 1987, WB Saunders.

65. Sigler BA: Solid neoplasms. In Jones DA, Dunbar CF, Jirovec MM: *Medical-surgical nursing: a conceptual approach*, New York, 1982, McGraw-Hill.

66. Sigler BA, Hooper JA: Nursing care of the head and neck cancer patient. In Myers EN, Suen JY, editors: *Cancer of the head and neck*, New York, 1989, Churchill Livingstone.

67. Singer MI: Surgical restoration of the voice after laryngectomy, *Advances in Otolaryngology–Head and Neck Surgery* 2:141-165, 1988.

68. Slavin RG: Recalcitrant asthma: could sinusitis be the culprit?, *The Journal of Respiratory Diseases* 12(2):182-194, 1991.

69. Surratt S et al: Troubleshooting a sump tube, *American Journal of Nursing* 93(1):42-47, 1993.

70. Thibodeau GA, Patton KT: *Anatomy and physiology*, ed 2, St Louis, 1993, Mosby.

71. Thompson JM et al: *Mosby's clinical nursing*, ed 3, St Louis, 1993, Mosby.

72. Tortorelli B: Acoustic neuroma: an overview of the disorder and nursing care of these patients, *J Neurosurgical Nursing* 170-171, August 1981.

73. Voke J: Aspects of hearing: functions of the cochlea, *Nursing Times* 22:60-62, August 1984.

74. Voke J: Aspects of hearing: physiology of the ear, *Nursing Times* 15:28-30, August 1984.

75. Westlake C: Commitment to function: microsurgical flaps, *Plastic Surgical Nursing* 11(3):95-101, 1991.

76. Wilson SF, Thompson JM: *Respiratory disorders*, St Louis, 1990, Mosby.

77. Yasko JM: *Care of the client receiving external radiation therapy*, Philadelphia, 1980, American Cancer Society.

Index